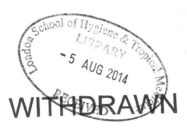
# Health professional mobility in a changing Europe

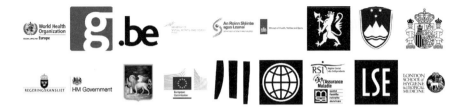

The European Observatory on Health Systems and Policies supports and promotes evidence-based health policy-making through comprehensive and rigorous analysis of health systems in Europe. It brings together a wide range of policy-makers, academics and practitioners to analyse trends in health reform, drawing on experience from across Europe to illuminate policy issues.

The European Observatory on Health Systems and Policies is a partnership between the World Health Organization Regional Office for Europe, the Governments of Austria, Belgium, Finland, Ireland, the Netherlands, Norway, Slovenia, Spain, Sweden and the United Kingdom; and the Veneto Region of Italy, the European Commission, the European Investment Bank, the World Bank, UNCAM (French National Union of Health Insurance Funds), the London School of Economics and Political Science, and the London School of Hygiene & Tropical Medicine.

# Health professional mobility in a changing Europe

New dynamics, mobile individuals and diverse responses

*Edited by*

**James Buchan, Matthias Wismar, Irene A. Glinos, Jeni Bremner**

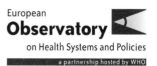

European
**Observatory**
on Health Systems and Policies
a partnership hosted by WHO

**Keywords:**
CAREER MOBILITY
HEALTH PERSONNEL
HEALTH POLICY
HEALTHCARE PROVIDERS
PERSONNEL MANAGEMENT
PUBLIC HEALTH

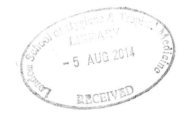

> Address requests about publications to: Publications, WHO Regional Office for Europe, UN City, Marmorvej 51, DK-2100 Copenhagen Ø, Denmark.
>
> Alternatively, complete an online request form for documentation, health information, or for permission to quote or translate, on the Regional Office web site (http://www.euro.who.int/pubrequest).

The designations employed and the presentation of the material in this publication do not imply the expression of any opinion whatsoever on the part of the European Observatory on Health Systems and Policies concerning the legal status of any country, territory, city or area or of its authorities, or concerning the delimitation of its frontiers or boundaries. Dotted lines on maps represent approximate border lines for which there may not yet be full agreement.

The mention of specific companies or of certain manufacturers' products does not imply that they are endorsed or recommended by the European Observatory on Health Systems and Policies in preference to others of a similar nature that are not mentioned. Errors and omissions excepted, the names of proprietary products are distinguished by initial capital letters.

All reasonable precautions have been taken by the European Observatory on Health Systems and Policies to verify the information contained in this publication. However, the published material is being distributed without warranty of any kind, either express or implied. The responsibility for the interpretation and use of the material lies with the reader. In no event shall the European Observatory on Health Systems and Policies be liable for damages arising from its use. The views expressed by authors, editors, or expert groups do not necessarily represent the decisions or the stated policy of the European Observatory on Health Systems and Policies or any of its partners.

This volume is part of the PROMeTHEUS research projecy which received funding from the European Community's Seventh Framework Programme (FP7/2007–2013) under grant agreement 223383.

**ISBN 978 92 890 5025 8**

Printed in the United Kingdom

Cover design by Dimitri Culot

# Contents

# Acknowledgements

This book, the second volume of the PROMeTHEUS project, could not have been written without the ground-laying work delivered by our colleagues from all over Europe contributing to the first volume as country informants, country correspondents and authors. As authors and editors of the second volume we are deeply indebted to their intellectual leadership, expertise and commitment!

The aim and concept of this book were substantially shaped and refined by insights gained from the interaction with policy-makers and senior officials in a continuous string of face-to-face meetings including policy dialogues in Prague, Venice, Stockholm (2009), Slovenia, Lithuania (2010), Hungary, the policy dialogues in Louvain/Leuven during the Belgian EU Presidency (2010), and the Baltic policy dialogue in Tallinn (2013), the joint workforce conference in Brussels (2011), parallel forums and workshops at the EHFG, Gastein (2009–2011), the event in the European Parliament (2011) and the discussion in the European Council 2011 in Gödöllő under the Hungarian EU Presidency. EHMA provided a platform for launching the first volume and discussing implications for the second at its annual conference in Porto, Portugal (2011). The editors presented preliminary results of this volume in a large number of talks and presentations, and we have to admit that we are unaware of all the presentations delivered by our authors. For all these events mentioned above we are most grateful for the funding, support and advice from the European Commission, the WHO Regional Office for Europe and all the governments and institutions involved. Particular thanks go to Willy Palm (European Observatory) for organizing, co-organizing and/or supporting all mentioned face-to-face meetings.

This book would not have been written without the European Commission. We are most grateful for the constant and active contents-related involvement of Katja Neubauer, Caroline Hager, Balazs Lengyel and Liz Kidd (now retired) from the European Commission DG SANCO. Their input and advice has been indispensable for keeping on track and getting the most out of the project for European policy development and implementation. Many thanks to Jürgen Tiedje and his team from the European Commission DG MARKT, for keeping us in the loop on developments updating the directive on the recognition of professional qualifications. And of course, it was the European Commission DG RESEARCH with its Seventh Framework Programme that has provided the funding for PROMeTHEUS to allow for international and comparative health systems research. Also EU funded were our 'sister projects' MoHProf and RN4Cast with whom we have collaborated on various occasions. Our thanks go to Walter Sermeus (University Leuven) and Roumyana Petrova-Benedict of the International Organization for Migration (IOM).

We would like to offer special thanks to our Belgian colleagues Daniel Reynders, Leen Meulenbergs (now WHO), Michel Van Hoegaerden, Riet De Kempeneer, Henk Vandenbroele, Lieve Jorens and Lieven de Raedt for their exemplary support during the Belgian Presidency (2011), their leadership of the Joint Action (as of 2013) and their generosity for involving us in their skill-mix event at the World Health Assembly (2013).

We would also like to send very warm thanks to Miklós Szócska and his teams in the Ministry and in Semmelweiss University, Budapest, Hungary, for their immense support and also for providing a live role model for bridging science and policy.

Over the years, Arne Petter Sanne, Otto Christian Rø and Bjørn Guldvog from the Norwegian Directorate of Health have supported and involved us whenever possible. Thank you for your trust and effective partnership.

There are so many individuals who have wholeheartedly supported this book by advice, support and input that we are necessarily bound to fail to mention all. Still we would like to mention our friend Marc Schreiner from the German Hospital Federation. We greatly benefited from his technical expertise, his political skills and his readiness to join our events on short notice. Many thanks also to Todorka Kostadinova and her team from Varna University, Bulgaria, for actively involving us in their work for the Joint Action. Paul Giepmans of EHMA, who has contributed as a co-author, has also been indispensable as an efficient and shrewd administrator and organizer. We are grateful to Claudia B. Maier and Gilles Dussault, co-editors of the first volume, for agreeing to fill two (difficult) gaps in this book by writing each a chapter at very short notice. Christiane Wiskow of the International Labour Organization (ILO) has reviewed the first volume and also the thematic chapters of the second volume with the same unparalleled technical competence and thorough scrutiny. Gilles Dussault has meticulously reviewed the entire second volume while chapters 1 and 2, updated and rewritten in December 2013, also benefited from a judicious review by Niamh Humphries.

We have benefited a lot from input of major European associations either as members of our advisory board, or as participants in policy dialogues and other events. Our thanks go to the European Federation of Nurse Associations (EFN), the European Federation of Public Service Unions (EPSU), the European Hospital and Healthcare Federation (HOPE), the European Hospital and Healthcare Employers' Association (HOSPEEM), the European Union of Medical Specialists (UEMS) and the World Medical Association (WMA).

Finally, we would like to thank our colleagues at the Observatory and WHO with whom we worked over the years and will keep working in the future. A heartfelt thanks to Jonathan North, Caroline White and Jane Ward for their dedicated, patient assistance in producing this volume; and, of course, many thanks to Josep Figueras for his steadfast support and advice. Our special thanks go to all the WHO country offices which have been extremely instrumental in helping us find suitable country contacts, correspondents and authors. Many of them have been actively involved in organizing policy dialogues and seminars. We have benefited greatly from this exceptional infrastructure. WHO headquarters in Geneva and the WHO Regional Office for Europe have been pushing vigorously for the implementation of the WHO global code of practice on the international recruitment of health personnel. This code has been key to this volume. We would like to express our gratitude to our Geneva colleagues for their excellent collaboration. Rüdiger Krech and Amani Siyam supported our input at the Oslo (Norway) preparatory meeting, the follow-up meeting of the 2008 Tallinn charter (2013) and the Third Global Forum on Human Resources for Health in Recife, Brazil (2013). At home in Europe Hans Kluge from the WHO Regional Office for Europe has always been very supportive during all events, discussions and projects. Finally we want to thank our colleague and friend Galina Perfilieva, WHO Regional Adviser for Human Resources for Health, for her unconditional and very engaged support for whatever initiative improves human resources for health. Thank you Galina.

# List of tables, figures and boxes

*Figures*

*Boxes*

# List of abbreviations

| | |
|---|---|
| **CPD** | continuous professional development |
| **EEA** | European Economic Area |
| **EPSU** | European Federation of Public Service Unions |
| **EU** | European Union |
| **EU12** | New Member States in May 2004 (10, the EU10) and January 2007 (2) |
| **EU15** | Member States before May 2004 |
| **EU27** | All 27 Member States as of 2013 |
| **GATS** | General Agreements of Trade in Services |
| **GDP** | Gross domestic product |
| **GP** | General practitioner |
| **HOSPEEM** | European Hospital and Health Care Employers' Association |
| **NCHD** | Non-consultant hospital doctors (Ireland) |
| **NGO** | Nongovernmental organization |
| **NHS** | UK National Health Service |
| **OECD** | Organisation for Economic Co-operation and Development |
| **WHO** | World Health Organization |

# List of contributors

**Linda Aiken**, Professor and Director, Center for Health Outcomes and Policy Research, School of Nursing, University of Pennsylvania, United States

**Posy Bidwell**, Research Assistant, Centre for Health Policy and Management, Trinity College Dublin, Dublin, Ireland

**Ruairi Brugha**, Head of Division of Population Health Sciences, Department of Epidemiology and Public Health Medicine, Royal College of Surgeons in Ireland, Dublin, Ireland.

**Luk Bruyneel**, Researcher, Centre for Health Services and Nursing Research, Katholieke Universiteit Leuven, Leuven, Belgium

**James Buchan**, Professor, School of Health, Queen Margaret University, Edinburgh, Scotland

**Reinhard Busse**, Professor, Department Healthcare Management, Berlin University of Technology, Berlin, Germany

**Carmen Mihaela Dolea**, Technical Officer, World Health Organization, Geneva, Switzerland

**Gilles Dussault**, Professor, International Public Health and Biostatistics Unit, Instituto de Higiene e Medicina Tropical Universidade Nova de Lisboa, Lisbon, Portugal, and Coordinator, WHO Collaborating Centre for Health Workforce Policy and Planning, Lisbon, Portugal

**Paul Giepmans**, Policy Analyst, European Health Management Association, Brussels, Belgium

**Edmond Girasek**, Assistant Professor, Health Services Management Training Centre, Semmelweis University, Budapest, Hungary

**Irene A. Glinos**, Senior Researcher, European Observatory on Health Systems and Policies, Brussels, Belgium

**Charlotte Humphrey**, Professor, Florence Nightingale School of Nursing and Midwifery, King's College, London, United Kingdom

**Niamh Humphries**, Senior Research Fellow, Department of Epidemiology and Public Health Medicine, Division of Population Health Sciences, Royal College of Surgeons in Ireland, Dublin, Ireland

**Elisabeth Jelfs**, Director of Policy, Council of Deans of Health, London, United Kingdom, previously Deputy Director, European Health Management Association, Brussels, Belgium

**Moritz Knapp**, Consultant, Freelance, previously Consultant at Andersson Elffers Felix, Utrecht, the Netherlands

**Eszter Kovacs**, Assistant Professor, Health Services Management Training Centre, Semmelweis University, Budapest, Hungary

**Dessislava Kuznetsova**, Programme Coordinator, Open Society Institute, Sofia, Bulgaria

**Emmanuel Lesaffre**, Professor, Leuven Biostatistics and Statistical Bioinformatics Centre, Katholieke Universiteit Leuven, Leuven, Belgium, and Professor, Department of Statistics, Erasmus Medical Centre, Rotterdam, the Netherlands

**Baoyue Li**, Researcher, Department of Statistics, Erasmus Medical Centre, Rotterdam, the Netherlands

**Claudia B. Maier**, Programme Analyst, UNAIDS, Geneva, Switzerland, previously Technical Officer, European Observatory on Health Systems and Policies, Brussels, Belgium

**Sherry Merkur**, Research Fellow, European Observatory on Health Systems and Policies, LSE Health, London, United Kingdom

**Charles Normand**, Edward Kennedy Professor, Centre for Health Policy and Management, Trinity College Dublin, Dublin, Ireland

**Diana Ognyanova**, Researcher, Berlin University of Technology, Berlin, Germany

**Žilvinas Padaiga**, Professor, Department of Preventive Medicine, Faculty of Public Health, Lithuanian University of Health Sciences, Kaunas, Lithuania

**Evgeniya Plotnikova**, Research Fellow, Global Public Health Unit, School of Social and Political Science, The University of Edinburgh, Edinburgh, Scotland

**Martynas Pukas**, Researcher, Department of Preventive Medicine, Faculty of Public Health, Lithuanian University of Health Sciences, Kaunas, Lithuania

**Anne Marie Rafferty**, Professor, Florence Nightingale School of Nursing and Midwifery, King's College, London, United Kingdom

**Walter Sermeus**, Professor, Centre for Health Services and Nursing Research, Katholieke Universiteit Leuven, Leuven, Belgium

**Liudvika Starkienė**, Associate Professor, Department of Preventive Medicine, Faculty of Public Health, Lithuanian University of Health Sciences, Kaunas, Lithuania.

**Steve Thomas**, Associate Professor, Centre for Health Policy and Management, Trinity College Dublin, Dublin, Ireland

**Ella Tyrrell**, Research Assistant, Centre for Health Policy and Management, Trinity College Dublin, Dublin, Ireland

**Koen Van den Heede**, Senior Researcher, Centre for Health Services and Nursing Research, Katholieke Universiteit Leuven, Leuven, Belgium, and Expert Health Services Research, Belgian Health Care Knowledge Centre, Brussels, Belgium

**Peter Wijga**, Consultant, Andersson Elffers Felix, Utrecht, the Netherlands

**Matthias Wismar**, Senior Health Policy Analyst, European Observatory on Health Systems and Policies, Brussels, Belgium

**Ruth Young**, Reader, Florence Nightingale School of Nursing and Midwifery, King's College, London

**Boyan Zahariev**, Programme Director, Open Society Institute, Sofia, Bulgaria

# Part I
# Setting the scene, key findings and lessons

# Chapter 1

# Introduction to health professional mobility in a changing Europe

*James Buchan, Irene A. Glinos and Matthias Wismar*

My paediatrician has moved to Texas, my dentist to Dubai and my optician to Stockholm.

Greek woman quoted by Symons (2012)

## 1.1 Introducing the changing context

Europe is faced with fundamental change affecting public policy priorities, health systems and labour market behaviour. Health professional mobility, already changing as a result of European Union (EU) enlargement, has more recently been impacted by the effects of the financial and economic crisis. This volume, which builds on and extends the analysis conducted in the first volume of the PROMeTHEUS study (Wismar et al., 2011), takes account of this changing context by looking in detail at the motivations and experiences of mobile health professionals, and by examining the characteristics, impact and potential of policies aimed at "managing" aspects of mobility. It does so at a time when health workforce issues have become even more significant on the agenda of most EU countries and at EU level (European Commission, 2012b; Jelfs, 2012).

This volume provides evidence for policy-makers, managers, observers and those responsible for the health professions. It highlights that health professional mobility will be a persistent dynamic of labour markets and health policy, and that our understanding of the phenomenon will have to adapt and adjust as quickly as mobility trends and patterns are changing. Most importantly, it reinforces the message for policy-makers in European countries that health professional mobility has not been ended, or even reduced, by the continuing impact of the economic crisis, which first hit in 2008. The underpinning dynamics continue to have an impact on individual health professionals' choice of job and location, and on the viability of local and national approaches to health workforce planning, recruitment and retention. Moreover, there is a continued need to balance the ethical and efficiency considerations that these issues give rise to. Health professional mobility will continue to be a significant element in European health care labour markets, and policy-makers and planners will have to maintain their capacity to capture its changing trends and impact. The present volume is designed to focus on potential policy responses, policy "solutions" and instruments at managerial, national and international levels.

The remainder of this chapter comprises six parts. Sections 1.2–1.4 focus on the changing economic context, policy context and EU context, respectively, highlighting how they interact with health professional mobility. Section 1.5 describes the methodology of the research, and section 1.6 notes its limitations.

## 1.2 The financial and economic crisis in Europe

In a Europe deeply, but also unevenly, affected by economic crisis and recession, there is a clear sense that the world is changing, that health systems are being impacted and will have to respond, and that health professionals themselves will have to adapt. Demographically driven change in health care demand and provision has been joined by economic change as the world struggles with the impact of the global financial crisis. This second volume examines the dynamics of health professional mobility in the context of the economic crisis.

The Organisation for Economic Co-operation and Development (OECD) has reported that growth in health spending per capita has slowed or fallen in real terms in almost all European countries since 2008, reversing a trend of steady increases in previous years (OECD, 2012a). Financial constraints and public sector cost-containment mean that, while health care demand continues to increase, health care funding in many countries is constrained or reducing. Health systems, organizations and service provision in many countries are under cost-containment scrutiny and reform. In a labour-intensive sector such as health care, staffing costs and productivity are the focus of much of this attention. In many countries, health professional pay is being "frozen" or reduced; in some, staffing levels are declining. Health professionals' job-seeking behaviour in some countries is changing, as they try to hold on to jobs in challenging labour markets (Bortoluzzi & Palese, 2010; Brewer et al., 2012; International Labour Organization, 2012; Staiger, Auerbach & Buerhaus, 2012; Buchan & Seccombe, 2013; Buchan, O'May & Dussault, 2013) or respond to reductions in their pay, status and job prospects by leaving the health sector, or their country of practice (European Federation of Nurses Associations, 2012). However, the financial crisis, while stimulating some workers to consider migration, has also led some countries to raise barriers to migrant workers. In response to economic decline and rising unemployment rates, these countries are tightening their immigration policies (OECD, 2012b), which is reducing the opportunities for mobile health workers to enter some countries and in some cases may be displacing "traditional" pre-crisis migration flows into and within Europe, creating new migratory patterns to other countries or regions that have been less affected by the financial crisis.

The overall impact of the economic crisis on EU health systems has been variable (Fahy, 2012), and the health sector may have been impacted less negatively than other areas of the economy in many OECD countries (OECD, 2011). The assessment of trends in overall migration (i.e. not just health worker movements) in OECD countries suggests that the slowdown in migration caused by the economic crisis was short term (OECD, 2012b). Mobility of health professionals in EU Member States continues to be a central issue for most countries, but the patterns of mobility have changed, and for some individuals it is the impact of the crisis that has been the motivation to move. Some countries have been affected more than others by the impact of the economic crisis. Health professional mobility has not "stopped" because of this crisis, but at the aggregate level its magnitude, directions and impact have changed and will be changing further, and the experiences and motivations of individual mobile health professionals may also differ in the new economic reality.

## 1.3 The policy conundrum: ethics versus efficiency?

The challenges of health professional mobility are not new: they have been identified and observed across decades (for example, Mejia, Pizurki & Royston, 1979; Pang, Lansang & Haines, 2002; Wright, Flis & Gupta, 2008; Connell, 2010). What has changed in Europe is the creation of a border-free labour market, and its expansion with the EU enlargements of 2004, 2007 and 2013, which endows health professionals with the right to provide services and to establish themselves in another EU Member State. This provided new mobility opportunities for health professionals and reduced options for Member States to limit or selectively contain these cross-border flows. In parallel, since 2008 the financial crisis has contributed to redefining opportunities for individual health professionals, the health systems in which they practise and the priorities of health professional regulators. Shifting opportunities and widening inequalities present a context where the ethical and efficiency implications of policy options are being redefined.

A deepening understanding of the complexities of health professional mobility and the related economic and policy context is emerging (Stilwell et al., 2003; Glinos et al., 2011; Maier et al., 2011). There is broad acceptance that we need to go beyond a simple linear "brain drain" argument to grasp the full implications of health professional mobility, although the potential for negative impact on source countries cannot be denied and continues to dominate the media discourse.

There has been growing recognition that other factors must be considered when assessing the impact of health worker migration. These include the rights of individuals to move, and the related debate about treating mobile health professionals differently from other skilled migrants because of their exceptional importance (Alkire & Chen, 2006), the possibility of international mobility acting as an escape valve for the unemployed or as a way of career development for individual health professionals, the possible financial benefit to source countries of remittances sent home by migrant health professionals and the benefits when mobile health professionals return home with skills acquired abroad. The first volume also highlighted that so-called "destination" countries vary markedly in their level of reliance on international health workers, and this level can also change over time. Not all countries are equally active in international recruitment, or equally dependent on international health workers. In addition, some countries have discovered that they are not as attractive to foreign health workers as they anticipated, which has forced them to change their workforce strategies (Albreht, 2011). However, the argument that there needs to be a more "ethical" approach to international recruitment to mitigate any negative effects of skills loss in developing and crisis-hit countries continues to resonate, and was a driving force in the adoption by the World Health Organization (WHO), in 2010, of the WHO *Global Code of Practice on the International Recruitment of Health Personnel.*

In the context of an ethical dimension to health professional mobility, the EU logic of free movement, however, presents a paradox: while migration from outside the EU is subject to national rules and international codes, intra-EU mobility is guaranteed by the treaties, and options to hinder it are limited. At a time when the gap between economic and labour market conditions is widening, as is the gap in unemployment rates, in the 28 Member States, new questions emerge on the ethics of destination countries relying on foreign inflows of health professionals to replenish their workforce, including from EU countries hit hardest by the crisis (Stuckler et al., 2011; Glinos, 2012; Mladovsky et al., 2012).

If the "ethical" dimension of health professional mobility has been its most obvious aspect in recent years, the issue of "efficiency" has also become more apparent. Partly as a result of the cost-containment pressure in many health systems, there has been increased policy emphasis on effective workforce planning, improved health workforce productivity, and, in some countries, an increased focus on best use of skills, or redeployment or re-skilling of health workers (e.g. the European research project MUNROS on the impact on practice, outcomes and cost of new roles for health professionals; Health Economics Research Unit, 2013). Health professional mobility is a factor that can be harnessed in support of these policy goals, but it can also undermine health workforce policy objectives if not properly assessed.

The *WHO Global Code of Practice* devotes considerable attention to the need for effective workforce planning and retention of health workers: for countries to aim for a sustainable approach to workforce planning, to reduce over-reliance on internationally recruited health workers and to promote ethical treatment of individual mobile health workers. The first report to the World Health Assembly on progress with implementation of the Code, in May 2013, has shown patchy progress, particularly in "source countries" that may be most impacted by outmigration of key staff; however, the report did highlight relatively high levels of engagement with the Code in countries of the WHO Europe Region compared with other regions (WHO, 2013). At the time of completing this book, the effective implementation of the WHO *Global Code of Practice* remains unfinished business (Edge & Hoffman, 2013).

The "efficiency" dimension relates both to organization/management level practice in effective recruitment and induction of mobile health professionals and to the existence of a system/national level policy, planning and regulatory framework that ensures that mobile health professionals are enabled to work at their optimum level. Both organization and national levels are considered in this volume.

The ethics and efficiency dimensions of health worker mobility are sometimes presented as two diametrically opposed and mutually exclusive policy challenges. However, no health system, country or region can risk ignoring either. The search for more effective health workforce planning and productivity, the current and forecast health workforce shortages in many countries in Europe and elsewhere (Ono, Lafortune & Schoenstein, 2013), the need for health workforce sustainability, the dynamic nature of health professional mobility, and the monitoring of recruitment practice related to the WHO *Global Code of Practice* all result in growing interdependence between countries and health systems. In this volume, aspects of both efficiency and ethics will be examined from a health system perspective, looking at the impact on, and integration of, international health workers, their effective management and retention, and policy responses and policy instruments in use at national and international level.

## 1.4 The EU legal basis and recent policy development

The primary focus of this volume is on mobility within, into and out of Europe, most notably the 32 countries of the European Economic Area (EEA) including Switzerland, where the legal and policy contexts at EU level greatly influence health professional mobility (Tjadens, Weilandt & Eckert, 2012).

The EU constitutes a unique legal environment for health professional mobility. The free movement of workers is an economic imperative and a civil right enshrined in the treaties and supported by secondary legislation. In relation to health professions, the most important is Directive 2005/36/EC on the recognition of professional qualifications, which in 2013 was being modernized by the European Commission, the European Parliament and EU Member States (European Commission, 2013a)[1]. This Directive ensures portability of qualifications of medical doctors, dentists, registered nurses and midwives and facilitates the mobility of these professionals within the EU. The process is an automatic procedure in which their qualifications are checked on the basis of the conformity of their qualification levels and training periods rather than by individual assessment of their skills and required competencies. Directive 2005/36/EC delineates the EEA as the largest region in the world with "free" mobility for health professionals.

Freedom to move has its benefits, but it also has some constraints. As noted above, the economic crisis has led to some countries tightening entry requirements for health professionals, but this national policy change has been directed at non-EU-trained workers. The end result is that there is now evidence of significant rebalancing of the magnitude of EU and non-EU health professional flows into some countries in the region, with a relative increase in EU flows, which cannot be controlled to the same extent at national level. Similarly, the relatively unrestricted ability to move within the EU also means that more health professionals from the countries hit hardest by the economic crisis may be moving, even if job prospects at the destination point within the EU appear less attractive than before. The key point here is the relative situation perceived by potential mobile health workers in different EU countries. Health sector employment opportunities, for example in the United Kingdom or Ireland, may be lower than before the economic crisis but remain at a higher level than in other parts of the EU, notably southern Europe.

Another, related, issue that has become more prominent in some countries is national policy concern about the patient safety implications of care being provided by mobile health professionals (Informal Network of Competent

---

1 Directive 2013/55/EU of the European Parliament and of the Council amending Directive 2005/36/EC on the recognition of professional qualifications and Regulation (EU No 1024/2012 on administrative cooperation through the Internal Market Information System was adopted on 20 November 2013. Legal text available at: http://eur-lex.europa.eu/LexUriServ/LexUriServ.do?uri=OJ:L:2013:354:0132:0170:en:PDF

Authorities for Doctors, 2010). Some of these are short-term and/or repeat "commuting" health professionals who cross borders to provide temporary and locum cover for established workers. This issue has been most prominent in media coverage and policy debate (e.g. in the context of the modernization of Directive 2005/36/EC) in relation to language proficiency of some of these mobile health professionals, and limitations placed by EU Directives on language tests by national regulatory authorities (Parkinson, 2011; Rimmer, 2011), but it also relates to broader issues of differences in training content, competencies and national regulatory approaches (de Vries et al., 2009).

At a policy level, there is recognition that health professional mobility needs to be understood within the wider strategies addressing general workforce issues in Europe. Against the background of economic, labour market and regulatory change, the EU has reaffirmed its interest in the health workforce as critical to sustained improvement in the health of the population. On 18 April 2012, the European Commission published its report *Towards a job-rich recovery*, which set out a range of measures to encourage employment and strengthen economic growth in Europe, with a focus on the demand side of job creation, and setting out ways for Member States to encourage hiring by reducing taxes on labour or supporting business start-ups more (European Commission, 2012b). The report identified the areas with the biggest job potential for the future: the green economy, information and communications technology and the health sector (European Commission, 2012b). Simultaneously, the European Commission published the *Action Plan for the EU health workforce* (European Commission, 2012a), which aimed to improve health workforce planning and forecasting, offer long-term job prospects in the sector and stimulate exchange on innovative and effective recruitment and retention strategies for health workers.

The *Action Plan* noted that health care is highly labour intensive and one of the largest sectors in the EU, accounting for about 17 million of all jobs (8%) in the EU. Despite the economic downturn, the *Action Plan* highlighted that the sector continues to grow and, with an ageing population and the rising demand for health care, emphasized that it will remain a key driver for jobs, with an estimated 8 million job openings between 2010 and 2020. It also noted that the sector faced major challenges "at a time of severe budget constraints, including health workforce shortages and skill mismatches in many countries", and reports that "There is recent and worrying evidence that the cost-containment measures to reduce public expenditure is profoundly affecting the recruitment and retention of health care staff and in particular nurses, the largest health profession, in almost half of EU28. Maintaining an adequate supply and quality of health care services under severe budget constraints is thus a key issue to be addressed by policy-makers." The European Commission estimates that, without further measures to meet these challenges, there will be a potential shortfall of around 1 million health care workers in the EU by 2020, and double that figure if long-term care and ancillary occupations are taken into account.

The *Action Plan* is intended to assist Member States in tackling these challenges and it sets out actions to foster European cooperation and sharing of good practice in order to help in improving health workforce planning and forecasting, to anticipate future skills needs and to improve the recruitment and retention of health professionals while mitigating the negative effects of migration on health systems.

The *Action Plan* has now formally been launched as a *Joint Action on Health Workforce Planning and Forecasting* (European Commission, 2013b), which highlights that demand, need and supply of the health workforce will be influenced by multiple factors such as the ageing population, the ageing workforce, rising care use and rising costs in a context of budget constraints. The general objective of the *Joint Action* is to establish and serve as a platform for collaboration and exchange between EU Member States to prepare the future health workforce. There are four core work packages in the *Joint Action*.

1. *Data for health workforce planning*. This provides the key building blocks of the planning and forecasting systems by providing better understanding of collected data at EU Member State and European level. Special attention will be given to migration and mobility data.

2. *Exchange of good practices in planning methodologies*. This will promote and support the use of quantitative model-based planning methodologies (both supply side and demand side) based on what is in use today, informed by "good practices" evaluation. The health professions in focus will be doctors, nurses, pharmacists, dentists and midwives.

3. *Horizon scanning*. This will document qualitative workforce planning in Member States by exchanging experience, practices, outputs and outcomes in horizon-scanning methodologies and will support the use of horizon scanning. It will also estimate future needs in terms of skills and competencies of the health workforce.

4. *Sustainability of the results*. This will consolidate the *Joint Action* experience and results with a view to continuation. It will identify partners to continue the activities and will develop a coherent plan for follow-up and reinforce the impact of health workforce planning and forecasting on policy-making.

Developing effective and sustained health workforce planning and policy is a critical issue at organizational, national and EU level, and the aim of this volume is to contribute to a better understanding of current policy practice and priorities.

## 1.5 Methodology

This volume takes a more in-depth look at current health workforce data and its utility for assessing health professional mobility, the experiences of mobile health professionals, management responses to health worker retention and current experience with policy instruments to track and manage health professional mobility. A range of methodologies are employed in the volume:

- the scoping review on the conceptual underpinnings of health professional mobility;

- a critical analysis of health workforce data, indicators and register methodologies;

- a literature review of the impact of the global financial crisis on health professional mobility;

- quantitative and qualitative methodologies on the experiences and motivations of the mobile health professional;

- expert interviews to capture the perspective of health care managers; and

- literature analysis and expert interviews on the impact of policy instruments.

These methodologies are explained in more detail in the individual chapters.

## 1.6 Limitations

The limitations of available data on health professional mobility constitute a constraint for effective policy and planning (Wismar et al., 2011). Data sets in different countries are often incomplete or out of date, and the data sets are not always compatible across national boundaries. This continues to be a limiting factor, despite recent and ongoing efforts by WHO, OECD, International Labour Organization and Eurostat at harmonizing data collection and analysis. In particular, it can be difficult to develop an up-to-the-minute assessment of the dynamics of changing patterns of mobility when data aggregation, verification and publication are often significantly "behind the curve" of change (Buchan, O'May & Dussault, 2013). This places some limitations on detailed analysis and interpretation, which are compounded by the additional time required to edit, quality assure and publish conclusions in a volume. Nevertheless, there remains an opportunity to make more effective use of the data sets that do exist and to harness them more effectively to support policy-making.

The variable impact of the economic crisis at individual and national level has already been identified. With limited space for detailed case studies of policy responses and mobile health professional experiences, it is not possible to provide a complete and detailed picture across all EU Member States. The case studies that are reported are selected to illustrate the breadth of experiences and responses that are evident in the region, and beyond.

## References

Albreht T (2011). Addressing shortages: Slovenia's reliance on foreign health professionals, current developments and policy responses. In Wismar M et al., eds. *Health professional mobility and health systems. Evidence from 17 European countries.* Copenhagen, WHO Regional Office for Europe on behalf of the European Observatory on Health Systems and Policies:511–537.

Alkire S, Chen L (2006). Medical exceptionalism in international migration: should doctors and nurses be treated differently? In Tamas K, Palme J, eds. *Globalizing migration regimes: new challenges to transnational cooperation.* Farnham, UK, Ashgate (Research in Migration and Ethnic Relations Series).

Bortoluzzi G, Palese A (2010). The Italian economic crisis and its impact on nursing services and education: hard and challenging times. *Journal of Nursing Management*, 18:515–519.

Brewer C et al. (2012). Original research. New nurses: has the recession increased their commitment to their jobs? *American Journal of Nursing*, 112(3):34–44.

Buchan J, Seccombe I (2013). The end of growth? Analysing NHS nurse staff. *Journal of Advanced Nursing*, 69(9):2123–2130.

Buchan J, O'May F, Dussault G (2013). The nursing workforce and the global economic crisis. *Journal of Nursing Scholarship*, 45(3):298–307.

Connell J (2010). *Migration and the globalisation of health care: the health worker exodus?* Cheltenham, UK, Edward Elgar.

de Vries H et al. (2009). *International comparison of ten medical regulatory systems: Egypt, Germany, Greece, India, Italy, Nigeria, Pakistan, Poland, South Africa and Spain.* Cambridge UK, RAND Europe (Report for the UK General Medical Council).

Edge JS, Hoffman SJ (2013). Empirical impact evaluation of the WHO global code of practice on the international recruitment of health personnel in Australia, Canada, UK and USA. *Globalization and Health*, 9:60.

European Commission (2012a). *Staff working document on an action plan for the EU health workforce. Towards a job-rich recovery*. Strasbourg, European Commission (http://ec.europa.eu/dgs/health_consumer/docs/swd_ap_eu_healthcare_workforce_en.pdf, accessed 2 January 2014).

European Commission (2012b). *Communication from the Commission to the European Parliament, the Council, the European Economic and Social Committee and the Committee of the Regions: towards a job-rich recovery*. Strasbourg, European Commission (COM(2012) 173 final) (http://ec.europa.eu/dgs/health_consumer/docs/towards_job_rich_recovery_en.pdf, accessed 13 January 2014).

European Commission (2013a). *Directive 2005/36/EC: policy developments* (http://ec.europa.eu/internal_market/qualifications/policy_developments/index_en.htm, accessed 13 January 2014).

European Commission (2013b). *Joint action on health workforce planning and forecasting*. Brussels, European Commission (http://euhwforce.weebly.com/, accessed 13 January 2014).

European Federation of Nurses Associations (2012). *Caring in crisis: the impact of the financial crisis on nurses and nursing. A comparative overview of 34 European countries*. Brussels, European Federation of Nurses Associations (http://www.efnweb.be/wp-content/uploads/2012/05/EFN-Report-on-the-Impact-of-the-Financial-Crisis-on-Nurses-and-Nursing-January-20122.pdf, accessed 5 December 2013).

Fahy N (2012). Who is shaping the future of European health systems? *British Medical Journal*, 344:e1712.

Glinos IA (2012). Worrying about the wrong thing: patient mobility vs. health professional mobility. *Journal of Health Services Research and Policy*, 17(4):254–256.

Glinos IA et al. (2011). Health professional mobility and health systems in Europe: conclusions from the case-studies. In Wismar M et al., eds. *Health professional mobility and health systems. Evidence from 17 European countries*. Copenhagen, WHO Regional Office for Europe on behalf of the European Observatory on Health Systems and Policies:67–85.

Health Economics Research Unit (2013). *MUNROS: health care reform – the impact on practice, outcome and costs of new roles for health professionals*. Aberdeen, Health Economics Research Unit, University of Aberdeen (http://www.abdn.ac.uk/munros/, accessed 13 January 2014).

Informal Network of Competent Authorities for Doctors (2010). *Berlin statement: European Commission's evaluation of Directive 2005/36/EC on the mutual recognition of professional qualifications.* London, General Medical Council (http://www.gmc-uk.org/Joint_Berlin_statement_28_Oct_2010_37914074.pdf, accessed 13 January 2014).

International Labour Organization (2012). *The impact of public sector adjustments in Europe.* Geneva, International Labour Organization.

Jelfs E (2012). Workforce issues in European Union health policy. *Health Service Management Research*, 25:48–49.

Maier CB et al. (2011). Cross-country analysis of health professional mobility in Europe: the results. In Wismar M et al., eds. *Health professional mobility and health systems. Evidence from 17 European countries.* Copenhagen, WHO Regional Office for Europe on behalf of the European Observatory on Health Systems and Policies:23–66.

Mejia A, Pizurki H, Royston E (1979). *Physician and nurse migration: analysis and policy implications. Report on a WHO study.* Geneva, World Health Organization.

Mladovsky P et al. (2012). *Health policy responses to the financial crisis.* Copenhagen, WHO Regional Office for Europe on behalf of the European Observatory on Health Systems and Policies (Policy summary 5) (http://www. euro.who.int/__data/assets/pdf_file/0009/170865/e96643.pdf, accessed 13 January 2014).

OECD (2011). *Health at a glance 2011: OECD indicators.* Paris, Organisation for Economic Co-operation and Development (http://www.oecd.org/health/ health-systems/49105858.pdf, accessed 1 October 2013).

OECD (2012a). *Health at a glance: Europe 2012.* Paris, Organisation for Economic Co-operation and Development (http://www.oecd.org/health/ health-systems/HealthAtAGlanceEurope2012.pdf, accessed 13 January 2014).

OECD (2012b). *International migration outlook 2012.* Paris, Organisation for Economic Co-operation and Development.

Ono T, Lafortune G, Schoenstein M (2013). *Health workforce planning in OECD countries: a review of 26 projection models from 18 countries.* Paris, Organisation for Economic Co-operation and Development (OECD Health Working Paper 62) (http://dx.doi.org/10.1787/5k44t787zcwb-en, accessed 13 January 2014).

Pang T, Lansang M, Haines A (2002). Brain drain and health professionals. *British Medical Journal*, 324:499–500.

Parkinson J (2011). Foreign GPs will face English language test – Lansley. *BBC online*, 4 October (http://www.bbc.co.uk/news/uk-politics-15164373, accessed 13 January 2014).

Rimmer A (2011). Doctors must be GMC-registered before language can be tested. *GPonline*, 20 December (http://www.gponline.com/News/article/1110100/Doctors-GMC-registered-language-tested/, accessed 13 January 2014).

Staiger D, Auerbach D, Buerhaus P (2012). Registered nurse labor supply and the recession: are we in a bubble? *New England Journal of Medicine*, 366:1463–1465.

Stilwell B et al. (2003). Developing evidence-based ethical policies on the migration of health workers: conceptual and practical challenges. *Human Resources for Health*, 1:8.

Stuckler D et al. (2011). Effects of the 2008 recession on health: a first look at European data. *Lancet,* 378:124–125.

Symons K (2012). Down and Out in London, Paris, Athens…. *Australian Financial Review*, 24–25 November, p. 15.

Tjadens F, Weilandt C, Eckert J (2012). *Mobility of health professionals: health systems, work conditions, patterns of health workers' mobility and implications for policy makers.* Bonn, Scientific Institute of the Medical Association of German Doctors.

WHO (2010). *WHO global code of practice on the international recruitment of health personnel.* Geneva, World Health Organization (Sixty-third World Health Assembly, WHA63.16) (http://www.who.int/hrh/migration/code/WHO_global_code_of_practice_EN.pdf, accessed 1 October 2013).

WHO (2013). *The health workforce: advances in responding to shortages and migration, and in preparing for emerging needs.* Geneva, World Health Organization (Report by the Secretariat for the Sixty-sixth World Health Assembly, Provisional Agenda Item 17.4) (http://apps.who.int/gb/ebwha/pdf_files/WHA66/A66_25-en.pdf, accessed 13 January 2014).

Wismar M et al., eds. (2011). *Health professional mobility and health systems. Evidence from 17 European countries.* Copenhagen, WHO Regional Office for Europe on behalf of the European Observatory on Health Systems and Policies.

Wright D, Flis L, Gupta M (2008). The "brain drain" of physicians: historical antecedents to an ethical debate, c. 1960–79. *Philosophy, Ethics, and Humanities in Medicine*, 3:24.

Chapter 2

# Health professional mobility in a changing Europe: lessons and findings

*Irene A. Glinos, James Buchan and Matthias Wismar*

The purpose of this chapter is twofold. First, it provides the reader with an in-depth and comprehensive analysis of the findings of the book. The lessons from the chapters have been distilled, analysed and regrouped into five themes representing the essence of the volume. Second, the chapter provides a detailed overview of each of the 14 subsequent chapters, highlighting the key points and illustrative findings.

## 2.1 Lessons from the evidence

### 2.1.1 Health professional mobility in Europe: a fast moving target

A message consistently emerging from the research is the rapidly changing, dynamic nature of health professional mobility, on the one hand, and its endurance on the other.

The constantly changing nature of mobility is a result of the multitude of factors influencing mobility. Factors playing a role in the decision to migrate and enabling the migration process include individual motivations, experiences and expectations (Chapters 3, 6–11); working conditions and general circumstances in the home and destination country (Chapters 3, 11, 15 and 16); and legal frameworks and policy instruments (Chapters 6, 12, 13, 14 and 16). Any change in this landscape of factors will affect the appeal of migrating, or that of staying. Health professional mobility reflects and responds to the factors and context that surround it.

Although the magnitude, directions and composition of migratory flows change, their importance does not diminish. The development of this volume coincided with the onset of the financial and economic crisis in Europe, at a time when it was not known what the downturn would mean for health professional mobility. The insights from the study show the persistence of mobility in turbulent and unpredictable times (Chapter 3), confirm its continued relevance and underscore the need to understand the dynamics of the phenomenon.

The changing and unpredictable patterns of health professional mobility and its enduring importance, together with the evolving context in which it takes place (explained in detail in section 2.1.3 below), mean that no country can disregard health professional mobility or consider itself "safe": it might benefit from inflows of health professionals today, but be losing health workforce tomorrow. "No health without a workforce" (Campbell et al., 2013) captures the exceptional importance of health professionals for the functioning of health systems, and the vulnerability of health systems to workforce fluctuations; countries have few certainties as to which health professionals will come, go or stay. The economic instability that many European countries face adds to the uncertainty. In the span of two decades, countries such as Ireland and Spain have gone from being exporters of health professionals in the 1990s to being importers around the mid-2000s to meet increasing demand, to then again experiencing outflows of doctors and/or nurses since around 2010 when the effects of the economic crisis hit (López-Valcárcel, Pérez & Quintana, 2011; Buchan & Seccombe, 2012). Other countries, such as Bulgaria, Greece, Portugal, Romania and the United Kingdom, are also witnessing changes in the directions and extent of mobility, not least in connection with the financial crisis (Galan, Olsavszky & Vladescu, 2011; Labrianidis, 2011; see also Chapter 3), suggesting the re-emergence of flows from poorer to wealthier countries, often going south to north, and widening asymmetries in Europe.

The second reason why mobility cannot safely be disregarded is that countries, in particular within the free mobility zone of the EU (Chapter 6), do not have complete control over flows. Measures taken by destination or source countries are but one of the many factors influencing mobility. For example, between 2006 and 2012 the number of nurses from Poland registering in the United Kingdom fell by more than 50%, while that of nurses from Portugal grew 10-fold, neither a result of a United Kingdom policy but rather a consequence of the wider economic situation improving and worsening, respectively, in the home countries (Chapter 3). Countries that previously attracted, or even relied on, foreign arrivals witness changing directions of flows as home countries attract returners – Polish medical doctors are known to be returning to Poland, while Swiss hospitals experience the return of German medical doctors to

Bavaria (Kautsch & Czabanowska, 2011; Altwegg, 2013; Bavarian Ministry of Economic Affairs and Media, Energy and Technology, 2013) – or as other destination countries exert a greater pull. The risks of relying on a foreign health workforce are thus exacerbated by the difficulty of predicting, let alone planning, flows and grow in line with the extent of reliance. In the 31 European and OECD countries studied, reliance on foreign medical doctors reported active on the registry exceeded 20% in Luxembourg, the United Kingdom, Sweden, Ireland, Switzerland, New Zealand, the United States, Australia and Canada, and on foreign nurses in Luxembourg, Ireland, New Zealand and Malta (Chapter 5). For countries witnessing outflows of health professionals, the challenges in predicting and steering flows are arguably even greater. Examples of EU Member States with dedicated policies to manage outflows are rare (Wismar et al., 2011; see also Chapter 12), which could be related to a lack of awareness. Few countries collect accurate outflow data, a situation made worse when health professionals do not deregister from national registries when leaving the (home) country (Chapter 5).

At a conceptual level, the volatility of flows means that our tools and understanding must be able to adapt as quickly as health professional mobility does. Established ways of thinking about the phenomenon are challenged. Categories such as "sending" and "receiving" countries become blurred or outdated not only because flows change but also because different groups of professions, and of health professionals, are affected differently: for example Ireland, which has experienced outflows of Irish-trained medical doctors but inflows of medical doctors trained in non-EU countries (Chapter 10). The return movements of health professionals to their home countries, and the frequent, itinerant or repeated movements of doctors and nurses commuting and travelling between countries, turn the categories on their head and call for new terms such as "expertise-gain" and "countries as stepping stones" to be considered in parallel with "brain drain", despite many of these movements often going unnoticed (Chapters 5 and 6). Finally, the implicit suggestion that countries actively "send" or "receive" health professionals neglects the fact that mobility often happens independently of any deliberate policy action; mobility, particularly within the EU, hinges on an individual's decision to move, and evidence suggests that the role of bilateral labour agreements may be waning (Chapter 14).

### 2.1.2 Often misunderstood and neglected: the mobile individual

A second key message emerging from the research is that one must look at the individual migrant in order to fully grasp health professional mobility and its diversity.[1] Several chapters (Chapters 6–11) in this volume focus on mobile individuals, their experiences and their migratory journeys. By zooming in, the approach complements the insights from the macro-analysis of health professional mobility (Chapters 3–5). Two observations in particular enrich the debate.

First, behind the statistics and aggregated data, health professional mobility is a phenomenon composed of different types of mobile health professional each having a particular set of motivations and behaviours. The *livelihood migrant, career oriented, backpacker, commuter, undocumented* and *returner* differ in terms of their purpose of migration (e.g. settling down or acquiring specialized training), length of stay, personal profile and direction of movement (Chapter 6). Identifying and distinguishing between the types is of relevance to policy-makers and managers who try to steer in- and outflows because it allows targeting health workforce measures to retain and recruit health professionals more effectively. A senior nurse looking for further career development opportunities will not be motivated by the same incentives as a recently graduated medical doctor curious to experience other health systems and cultures. The individual decision to stay or leave is a complex process influenced by considerations endogenous to the health systems (e.g. training opportunities and job satisfaction), and by factors lying outside of those systems (e.g. work–life balance or political stability) (Chapter 10), but is often also an ongoing, gradual process as individuals more or less continuously decide whether to remain or to move on (Chapter 8). It also seems to suggest that the likelihood of further mobility is higher among migrants than among those who have never moved – "once a migrant, always a migrant".

Second, and much in line with the findings of the first PROMeTHEUS volume, health professional mobility is far from always an easy or "happy" experience for the individual, with implications for the systems involved. As for all types of migration, the accounts of health professionals who in some way have experienced migration are littered with difficult choices, frustration of having to leave to find something better and challenging circumstances in the new country, but also in the old, for those who return or those who stay behind (Chapters 7–11). Integration into the new system and the role that the migrant health professional has within that system play a key role in the migration experience. There is compelling evidence that migrant health professionals are at greater risk of being required to work below their skill level, which can then lead to disappointment for the individuals involved and to suboptimal wasteful situations in the health systems (Chapters 10 and 11). Discrimination and unfavourable working conditions also appear to disproportionally affect foreign

---

1 In this chapter, the terms "mobility" and "migration", as well as "mobile individual" and "individual migrant", are used interchangeably. Chapter 6 has a detailed discussion of terminology.

trained health professionals (Chapters 9 and 10) and is especially problematic for the "undocumented" health professionals working on an informal basis (Chapter 6). Yet going back to the home country is not necessarily easy either, as the returning health professional may find that qualifications and competences acquired abroad are not recognized or cannot be put to use through a lack of medical equipment. Better skills also translate into higher pay expectations, which may reduce employment opportunities when health professionals return home (Chapter 8). For the individual migrant, mobility may be voluntary but it is rarely uncomplicated.

### 2.1.3 Determinants of change: increasing health systems interdependence

The complexity of health professional mobility is reinforced by wider ongoing developments in the socioeconomic and geo-political context, which shape the factors and alter their relative weight. First, the EU enlargements of 2004, 2007 and 2013 meant that the European zone of free mobility and the labour markets of existing EU Member States gradually opened up to 13 new countries and their 100 million citizens. The enlargements have increased the scale of mobility flows in the EU, as well as the relative importance of intra-EU movements contributing to a pattern of east-to-west movements, but there is consensus that the overall "enlargement effect" has been moderate, and less than expected (Chapter 4). Moreover, countries such as the United Kingdom, Ireland and Finland continue receiving health professionals from non-EU countries (Kuusio et al., 2011; see also Chapters 8 and 10).

The second contextual development is the economic and financial crisis that Europe has been going through since around 2009 (depending on the country). Results of reasearch are only just emerging but there is evidence that the westwards movements in the EU have been joined by south-to-north flows as health professionals from crisis-hit countries migrate to countries with stronger economies. While all EU Member States have seen their room for manoeuvre reduced since the rules on EU economic governance came into force in late 2011 (European Commission, 2013a), countries receiving bailouts from the "troika" of the European Commission, International Monetary Fund and the European Central Bank face even stricter conditions with imposed spending cuts. Austerity measures and budgetary restrictions impact on the health care sector, for example in the form of pay cuts, recruitments freezes, early retirement schemes, staffing reductions, underemployment, unemployment, increased workloads and lower work morale; all of these can and do encourage emigration (Chapter 3). Outside the health system, tax increases, lower service levels, social unrest and wider unemployment may also spur the decision to leave as living standards fall or spouses and partners lose jobs. While it is impossible to isolate the causes of migration, it is conceivable that the effects of the economic crisis on health professional mobility will surpass the "enlargement effect" given the scale and duration of the crisis.

Third, the global demand for health workforce is increasing but is not being matched by a similar growth in supply. On the demand side, pressures stem mainly from a growing world population (Campbell et al., 2013). The WHO estimates the current global health workforce shortage at 7.2 million professionals, up from 4.3 million, and forecasts a shortage of 12.9 million by 2035 (Campbell et al., 2013). When countries do not produce sufficient numbers of health professionals but have the resources, international recruitment and mobility can become a way to fill vacant posts. Policy decisions and policy changes on international recruitment, especially in countries with attractive working conditions and labour markets that have the capacity to absorb large numbers of migrant health professionals, may have almost instant knock-on effects on countries with less favourable conditions. Global competition for qualified health professionals is likely to increase against this backdrop of projected increases in shortages of skilled health workers and as the internationalization of practice standards and of health profession curricula make the skills and competences of health professionals increasingly portable (Cortez, 2009).

Fourth, demographic factors play an important role. The population of Europe is ageing and so is its workforce. The European Commission talks about the "retirement bulge": around one-third of medical doctors in the EU were over 55 in 2009, and by 2020, 3.2% of all European doctors are expected to retire *annually* (European Commission, 2012). The situation might be even more alarming for nurses (OECD, 2013; Buchan, O'May & Dussault, 2013). As Europe's active workforce is shrinking, not only will countries be competing for health workforce but also different sectors of the economy will be competing to attract sufficient recruits. Decisions on what is the right number of doctors, nurses, but also of school teachers and engineers, are likely to get increasingly thorny.

The result is that health workforce policy can no longer be regarded as an isolated or a purely domestic issue. On the one hand, national efforts to plan, produce, retain and attract health professionals are exposed to, and may be undermined by, the pay levels, job opportunities and workforce policies in other countries, or indeed in other sectors. On the other hand, public and private employers, recruitment agencies and health care managers increasingly fish from the same pool of a global, but finite, health workforce. In a context where decisions taken in one health system have repercussions elsewhere, countries become increasingly *interdependent*.

### 2.1.4 Policy implications: unfinished homework, improving EU workforce intelligence

Attention around health professional mobility is mounting as observers and policy-makers gradually recognize its role in supplying many health systems with the workforce they need to function, while stripping other systems of scarce health professionals.

Health systems cannot afford to ignore health professional mobility, whether because they rely on foreign inflows to replenish the workforce or because health professionals choose to leave the country. But acknowledging that inflows and outflows are taking place is not enough. Countries experiencing large inflows must understand *why* they rely on international recruitment of health workforce. Taking effective policy measures will depend on whether domestic underproduction or geographical maldistribution is the cause, or whether difficulties in retaining a domestic health workforce mean that foreign inflows replace national outflows. Similarly, countries witnessing large outflows must understand whether these are the result of a structural overproduction of health professionals; an inability to meet the costs of employing these professionals; or unsatisfactory or worsening working and living conditions that stimulate attrition to other sectors and migration to other countries. The first signals that public resources may not be used to greatest effect; the second that there is a mismatch between training capacity and funded demand, and the third that the country could be running short of qualified health workforce. As health professional mobility frequently is a symptom of deeper health system problems in sources and destinations (Wismar et al., 2011), ignoring mobility, or using it as a "solution", only delays tackling the real issues.

Without information about the causes and drivers of migration, policy responses cannot address the underlying problems. If countries wish to retain their workforce, they need to pay attention to the different motivations of mobile individuals. Frustration over stagnant career progression will not be solved, for example, by easing doctors' workloads. While the collection of quantitative data on mobility is necessary for countries and international organizations to monitor flows, acknowledging and identifying the different types of mobile health professional and the related motivations (see section 2.1.2) not only complements the numbers but shed light on what action to take in the face of health professional mobility. Apart from a handful of notable exceptions (Eke, Girasek & Szócska, 2011; see also Chapters 7–10), systematic large-scale enquiry into the motivations of mobile and potentially mobile health professionals remains rare.

The unwavering need for more accurate information and more effective policies is closely connected to the issue of how to make better use of the increasingly scarce resource that is the health workforce. Growing interdependence (see section 2.1.3) implies that countries must find ways to get the best out of each health professional and avoid "brain waste" (Chapter 10). This can involve one or more of a number of initiatives: reducing time spent on performing tasks below skill levels, whether medical or administrative (Chapters 7, 10 and 11); improving employment terms and conditions, training opportunities, career progression, and the transparency and fairness of job-related processes (Chapter 10); improving retention at organization level through measures such as giving staff ownership over their work, providing childcare facilities, or competitive remuneration (Chapters 12 and 15); deploying the health workforce to rural and remote areas by introducing clinical nurse consultants (e.g. as in Samoa and Vanuatu); or by earmarking funds specifically for contracting health professionals to work in underserved regions (e.g. in Senegal) (Chapter 16). This illustrates the breadth of possible measures and their global applicability. Awareness is also growing that a satisfied health workforce can lead to better patient outcomes (Aiken et al., 2012).

As the health system context is undergoing profound changes and is affecting the determinants of mobility, the need for accurate health workforce data is growing. Yet little is known about how health workforce recruitment, retention and mobility across the next 20 years will be affected by the changing roles of the health profession, hospital budget cuts, salary levels, recruitment freezes, raised retirement ages or training post caps. The reactions to, and consequences of, the economic crisis, demographic pressures and the global health workforce shortage are likely to be of long-term relevance. Yet countries are in no better shape today than 10 years ago with regards to monitoring and collecting data on health professional mobility. As outflow data are the hardest to collect, source countries are probably even worse off in terms of knowing what is happening to their workforce (Chapter 5).

Although health professional mobility has reached the international policy agenda, there is still a need for more concrete action. Positive developments include the commitment to improved monitoring efforts undertaken by the WHO since 2010 as part of the *Global Code of Practice*, the sharing of best practices within the European *Joint Action*, and structured collaboration between the three main international data holders (WHO, OECD and European Commission). However, data collated at the international level can only be as good as the data provided by national bodies. Unless countries invest time and money in better workforce intelligence systems, large gaps in our understanding of health professional mobility will remain. Crisis-hit countries with least capacity to improve information systems may, however, be those who most urgently need them (Chapter 5).

### 2.1.5 The ethical dimension of health professional mobility: a new map of Europe?

The changing dynamics brought about by the economic downturn and global shortages affect the balance of power between countries as it becomes increasingly difficult for poorer systems to retain, and compete for, health professionals. Again, the EU provides a particular setting where the Treaty-based individual right to move freely within the EU prevails over the principles of ethical international recruitment established by the *WHO Code of Practice* (WHO, 2010). Yet with disparities in the EU on the rise, ethical and policy questions emerge on what are the responsibilities of both source and destination countries in planning, training and retaining health workforces (Glinos, 2012). Crisis-hit, resource-strained countries will have less policy capacity to act, and less means to invest, but there is mounting evidence to show that cutting the means allocated to the health system and its workforce is short-sighted and can have dramatic unwanted effects (Kentikelenis et al., 2011; McKee et al., 2012; Mladovsky et al., 2012; see also Chapter 3). For wealthier countries, being in a better situation and able to attract health professionals from abroad does not justify ignoring health professional mobility and its effects either. It must also be recognized that different countries will have very different levels of impact on international labour markets, in part dependent on the size of their workforce and of any current shortages, as well as the level of active recruitment. Countries with larger labour markets and bigger workforce needs have the potential for a much bigger impact on international labour markets. They must be aware of the consequences of their actions on smaller or less well-resourced neighbours and other countries. Although countries such as Luxembourg and the United Kingdom show similar levels of reliance on foreign medical doctors (representing around 35–40% of the total medical workforce in each country), the effect that Luxembourg, with its 605 foreign medical doctors, might have in terms of impacting on the health workforce of source countries is dwarfed when compared with a larger labour market such as that in the United Kingdom, which has 91 000 internationally trained medical doctors on its registry (Chapter 5).[2]

There is good reason to believe that the economic crisis and the austerity measures imposed are leading to widening disparities in Europe (e.g. European Commission, 2013b). For countries such as Bulgaria and Romania, the situation

---

2 United Kingdom data based on the total number of doctors on the General Medical Council's List of Registered Medical Practitioners (259 719 as of December 2013; General Medical Council, 2013). It is important to note that the United Kingdom no longer actively recruits from developing countries.

seems to be deteriorating, not improving, since accession to the EU in 2007. Other older Member States such as Greece are also facing enormous difficulties in pulling out of the crisis, while Ireland is still able to attract medical doctors from non-EU countries. At the same time, some destination countries may "benefit" from the crisis elsewhere as their large labour markets need qualified professionals and they are able to offer opportunities to the young and the brightest health professionals escaping crisis-hit countries. As the gap between wealthier and poorer EU Member States is widening, a new map of Europe and of its mobility flows may be emerging based on the relative strength of countries' economies and their ability to train, attract and retain health professionals. For the EU as a political entity, built to foster prosperity and reduce asymmetries between its members, a changing map raises new ethical and policy questions in terms of the relationship between Member States and whether there is, or should be, any scope for intra-EU solidarity.

## 2.2 Chapter findings

The volume is organized into four parts and includes 16 individual chapters. Part I comprises the introduction (Chapter 1), which presents the rationale of the book, its policy context, the research questions and methods, and this chapter.

Part II traces the changing dynamics of health professional mobility. Chapter 3 analyses health professional mobility in the financial and economic crisis. While there are wide variations in how countries have been affected by and have responded to the financial crisis, the chapter shows that many of the pull and push factors of health professional mobility have been profoundly affected, resulting in changing magnitudes and directions of mobility, although a reduction of mobility is not observed.

Chapter 4 summarizes the effects of the EU enlargements of 2004 and 2007. The accession of 12 new Member States with a population of over 100 million citizens expanded the labour market considerably. The chapter puts the enlargement in the context of the overall mobility and traces inflows and outflows in sending and receiving countries. The chapter concludes that mobility has become more diverse and that overall outflow from the new Member States has remained moderate, although some countries have lost considerable numbers of health professionals. Negative impact was observed particularly in remote and already underserved areas.

Chapter 5 presents an analysis of the reliance on foreign health professionals and mobility trends. It is a data-critical chapter that explores indicator availabilities, definitions and registry methodologies. Based on this review, the chapter defines a "yardstick" outlining key criteria for useful data collection, including coverage, timeliness, indicators, lines of accountability, data triangulation and international collaboration and exchange of data. This yardstick is to be used in countries when trying to improve data quality, not only for monitoring cross-border mobility but also for health workforce forecasting.

Chapter 6 questions who are the mobile individuals. At aggregate level, a statistical analysis of the data suggests that mobile health professionals are a homogeneous group, which would imply that they leave, return and stay for the same reasons. This is not an accurate representation, and the chapter distinguishes six types of mobile professional: the livelihood migrant, the career oriented, the backpacker, the commuter, the undocumented and the returner. The chapter discusses the important implications of this typology for retention strategies but also for documenting cross-border mobility.

If we are to find effective responses to health professional mobility in a changing Europe, we need to better understand these individuals regarding their motivations and experiences. Part III contains five chapters that explore the mobile individual. Chapter 7 presents a differentiated account of what makes Lithuanian health professionals leave and what makes them stay. Motivations and experiences of Lithuanian doctors, nurses and dentists were gathered through interviews conducted in Lithuania and Sweden. While remuneration issues were key to justifying mobility, they were not sufficient and a host of health system-related issues were raised, ranging from recognition to hospital management, training and the availability of technologies.

Chapter 8 takes a slightly different perspective in so far that health workers from other EU countries were interviewed to learn about their motivations, experiences and plans regarding cross-border professional mobility. The chapter explores policy implications for the United Kingdom regarding the integration of the foreign health workforce, language standards and language testing, and exchange of regulatory information between countries. The chapter also presents some counter-intuitive experiences, for example that some health professionals find it difficult to return to their country of origin because the experience abroad is not considered of value at home.

Chapter 9 deals with a slightly different sample of mobile health professionals including German and foreign health workers that have moved to Germany, returned from abroad or are planning to leave the country. The findings demonstrate that foreign medical doctors face a number of difficulties, including language and cultural barriers, bureaucracy and increased documentation requirements. Integration courses providing language skills, as well as cultural, organizational and medical knowledge, are a crucial factor facilitating migration and the successful integration of foreign health professionals. The chapter sheds light on a series of successful retention strategies targeting German medical doctors and nurses.

Chapter 10 explores why foreign medical doctors came to Ireland, stayed there or were planning to leave. The focus is on non-EU medical doctors. Many of the migrant doctors interviewed were planning onward migration because of their working conditions in Ireland. The chapter demonstrates that Irish-trained and foreign-trained doctors were motivated by much the same factors, as dissatisfaction with the postgraduate training environment for non-consultant hospital doctors is a key motivation for leaving the country. The chapter concludes that, without thorough reform, it is likely that Ireland will continue both to have a high dependency on non-EU migrant doctors and also to experience a high turnover of Irish-trained doctors.

Foreign-trained nurses are often not optimally integrated in the domestic health workforce. Chapter 11 analyses whether there is a difference between domestically trained and foreign-trained nurses from developing countries with regards to performing tasks below their skill level. The analysis is based on a large data collection from a cross-sectional study including 12 countries. The chapter concludes that high proportions of foreign-trained nurses from developing countries perform tasks below their skill level. The extent to which this is a matter of different "imported" work cultures, different curricula or discrimination remains unclear. Policy implications for better realizing the potential of foreign nurses from developing countries refer to the need for continuous professional training, to improve language skills, and a better understanding of skills and task profiles of foreign nurses.

Part IV includes five chapters devoted to policy responses. Chapter 12 sets the scene by looking at how governments, states, regions and health care providers try to manage the mobility of health professionals in order to address health workforce challenges. Presenting a broad overview of interventions, the chapter first describes *general* health workforce policies that indirectly affect the mobility of health professionals (i.e. covering self-sufficiency, retention and health workforce planning); it then goes on to explain health workforce *mobility* policies (e.g. international (ethical) recruitment), bilateral agreements (classified by their primary aim: ethical recruitment, international development, common labour markets and optimization of health care in border regions) and the role of recruitment agencies in health workforce mobility.

Chapter 13 focuses on national and international instruments and in particular on the use of so-called codes of practice for international recruitment, on potential effects of the General Agreements of Trade in Services (GATS; WHO,

1995) and on Directive 2005/36/EC on the mutual recognition of professional qualifications (European Commission, 2005). This chapter on codes of practice acknowledges a surge in the use of these instruments and their utilization for specifying career pathways, with an emphasis on the self-sufficiency or workforce sustainability that comes with the codes. It also shows, however, the need for monitoring and accountability if these codes are to have any real impact. Regarding the European Community Directive on the recognition of professional qualifications, the policy process has shown how important and at the same time difficult it is to include calls for cross-border continuous professional development (CPD) in the Directive.

Chapter 14 presents an analysis of the role of bilateral agreements as a policy response to health professional mobility and migration. The chapter gives an overview on the motivation and uses of bilateral agreements in cross-border health professional mobility. It details the United Kingdom practice of using those agreements in the form of both memoranda of understanding and contracts. The chapter concludes that the role of bilateral labour agreements has gradually transformed since the 1960s from primarily tools for labour recruitment to tools with a broader potential array of functions. As bilateral agreements can be costly and face competition from the more flexible practices of private recruitment agencies, their continuation is in doubt, although they might remain a component of diplomatic etiquette.

Chapter 15 switches from the national to the organizational perspective. It focuses on retention strategies in health care organizations. It presents case studies from hospitals in the Netherlands, Austria and Lithuania, reviewing the health workforce situation, the wide variety of retention approaches, and the characteristics of the strategies employed, including employment quality, work quality and organization quality. The chapter concludes that the organizational level has a key role for implementing retention strategies, although there are domains where regional and national level has primary importance.

In some other regions of the world, notably parts of Africa and Asia, health workforce shortages and migration have been a more focused subject of policy debate for longer than in Europe. To benefit from these experiences, Chapter 16 presents lessons from a global focus on health worker retention strategies. The chapter presents an evidence-based policy framework of 16 retention strategies relating to education, regulation, financial incentives and personal and professional support. A key message coming out of this work is that policy interventions are more effective when they are implemented in synergetic/complementary bundles rather than in isolation.

## References

Aiken LH et al. (2012). Patient safety, satisfaction, and quality of hospital care: cross-sectional surveys of nurses and patients in 12 countries in Europe and the United States. *British Medical Journal*, 344:e1717.

Altwegg J (2013). Nichts wie weg! *Frankfurter Allgemeine*, 8 October (http://www.faz.net/aktuell/feuilleton/deutsche-in-der-schweiz-nichts-wie-weg-12609351.html accessed 13 January 2014).

Bavarian Ministry of Economic Affairs and Media, Energy and Technology (2013). *Return to Bavaria*. Munich, Bavarian Ministry of Economic Affairs and Media, Energy and Technology (http://www.work-in-bavaria.de/en/employees/work/return-to-bavaria/, accessed 13 January 2014).

Buchan J, Seccombe I (2012). *Overstretched, under-resourced: the UK nursing labour market review 2012*, London, Royal College of Nursing (http://www.rcn.org.uk/__data/assets/pdf_file/0016/482200/004332.pdf, accessed 5 December 2013).

Buchan J, O'May F, Dussault G (2013). The nursing workforce and the global economic crisis. *Journal of Nursing Scholarship*, 45(3):298–307.

Campbell J et al. (2013). A universal truth: no health without a workforce. *Third Global Forum on Human Resources for Health, Recife, Brazil*. Geneva, Global Health Workforce Alliance and World Health Organization (Forum Report).

Cortez N (2009). International health care convergence: the benefits and burdens of market-driven standardization. *Wisconsin International Law Journal*, 26(3):646–704.

Eke E, Girasek E, Szócska M (2011). From melting pot to laboratory of change in central Europe: Hungary and health workforce migration. In Wismar M et al., eds. *Health professional mobility and health systems. Evidence from 17 European countries*. Copenhagen, WHO Regional Office for Europe on behalf of the European Observatory on Health Systems and Policies:365–394.

European Commission (2005). *Directive 2005/36/EC on the recognition of professional qualifications*. Brussels, European Commission (http://ec.europa.eu/internal_market/qualifications/policy_developments/legislation/index_en.htm, accessed 5 August 2013).

European Commission (2012). *Staff working document on an action plan for the EU health workforce. Towards a job-rich recovery*. Strasbourg, European Commission (http://ec.europa.eu/dgs/health_consumer/docs/swd_ap_eu_healthcare_workforce_en.pdf, accessed 2 January 2014).

European Commission (2013a). *EU economic governance*. Brussels, European Commission (http://ec.europa.eu/economy_finance/economic_governance/index_en.htm, accessed 13 January 2014).

European Commission (2013b). *Health inequalities in the EU: final report of a consortium (Consortium lead: Sir Michael Marmot)*. Brussels, Directorate-General for Health and Consumers (http://ec.europa.eu/health/social_determinants/docs/healthinequalitiesineu_2013_en.pdf, accessed 13 January 2014).

Galan A, Olsavszky V, Vladescu C (2011). Emergent challenge of health professional emigration: Romania's accession to the EU. In Wismar M et al., eds. *Health professional mobility and health systems. Evidence from 17 European countries*. Copenhagen, WHO Regional Office for Europe on behalf of the European Observatory on Health Systems and Policies:449–478.

General Medical Council (2013). *List of registered medical practitioners: statistics*. London, General Medical Council (http://www.gmc-uk.org/doctors/register/search_stats.asp, accessed 13 January 2014).

Glinos IA (2012). Worrying about the wrong thing: patient mobility vs. health professional mobility. *Journal of Health Services Research and Policy*, 17(4):254–256.

Kautsch M, Czabanowska K (2011). When the grass gets greener at home: Poland's changing incentives for health professional mobility. In Wismar M et al., eds. *Health professional mobility and health systems. Evidence from 17 European countries*. Copenhagen, WHO Regional Office for Europe on behalf of the European Observatory on Health Systems and Policies:419–448.

Kentikelenis A et al. (2011). Health effects of financial crisis: omens of a Greek tragedy. *Lancet*, 378:1457–1458.

Kuusio H et al. (2011). Changing context and priorities in recruitment and employment: Finland balances inflows and outflows of health professionals. In Wismar M et al., eds. *Health professional mobility and health systems. Evidence from 17 European countries*. Copenhagen, WHO Regional Office for Europe on behalf of the European Observatory on Health Systems and Policies:163–180.

Labrianidis L (2011). *Investing in leaving: the Greek case of international migration of professionals in the globalization era*. Athens, Kritiki.

López-Valcárcel BG, Pérez PB, Quintana CDD (2011). Opportunities in an expanding health service: Spain between Latin America and Europe. In Wismar M et al., eds. *Health professional mobility and health systems. Evidence from 17*

*European countries.* Copenhagen, WHO Regional Office for Europe on behalf of the European Observatory on Health Systems and Policies:263–294.

McKee M et al. (2012). Austerity: a failed experiment on the people of Europe. *Clinical Medicine*, 12:346–350.

Mladovsky P et al. (2012). *Health policy responses to the financial crisis.* Copenhagen, WHO Regional Office for Europe on behalf of the European Observatory on Health Systems and Policies (Policy summary 5) (http://www.euro.who.int/__data/assets/pdf_file/0009/170865/e96643.pdf, accessed 13 January 2014).

OECD (2013). *Health at a glance 2013: OECD indicators.* Paris, Organisation for Economic Co-operation and Development (http://www.oecd.org/els/health-systems/Health-at-a-Glance-2013.pdf, accessed 13 January 2014).

WHO (1995). *General agreement on trade in services (GATS).* Geneva, World Health Organization (http://www.who.int/trade/glossary/story033/en/index.html, accessed 3 January 2014).

WHO (2010). *WHO global code of practice on the international recruitment of health personnel.* Geneva, World Health Organization (Sixty-third World Health Assembly, WHA63.16). (http://www.who.int/hrh/migration/code/WHO_global_code_of_practice_EN.pdf, accessed 1 October 2013).

Wismar M et al., eds. (2011). *Health professional mobility and health systems. Evidence from 17 European countries.* Copenhagen, WHO Regional Office for Europe on behalf of the European Observatory on Health Systems and Policies.

# Part II
# The changing dynamics of health professional mobility

# Chapter 3

# The economic crisis in the EU: impact on health workforce mobility

*Gilles Dussault and James Buchan*

## 3.1 Introduction

Economic conditions rank high in the list of factors that influence the mobility of health professionals. Studies of mobility flows in the EU and elsewhere tend to show that health professionals move from poorer to richer environments. This is the case in times of economic stability, but is it also the case in times of economic crisis when the conditions in traditional destination countries are also difficult? The PROMeTHEUS project was commissioned in advance of the global financial crisis that first hit in 2007–2008 and which continues to be a dominant feature of the policy and labour market context across EU Member States. This chapter gives consideration to the ways in which the crisis has manifested itself in the health sector, with a specific focus on health workforce mobility. The chapter sets the economic context of expenditure on health systems, reports on how EU Member States have responded to the crisis as it has impacted on health system funding, considers evidence on changes in mobility drivers and trends, and looks at the consequences, now and in the future, for health professionals and EU health systems.

Developing an accurate country perspective or regional overview of the impact of the crisis on health workforce mobility is complex for various reasons. First, aggregation of, often incomplete, national or regional data takes time, and some effects will become "visible" to data analysis only after the event. Second, there are important variations in how the crisis has affected specific countries and in how these have responded, making it challenging to generalize. Third, as noted elsewhere in the book, the available data on the health workforce are fragmented, with more data on public sector employment, variable data on private sector/nongovernmental organization (NGO) employment, and often poor data on informal health workers, such as some of those employed in private homes. It is virtually impossible to assess if the crisis may have pushed more workers into the last category of employment. Finally, there is also a more technical point: it can be difficult to separate out the effects of the crisis on the health workforce and, therefore, to attribute causality to the impact of any specific economic and labour market changes on health workforce mobility.

This chapter works within these constraints, specifies what can be determined about the impact of the crisis on health professional mobility and considers some of the likely major implications for future policy development and planning. The chapter serves as both an update and a summary of a changed economic and labour market context for health professional mobility since the first book on the PROMeTHEUS project was published, and as a reminder that without a clear sense of this context and of the challenges it generates, policy-makers will not be able to respond adequately.

One obvious indicator of change as a result of the crisis is that real growth rate in gross domestic product (GDP) in many EU Member States has declined since 2007, with a sharper fall in 2009. Table 3A.1[1] provides Eurostat data for the 27 EU Member States as of 2013 (EU27). Some countries have fared better than others (e.g. Germany, Slovakia, Sweden), and some have suffered more than others (e.g. Greece, Ireland, Italy, Spain, Portugal). Others, mostly small countries, were severely hit by the crisis in 2009 and have shown signs of recovery afterwards (the Czech Republic, Finland, Estonia, Latvia and Lithuania).

Against this backdrop of economic decline, there can be a range of direct and indirect effects on EU populations, their quality of life, their economic well-being and their health status (Commission on Social Determinants of Health, 2008; Stuckler et al., 2009; McKee, Basu & Stuckler, 2012). However, this chapter will narrow the focus to examine the crisis in relation to health care labour markets and the health workforce. First, a framework of the links between the crisis, the health sector and the health workforce will be presented; the following sections will present data sets on trends and changes that have occurred as the crisis has developed. Health professional labour market and mobility issues and policy responses will then be examined and discussed.

---

1 Tables 3A.1 to 3A.8 are in the Annex to this chapter.

## 3.2 Methods

This chapter is based on a desk review of published and "grey" documentation on the various dimensions of the effects of the crisis on the health sector. It focuses on health workforce and mobility issues. The Cochrane Library, PubMed and Google Scholar databases were searched using combinations of the following key words: economic, financial crisis, effects, impacts, health sector, health workforce, European countries, plus the names of EU Member States. Documents included in the analysis come from scientific literature, media and opinion articles and from grey literature (e.g. reports, open letters, discussion papers and conferences, national statistics institutes and professional associations, among others). The aim was to develop a rapid overview of the issues and implications, and as such we have made use of recent media articles from reputable sources. It includes publications in English, French, Spanish and Portuguese from 2008 to the end of 2012. Statistical data were extracted from the OECD database and the WHO Health for All databases.

## 3.3 How the crisis affects the health sector

In relation to the impact of the economic crisis, the health sector across the EU has been a "victim" of a "shock": "an unexpected occurrence originating outside the health system that has a large negative effect on the availability of health system resources or a large positive effect on the demand for health services" (Mladovsky et al., 2012). Since 2008, it has had to deal with the consequences of events that originated elsewhere in the economy.

These consequences and their effects on the sector as a whole are better understood by reconstituting the pathways through which they are created, as illustrated by Fig. 3.1. The figure highlights the linkages between broader economic circumstances, different sectors of the economy including health, impact on labour markets and the health workforce and impact on health worker mobility.

While the primary focus of the chapter is on mobility, this cannot be considered in isolation from broader economic health system and workforce/labour market factors. This was a key message from the first book on the PROMeTHEUS project and is equally relevant when examining the impact of the crisis on health workforce behaviour, as clearly illustrated in Fig. 3.1. This impact could be manifested in changes in the total stock of workers, skills-mix and distribution, and in changes in internal mobility, motivation and productivity, working conditions (workload, salary and benefits, retirement age) and labour relations. All can be affected by decisions taken at health sector level but also by policy choices in other sectors, such as education, employment, labour law,

**Fig. 3.1** *Pathways of the impact of the economic crisis on the health workforce*

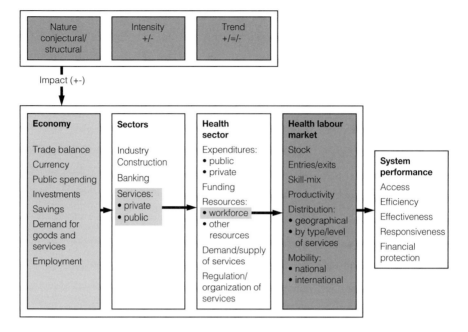

public administration and finance. Fig. 3.1 also highlights that the "end point" is how the crisis is affecting the various dimensions of the performance of health services systems, for example equity of access to services; service effectiveness, efficiency and responsiveness; and the capacity to protect citizens against the impoverishing effects of ill health.

To capture the variations between countries, the nature (conjectural or structural) and the intensity of the crisis must be considered. In some heavily indebted countries (e.g. Greece, Ireland, Italy, Portugal, Spain), the crisis hit more severely because of pre-existing structural economic weaknesses, such as high balance of payment deficits or low household saving rates, and therefore less resilience. The dependency of these countries on external borrowing has forced them to apply austerity measures negotiated with (or imposed by) lenders, mainly the European Central Bank, the European Commission and the International Monetary Fund. Another variable is the direction of the evolution of the crisis, whether it appears to be worsening (e.g. Greece, Spain) or easing off (e.g. Estonia, Ireland) or remains stable.

The most common and visible signs of the crisis have been higher costs of borrowing, more difficult access to credit for individuals and for companies, reduction in investments, higher unemployment and underemployment as a result of the contraction of demand for goods and services, reduction of imports, currency depreciation and even recession. Governments have used an array of strategies to reduce their budget deficit in order to bring down borrowing interest rates to manageable levels: public spending cuts, tax increases, labour market reforms and deregulation, and incentives to improve productivity and to make the allocation of financial resources more efficient. The effects on the various sectors of the economy may differ depending on political/ideological choices and on the capacity of interest groups to "protect" their sector.

Specific effects on the health sector are shown in the third column of Fig. 3.1. They can be grouped by the area affected: funding and expenditures, regulation and organization of the sector, sector costs, demand for and supply of services, and the workforce itself.

Looking first at data on expenditure on health as a broad indicator of available funding (Table 3A.2), there is less sign of a crisis than might have been expected. Total expenditure on health, as a percentage of GDP, remained relatively stable in most EU27 Member States. In 23 countries, it was even higher in 2010 or 2011 than in 2006 before the crisis set in. The four other countries, Bulgaria, Cyprus, Hungary and Latvia, experienced very small reductions. On average, EU Member States spent 8.95% of GDP on health in 2006 and 9.88% in 2010. However, when data on annual growth rates of total expenditure on health in real terms are examined (Table 3A.3), a more negative picture emerges. Expenditure in real terms declined after 2006 in all EU Member States except Germany (data not available for Bulgaria, Cyprus, Latvia, Lithuania and Malta). Most EU Member States may have proportionally spent the same or more of GDP on health across the period of the crisis but this was against a backdrop of diminishing overall GDP size. The average rate of expenditure was negative (−4.4%) in 2009–2010 in comparison with the previous year; at country level it varied significantly, with some countries (e.g. Germany, Netherlands, Slovakia and Sweden) reporting growth rates above 2%, while others reported significant declines (e.g. Estonia, 7.3%; Greece, 6.5%; Ireland, 7.6%).

Some countries experienced sharp decreases between 2008–2009 and 2009–2010, perhaps because the crisis had hit later or because of a policy implementation lag effect: the Czech Republic (from 11.7% to −4.1%), Denmark (from 5.9% to +1.7%), Poland (from 6.5% to 0.6%), Slovakia (from 8.5% to 2.6%), and the United Kingdom (from 7% to 0.2%).

Finally, when public expenditure is measured as a percentage of total expenditure on health, there has been little evidence in the data of a "withdrawal" of public expenditure on health across the period, with the exception of two countries. For most countries, the percentage of the total has remained relatively constant overall (Table 3A.4). In 11 countries, it slightly increased between 2006 and 2010; decreases were less than 1% in three countries, and in the others the range was from 1.2% to 5.6%, the outliers being Hungary (−5.0%) and Ireland (−5.6%).

How does this variable pattern of changes in level of funding impact on health services? The analysis of data on expenditure on health shows a varied pattern across the EU (Morgan & Astolfi, 2013) has an overview of OECD countries that reaches similar conclusions). Based on the observation of previous episodes of economic crisis, demand for health services should decline as a result of higher costs, reduced expenditure and reduced household incomes. This would be observed initially and principally in the private sector, as patients defer care or use public services as they are less able to afford private ones (WHO, 2009). There are no regional data on changes in demand for public services. In Greece, where this has been monitored, the number of admissions to public hospitals was 24% higher in 2010 than in 2009, and 8% higher in the first half of 2011 than in the same period in 2010; ambulatory visits to public health centres increased by 22% in 2011 compared with 2010 (Kaitelidou & Kouli, 2012).

## 3.4 National policy responses to the crisis

The previous section has highlighted how the crisis has manifested itself in changes to the pattern of expenditure on health. This section looks at how policy responses have impacted on the health sector, recognizing that there are important variations in how the crisis has affected specific countries and in how these have responded (Mladovsky et al., 2012). Most EU Member States were already facing important health sector challenges before the crisis started in late 2007 and most were engaged in some sort of reform. As it became clear that the crisis was going to last and to hit harder, the WHO Regional Committee for Europe, at its 2009 meeting, called for the "protection" of the health sector by governments in the following terms: "Investing in health and health systems is more than ever a must in times of crisis and should be an essential component of the societal response to the crisis". "Health leaders … were unanimous in advocating the protection of health budgets to be able to address public health threats effectively, widen access to essential health services, reduce inequalities in health and improve the performance and efficiency of health systems" (WHO, 2009, p. 1).

EU Member States responded to the crisis with a mix of cost-containment and "protection" measures. Examples of austerity measures have included budget cuts (targeted or not), increase of co-payments, reduction of public provision of some services, salary freeze or decrease for workers in the sector, personnel reductions, closure of facilities or a mix of these.

Specific country examples include Estonia, which cut its health budget by 24% and introduced a 15% co-payment for nursing inpatient care (Habicht, 2012); Greece, where the reduction of public expenditure has included a budget cut of €1.4 billion in the health sector in 2011, mainly in salary and benefits and in hospital costs, including medicines and equipment reductions (Kaitelidou & Kouli, 2012); Ireland, where the health budget was cut by €1 billion in 2010 and €746 million in 2011, and co-payments for medical services have increased; and Portugal, where measures have included reduction of the budget of public hospitals, doubling of user fees for some households and exclusion of services such as transportation of non-urgent patients (*Expresso*, 2012).

## 3.5 The impact of the crisis on the health workforce

The sections above have outlined the overall impact on the health sector and summarized key crisis-induced policy responses from within the health sector. This section considers what is known about the impact on the health workforce. First, comparative data on changes in the size ("stock") of the health workforce in different countries are examined before looking at specific examples of changes at country level in the size and shape of the health workforce.

The first workforce indicator to examine is the "stock" or size. The definition can vary in different data sets: some measure all who are registered, whereas others measure only those currently practising. An analysis of OECD data on physicians (Table 3A.5) and WHO/EU data on nurses (Table 3A.6) gives some sense of the evolution of the health workforce across the period under examination. Five EU Member States (France, Hungary, Italy, Latvia and Malta) report a slight decrease in the total number of physicians between 2006 and 2010. However, the EU average physician to population ratio increased from 312 per to 334 (Table 3A.5) and the nurse to population ratio increased from 792 to 834 (Table 3A.6). Estonia, Latvia and Lithuania are the only countries that reported a decrease in the ratio of nurses to population.

As noted in the introduction to this chapter, one of the limitations in using comparative data from OECD, WHO and other such sources is that there is an inevitable lag before these data are published, and as such the information will be months or even years behind the current "reality". By accessing data directly from sources in selected EU Member States, it is possible to develop a more recent picture of changes in the stock of doctors and nurses (Tables 3A.7 and 3A.8). These data, from Ireland, Italy, Portugal and Spain, present a more up-to-date and specific picture of changes in physician and nurse employment. Analysis across three time points, covering the period before and during the impact of the crisis, shows a variable change in the different countries but actual reductions in the stock of physicians in Portugal, and nurses in Italy and Ireland.

The reasons for staffing reductions that are apparent in some health systems are at least partly related to the impact of the crisis. Health care is labour intensive; the workforce is a major cost and when there is a need to contain costs there are "temptations to restrict it in its growth or even achieving its contraction as that can bring about significant savings" (Albreht, 2011, p. 1). This can be achieved by direct reductions in staffing, by changing skill-mix to a less costly one, by reducing pay and conditions of employment and by reducing pension entitlements, among other responses. All these responses have been noted in Europe. The European Federation of Nurses Associations conducted a survey of 34 European countries, including the EU27, on the impact of the economic crisis on nurses and nursing: over half of its member organizations reported pay cuts, pay freeze and rising unemployment for nurses; over a third of its member organizations reported concerns about quality of care and patient safety; and over one-fifth of its member organizations report downgrading of nursing and substitution of nurses with unskilled workers (European Federation of Nurses Associations, 2012).

Specific country examples include Bulgaria, where nurses' salaries were cut by 10–25% in 2009; Greece, which has cut salaries of all health care personnel (Kaitelidou & Kouli, 2012); Ireland, which put a moratorium on recruitment and promotion of health care personnel, cut positions, reduced fees for contracted professionals (e.g. general practitioners (GPs)) and initiated early retirement and voluntary redundancy schemes (Thomas & Burke, 2012); and England, where the National Health Service (NHS) has reduced the number of nurses it employs, reduced training levels, "frozen" vacant posts, increased pension contributions and "capped " any increases in public sector pay (Buchan & Seccombe, 2013).

## 3.6 The impact of the crisis on health workforce mobility

The previous section looked at the impact on numbers of health workers by examining data on "stock" at different points in time; it highlighted some of the policy responses that were focused specifically on reducing staffing costs within the health sector. Some of these policies will also impact on the mobility of health workers, either because the policy is targeted deliberately at changing the level of mobility or because a change in mobility patterns was an unintended consequence of the implementation of the policy.

To illustrate the impact on health worker mobility a simple "stock-flow" model (Fig. 3.2) was used as a starting point. This shows the main types of mobility

**Fig. 3.2** *One-box stock-flow model*

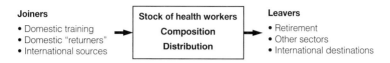

(flows) that, in combination, will act to affect the total number (stock) within the health workforce. The first book examining the PROMeTHEUS project (Wismar et al., 2011), and other chapters in this second book, illustrated how the magnitude and net direction of these different flows can change over time as a result of policy changes, as result of changed financial and labour market conditions and because of broader societal and cultural change. This model can also help to develop a better understanding of the possible impact of the crisis on health worker mobility.

If we recognize that trends and patterns of mobility will change over time, we can then make an assessment of how the crisis has impacted on the different flows in a specific country or system context. The key is to recognize that the actual impact on different flows may be in different directions in different countries, and that it is important to consider the impact – if any – on each component flow in order to make an overall assessment. Table 3.1 identifies each of these main joiner and leaver flows and highlights how the economic crisis may impact either to increase or reduce that flow, depending on the specific circumstances of the health services system or country.

While most assessments of the impact of the crisis focus understandably on negative effects and changes, it must not be assumed that the crisis only has negative effects on flows. There can also be positive effects if the right policy responses are implemented, such as the adoption of measures to improve productivity, to adjust regulation of the economy, to eliminate unnecessary or unproductive expenses, to stimulate savings and generally to make the allocation of financial resources more efficient. There may also be unplanned or unintended positive effects, such as moderating flows to and from the country, or even a "recession dividend" if health sector jobs and careers become more attractive to labour market entrants because alternative careers are perceived to have become less attractive or available. Within the health sector, access, quality and efficiency may improve in spite of difficult economic circumstances, depending on policy responses. For example, the development of primary care and ambulatory services or the better integration of the various levels of care can produce positive effects.

Table 3.1 highlights the extent to which there can be varying and sometimes countervailing pressures on mobility arising from the crisis and related policy

**Table 3.1** *Joiner and leaver flows in the economic crisis*

| Joiner flows: possible impacts of crisis | | Leaver flows: possible impacts of the crisis | |
|---|---|---|---|
| From domestic training | May *increase*, if health sector employment remains relatively stable and attractive | To retirement | May *increase* if "early retirement" policies stimulate workforce reductions |
| | May *reduce* if public sector funding for training is reduced, and training intakes subsequently decline | | May *reduce* if workers postpone retirement in response to economic uncertainty |
| | | | May *reduce* if country initiates policy of extending retirement age to reduce pension costs burden |
| From domestic "returners" | May *increase*, if employment opportunities in other sectors reduce; those with health sector qualifications may try to return to health sector | To other domestic sectors | May *increase* if there are fewer employment opportunities in health sector as a result of cost-containment and of redundancies |
| | May *reduce* if employment opportunities in health sector decrease | | May *reduce* if employment opportunities in other sectors decline and/or if conditions in health sector improve |
| From international sources | May *increase*, if the economy remains sufficiently strong to attract immigrants | To international destinations | May *increase* if reduced employment opportunities at home stimulate more workers to look abroad |
| | May *reduce*, if demand for new health workers slows down | | May *reduce* if employment opportunities in health sectors in usual destination countries diminish |
| | May *reduce* if country introduces more restrictive policies to reduce immigration to "protect" domestic workforce/ economy[a] | | |

[a] EU countries will not be able to target policies at reducing flows of doctors, nurses and midwives from other EU countries as freedom of movement is guaranteed.

responses. As such, there is no simple overall answer to the question of how the crisis has impacted on the mobility of health professionals in the EU. The impact has varied in different countries and across time.

In the first book examining the PROMeTHEUS project, it was noted that "the global financial crisis may have intensified motivations for migration or may have slowed them if fewer job opportunities were available in destination countries. While there are no concrete data, income related incentives to migrate and the perception of better opportunities can be expected to change considerably in the new economic environment" (Wismar et al., 2011, p. 46). This uncertainty about the overall impact of the crisis still exists in 2012, in part also because little has been done at a regional level to systematically monitor mobility itself or the factors that may influence it.

However, it is possible to assess mobility changes at a national level and to link these changes to the impact of the crisis. Several published studies point to a growth in outflow of health workers from countries that have been impacted negatively by the crisis (e.g. Saar & Habicht (2011) and Tjadens, Weiland & Eckert (2012)). This section also uses country case studies to develop a narrative-based analysis of available data and to track policy implementation across time, which can also highlight the shifting impact of different policies. Four country narratives are used to illustrate varying experiences and trends.

The first case study is Bulgaria (Box 3.1) which highlights how the ageing of the workforce and relatively low pay rates have contributed to labour market instability in the health sector. Box 3.2 covers Portugal and highlights a deepening impact of the crisis on the health system, including reduced staffing and employment conditions for health workers, and indications of increased migration of health workers to other countries, including some, such as the United Kingdom, which have not been "traditional" destinations. The third case study, Spain (Box 3.3), illustrates a sequence of policies to reduce pay rates, "freeze" vacancies and increase working hours; this has impacted on health workforce projections, calling into question planning outcomes developed in earlier years. There are also reports of increased outflow to other EU Member States and, in a reverse from the previous direction of flow, to Ecuador. The fourth case study, from the United Kingdom (Box 3.4), also reports on staffing reductions and pay freezes, plus a tightening of immigration controls, leading to an overall change in net migration patterns for nurses, with increased outflow and reduced inflow from non-EU countries, but increased inflow from elsewhere in the EU, a flow over which the United Kingdom Government has limited control.

These four country case studies serve to illuminate the variations in impact and policy response which have occurred in different EU Member States since the first impact of the crisis in 2008. They show that the crisis has led directly or indirectly to policy responses that have impacted on the workforce and its predilection to mobility. Where a feasible end-destination exists, this has meant that the flow has been towards perceived "better" employment and career prospects. As such, this is no different from other periods. What the crisis has done is sharpen the relative differences between prospects in the current location and the potential destination, and to increase the "push" factors to motivate individual health workers to move. The ability to actually then make

**Box 3.1** *Country case study: Bulgaria*

The health sector in Bulgaria is facing serious demographic challenges for human resources for health deriving from the ageing of the health workforce. Based on the professional registers maintained by the organizations for doctors and nurses and other health professionals in Bulgaria, medical professionals are characterized by a high mean age: 51 years for doctors and 49 years for nurses. The mean age for GPs is 52 years.

The mobility of health professionals is also an emerging issue in human resources for health, which is compounded by poor planning and the lack of a strategy to overcome these problems. The outflows of Bulgarian health professionals have been gradually increasing since EU accession. For the period 2009–2012, the professional organization of doctors issued 1 441 certificates for outstanding practice for doctors considering applying to work in other countries. In 2012 alone, this included 440, up from 260 in 2009. For the same period, 1 717 nurses and other health professionals obtained their certificates. This number represents approximately 5% of the health workforce.

According to a representative survey among medical professionals held in 2011, 22% of the medical professionals in the system are considering migration to other countries. The main factors that influence these migration decisions were reported to be remuneration, lack of professionals in specific specialties that burdens working, lack of funding for materials and expendables, and lack of modern equipment (Kuznetsova, 2012; Zahariev, 2012).

The first government reaction to the economic crisis was a general cut of 20% to the public budget in mid-2010. This directly affected the budgets of medical universities in Bulgaria. The universities successfully reached a compensation agreement with the government, allowing allocation of up to 5% of the student capacity of the university to for-profit students (who are not supported with state funding). In the same period (2009–2012), state funding provided per student decreased by 30%. In 2012, the guaranteed amount per student was 6 514 lev (€3 330) for a doctor and 3 465 lev (€1 770) for a nurse.

An additional problem that negatively affected medical students was the closure of state-funded places for resident doctors for the period 2005–2008. After 2008, a limited number of state-funded places for resident doctors were opened annually but most resident doctors have to pay for their specialization. In 2011, only 100 state-funded places were opened. This resulted in increasing numbers of young medical doctors migrating and, according to experts, currently approximately 37% of students are planning to specialize abroad without looking for opportunities in Bulgaria. In November 2012, it was announced that there would be 254 state-funded places opened for 2013, together with the launch of a project co-funded by EU structural funds that would ensure 1 000 additional places, but it is now reported that there are not sufficient candidates.

**Box 3.1** *contd*

Another impact of the crisis was that the full budget of the National Health Fund (funding for medical activities for hospital and out-of-hospital services) was not spent, and in the period 2009–2012, the government redirected approximately 1.6 billion lev from the fund to the national budget. This negatively affected the system and led to poor funding for medical activities, affected access to services and had a negative impact on management strategies for human resources for health. In 2012, the government reacted inconsistently to separate protests from health professionals who were funded directly by the Ministry of Health, such as emergency room staff and the staff in haematology units by ensuring a salary increase for emergency staff of 18% (mean salary, approximately 650 lev (€332)) but refusing national funding for raising salaries for haematology staff[2]. For the latter, municipality funds were allocated to prevent the mass exodus of the haematology unit staff in the town of Varna, ensuring a mean salary of 700 lev (€357).

Bulgaria lacks strategic vision and policies on how to address human resources for health-related problems. The economic crises have extended these problems and the health system will face serious obstacles in the near future.

*Prepared by Dessislava Kuznetsova and Boyan Zahariev*

**Box 3.2** *Country case study: Portugal*

In early October 2010, the Portuguese Government adopted the budget for 2011, the most restrictive in 25 years (European Hospital and Healthcare Federation, 2011). In 2012, the expected "savings" in the health sector were estimated at 8.2% (€710 million) compared with the previous year. The new budget for 2013 proposes a further cut of 19.6% in the National Health Service and 17% in the total health sector (Portuguese Ministry of Finance, 2012).

One of the main austerity measures in 2012 was to raise user fees in the National Health Service; for example, the fee for a visit to the emergency room went from €9.6 to €20 (Portuguese Ministry of Finance, 2012). In the pharmaceutical sector, the government expanded the utilization of generic drugs, introduced an electronic prescription system, raised the prices of some vaccines, and reduced reimbursement

2 03.10.2012 Most employees in emergency rooms are not motivated by the June salary growth http://www.mediapool.bg/povecheto-zaeti-v-barza-pomosht-ne-sa-motivirani-ot-yunskiya-rast-na-zaplatite-news197949.html

14.08.2012 Conflicts ripen in Emergency because of unclear rules for wages http://www.zdrave.net/Portal/News/Default.aspx?page=1&evntid=55887

27.11.2012 Hematologists in Varna remain on their job http://bulgaria.actualno.com/Hematolozite-vyv-Varna-ostavat-na-rabota-news_408247.html

13.12.2013 Salaries for hematologists are secured by taking money from orphanages http://bulgaria.actualno.com/Osigurjavat-zaplatite-na-hematolozite-s-parite-na-domovete-za-siraci-news_410110.html

19.11.2012 Salaries in Varna hematology units will be increased by another 20% http://btvnews.bg/article/bulgaria/zaplatite-na-hematolozite-ot-varna-shche-bdt-uvelicheni-s-oshche-20.html

**Box 3.2** *contd*

for some drugs and products. As a result, many pharmacies are now operating with negative margins, which will likely lead to the closure of many small ones (Pita Barros, Martins & Moura, 2012). Hospitals were also targeted; the government proposed the merger of several hospital centres and services, and the reduction of the number of managers and of nurses per shift (European Federation of Nurses Associations, 2012). Cuts in public sector employment were implemented to reduce the public deficit, in addition to pay cuts, which ranged from 5% to 10% in 2011, for public servants with a monthly salary above €1 400; in 2012, 2 of the 14 salary payments per year were cut, and a further reduction of 4.5% took place in 2013. This was a total of more than 30% in three years. Salaries and promotions have been frozen since 2010, and only one in two staff members who leave are being replaced (European Hospital and Healthcare Federation, 2011). Workloads were increased and the number of days of leave reduced. In 2010, planned changes in penalties for early retirement triggered a major increase in early retirement of physicians. Many of these early retirees went to the private sector, where salaries did not suffer the same reductions (Portuguese Observatory on Health Systems, 2012). There is some evidence of increased emigration of nurses (Buchan & Seccombe, 2012), and, more recently, of physicians. For example, data from the United Kingdom Nursing and Midwifery Council indicate that the number of Portuguese nurses admitted to their register had grown from 20 in 2006–2007 to more than 550 in 2011–2012. The Portuguese Nursing Council (*Ordem dos Enfermeiros*) reported that, on average, it receives 10 requests per day for the documentation needed to work abroad. In the first 10 months of 2012, the Council received 3 202 requests, compared with 1 724 for the whole of 2011 (*Sol*, 2012). The Medical Council (*Ordem dos Médicos*) has also reported an increase in physicians leaving the country, which it attributes to active recruitment by countries such as France, Germany and the United Kingdom (Statistics Portugal, 2012). Meanwhile, the *numerus clausus* for entry in medicine or nursing has not changed.

The number of new physicians has, in fact, been augmented as new programmes have started to produce graduates (Government of Portugal, 2012). The Medical Council and medical students associations have pleaded for a reduction in the number of entries in medical schools (*Radio Renascença*, 2012), on the basis that access to specialty training is not sufficient and that some graduates face unemployment. There is also concern resulting from the increase in young people studying medicine in foreign universities, a number estimated at around 1 400 (Government of Portugal, 2012).

The current economic crisis will not end soon in Portugal, but so far no mechanism has been set up to monitor and assess its effects on health services or on the workforce.

**Box 3.3** *Country case study: Spain*

In Spain, the pressure to reduce the deficit started a wave of constitutional reforms and significant public budget cuts (OECD, 2011), affecting the role of the state as employer, funder and provider of health care. The National Health Service has shifted from providing universal coverage through general taxation to a system funded through social security contributions. Now, only the unemployed not receiving unemployment benefit and retirees on the minimum pension will have access to free medicines (López-Valcárcel, 2011). Immigrants will only be entitled to emergency medical care and assistance with pregnancy and childbirth (López-Valcárcel, 2011). New legislation opens the possibility for private insurance to cover services previously reserved to the public system. In the community of Madrid, six hospitals and 10% of health centres are planned to become private, a measure strongly opposed by health workers and managers.

Public staff salaries were first reduced by 5%, followed by a pay "freeze" in 2011, as well as a limitation of replacement rate of 1 for every 10 leaving (European Hospital and Healthcare Federation, 2011; Gené-Badiaa et al., 2012). Surgical and clinical activities also suffered significant reductions (*Revista Redaccion Médica*, 2012). Another consequence has been that family and community medicine has become less attractive as it does not allow lost revenue to be made up by seeing patients privately, as would be the case for most other specialties.

As a consequence of these measures, the debate on the deficit in the number of health professionals has become irrelevant. Perceptions regarding issues such as the need for more physicians changed with decreases in the population, resulting from migration from regions such as Andalucia (Junta of Andalucia, 2012), increases in working hours from 35 to 37.5 hours per week and the interruption of programmes and projects (*El Pais*, 2012). Current projections suggest a surplus of 2000 new health professionals a year that the National Health Service will not be able to integrate (*El Correo*, 2012). Figures for mid-2012 indicated that 2402 physicians and 13 386 nurses were registered as unemployed; this is 44% and 27%, respectively, more compared with the same period in 2011 (Sahuquillo & Sevillano, 2012).

With regard to health professional mobility, the Medical Council (*Organización Medica Colegial*) reported that 948 physicians requested a competence certificate, required to work abroad, during the first six months of 2012 (*Revista Redaccion Médica*, 2012). The most common destinations are the United Kingdom, France, Portugal and Germany. There is also some anecdotal evidence of Spanish health professionals going to Latin America. For example, Ecuador, which exported approximately 3 000 dentists, nurses and physicians to Spain, is now experiencing rapid economic growth and is actively recruiting health professionals for the expansion of its public services network. The conditions are particularly attractive, including long-term contracts and annual salaries above €50 000, in a country where the cost of living is three times lower than in Spain (*Levante*, 2012).

**Box 3.4** *Country case study: United Kingdom*

In the United Kingdom, the economic crisis has impacted on health professional mobility by reducing employment opportunities, reducing funding for domestic training and increasing entry barriers for non-EU health professionals.

Most health care in the United Kingdom is delivered by the National Health Service (NHS), which has been the target of public sector funding constraint. In terms of NHS *funding,* there will be little or no growth in real terms in the period to 2016 (National Audit Office, 2012). This has impacted on the NHS both as an employer and as a funder of training.

In terms of its role as an *employer* of health professionals, the NHS has implemented national pay "freezes", with no pay increase for NHS nurses, allied health professionals and other staff; along with other parts of the public sector, it has reduced pension benefits for new staff, increased pension contributions from staff and increased the retirement age. There have also been localized reductions in staffing in employing organizations, which at the aggregate national level has led to a reduction in NHS nurse staffing and growth in employment of doctors (Royal College of Nursing, 2011; Ramesh, 2012). There is also an increased emphasis on "productivity improvements" through changed working methods and flexibilities.

In terms of supporting the *education* and *training* of new health professionals, cost-containment has led to reductions in the numbers of new health professionals being trained. For example, in nursing in 2011–2012 there were approximately 22 640 funded training places available across the four countries of the United Kingdom, compared with 24 800 the previous year (Buchan & Seccombe, 2012). Available figures suggest this number will reduce by about 5.6% (1 260 fewer places) in 2012–2013, to a total of around 21 380 (Snow, 2012). While reduced funding availability is leading to reductions in the number of health professionals being trained, applications for training are actually increasing, perhaps reflecting relatively reduced employment opportunities elsewhere. In 2012, there was a substantial rise in applications for nursing degree courses (up 24.6% to 197 980 compared with 156 719 in 2011; UCAS, 2012).

In terms of *immigration policy*, the policy of the government has been to raise the entry requirements, which has significantly reduced the number of health professionals moving to the United Kingdom from non-EU countries (Buchan & Seccombe, 2012); at the same time, there has been a growth in inflow from EU countries, which are not covered by the immigration policy changes. There has been a marked increase in nurses registering in the United Kingdom from EU countries such as Spain and Portugal, which have experienced extreme labour market problems in the Eurozone economic crisis. For example, the number of nurses admitted to the United Kingdom Register from Portugal grew from 20 in 2006–2007 to more than 550 in 2011–2012 (Howie, 2011; Williams, 2012).

a geographical move continues to be enabled within the EU by free mobility, while moves out of the EU are likely to be channelled towards countries that have suffered less from the crisis, such as Australia and Ecuador, and which have an "open door" policy to recruit health workers.

The OECD in its review of migration trends in 2012 reported that the slowdown in overall migration into OECD countries caused by the global economic crisis "seems to have come to an end", having fallen across the period 2008–2010; that many governments had introduced more restrictive migration policies; and that for the future, population ageing in the OECD area is likely to have a significant effect on migration trends. It also noted that 2011 was marked by a worsening of economic conditions in some Eurozone countries, in particular Greece, Ireland, Italy, Portugal and Spain, and that the evidence available to that date suggested that emigration from these countries had increased modestly (OECD, 2012).

This OECD overview is based on an assessment of all types of migration, all types of worker and all OECD countries. This chapter focuses on one group of workers, working in one sector, in one geographical region with free mobility for key personnel. While the focus is narrower, the analysis conducted in this chapter has highlighted that the impact of the crisis on health worker mobility has manifested itself in a range of ways, and that the overall impact has varied between countries and times. However, it is possible to distil down the evidence and analysis to a few key messages for policy-makers.

1. *The crisis has not constrained overall net health workforce mobility.* First, there is more evidence suggesting that the impact of the crisis has been a net increase in health worker flows at national level, rather than reduced flows. In part, this reflects free mobility for doctors, nurses and midwives across the EU, which cannot be constrained by governments, who may increase barriers to entry for non-EU health workers. In part, it reflects diminishing job and career prospects and a related increase in "push" factor for health workers in some health systems, most notably in countries of the south and east of the EU. Some EU Member States that are implementing austerity measures are also continuing to use "pull" factors to encourage inflow of health workers to fill vacancies that remain unattractive to domestically trained workers, such as the so-called "medical deserts" in France.

2. *The crisis has not ended the need for effective policy responses to health workforce mobility.* Health workforce mobility continues to be a feature of EU Member States. This emphasizes once more that there is a need to develop a more accurate picture of health worker mobility across the EU through regular and systematic monitoring in order to give early warning of any changes in

flows at a subregional level, and how these may contribute to oversupply or shortage. It also suggests that health systems and organizations will have to continue to develop more effective policies and management approaches to ensure that recruitment and employment of internationally mobile health workers are effective, and that their retention strategies are sufficiently robust to try to counter any unnecessary outflow of their staff. The crisis has redirected or changed the magnitude of some flows, but mobility will continue to be a feature of health care labour markets at country level, at EU level and beyond.

3. *The impact of the crisis has exposed current health workforce data limitations.* The impact of the crisis on the health sector, on the health workforce and on health mobility is a major policy challenge for all EU Member States and the EU itself. This chapter has highlighted that the continued inadequacies in health workforce data have hampered understanding of how the crisis has impacted on health workforce mobility, and have, therefore, also constrained the identification of appropriate policy responses. For example, little information is available on types of mobility flow that may have increased as result of the crisis, such as cross-border work, weekend work and short-term contracts. In addition, at times of budget restriction, governments may resist the idea of investing in information systems, but without them, planning and policy development are more amenable to political influence and may be less rational and evidence-informed. Spending on monitoring the effects of the crisis on the health workforce, including on mobility flows, may be an investment that will make it easier to produce a workforce that will meet system objectives such as equity of access to health services.

4. *The crisis may increase some aspects of health worker shortages in some EU Member States in the midterm.* Employment in the health sector in many countries has become less attractive as crisis-driven policy responses have reduced pay and career prospects. Health worker retention has, however, increased in many health organizations and systems, reflecting a relative lack of other opportunities, crisis-related extension of retirement age or diminishment of retirement benefits. Crisis-related measures have also led to reduced numbers of "new" health professionals being trained in some countries where training is publicly funded. As countries emerge out of crisis, and other sectors of their economy become more financially viable, the health sector will run the risk of seeing increased competition for staff plus increased turnover and mobility of staff at a time when it is also experiencing reductions in flows of new staff from training.

5. *The EU could become increasingly a single "protected" labour market for health workers.* Health worker flows from non-EU countries to the EU may have slowed because fewer job opportunities exist in the crisis, because some EU

Member States have tightened immigration controls and possibly because of increased international pressures to limit recruitment from developing countries and adopt the *WHO Global Code of Practice on the International Recruitment of Health Personnel* (WHO, 2010). Some EU Member States have actively promoted the implementation of the Code and encouraged employers to abide by its principles. A clearer picture of the impact of the Code, so far, should be available as the WHO Regional Office for Europe is monitoring this process and will report to the World Health Assembly in May 2013 (Dussault, Perfilieva & Pethick, 2012). A pattern of relatively more inter-EU mobility combined with lower levels of into-EU mobility could be continued. This raises implications for mid- to long-term health workforce planning, attaining policy objectives of self-sufficiency or sustainability in health workforce and "knock-on" effects on health labour markets in other regions.

6. *The short-term impact of the crisis masks longer-term health system and workforce challenges for Europe.* The health systems in most EU Member States are coming under increased pressure as a result of population demographic changes, while the health workforce itself is ageing in many EU countries. This will exacerbate any existing shortages, as demand increases and more of the current workforce reach retirement age. If EU Member States focus only on the short term and on cost-containment in response to the crisis, such as non-replacement of retirees and restricted recruitment, they may miss other looming health workforce challenges. In announcing a Joint Action on Health Workforce Planning across the EU, a recent EU document noted that "maintaining an adequate supply and quality of health-care services under severe budget constraints is thus a key issue to be addressed by policy makers" (European Commission, 2012).

## 3.7 Conclusions

There is scope for policy support at EU level to address these issues emerging from the impact of the crisis on health systems and health worker mobility. The EU has an underpinning Health Strategy, and the European Commission can help, through the Joint Action Plan, by supporting countries to develop solid data collection mechanisms, analyse regional trends and identify and disseminate good practices. It can also caution against measures that may bring some short-term benefits but at the expense of long-term costs.

A report by the European Commission and the Economic Policy Committee (2010) warned EU Member States that reductions in families' disposable income and higher unemployment rates may lead to a deterioration of health indicators and to an increase in demand for health services, which would call for scaling-up spending in health, including for hiring more personnel. At the time, it recommended actions such as creating an "anti-crisis unit" in each ministry of health to monitor the situation, identify strategic options that protect equitable access to health services, maintain health service quality and, at the same time, improve health service efficiency. The ministries should also mobilize stakeholders to advocate these options, particularly to the ministries of finance.

There is a continued risk that the crisis and its aftermath will continue to push countries to develop short-term "protective" measures for their own health systems without a proper understanding of either the aggregate impact of different policy interventions or the connection they have with other countries whose own policy changes will have ripple effects across national borders. In this context, health worker mobility will continue to be shaped and directed by broader health system policies and will continue to be a factor that policy-makers must understand in developing effective health workforce policies and planning.

## Annex

GDP is a measure of economic activity, defined as the value of all goods and services produced less the value of any goods or services used in their creation. The calculation of the annual growth rate of GDP volume is intended to allow comparisons of the dynamics of economic development both over time and between economies of different sizes. For measuring the growth rate of GDP

**Table 3A.1** *Real growth rate in GDP as a percentage change on the previous year, EU27*

| Country | 2000 | 2006 | 2007 | 2008 | 2009 | 2010 | 2011 | 2012[a] |
|---|---|---|---|---|---|---|---|---|
| Austria | 3.7 | 3.7 | 3.7 | 1.4 | −3.8 | 2.1 | 2.7 | 0.8 |
| Belgium | 3.7 | 2.7 | 2.9 | 1.0 | −2.8 | 2.4 | 1.8 | −0.2 |
| Bulgaria | 5.7 | 6.5 | 6.4 | 6.2 | −5.5 | 0.4 | 1.7 | 0.8 |
| Cyprus | 5.0 | 4.1 | 5.1 | 3.6 | −1.9 | 1.1 | 0.5 | −2.3 |
| Czech Republic | 4.2 | 7.0 | 5.7 | 3.1 | −4.7 | 2.7 | 1.7 | −1.3 |
| Denmark | 3.5 | 3.4 | 1.6 | −0.8 | −5.8 | 1.3 | 0.8 | 0.6 |
| Estonia | 9.7 | 10.1 | 7.5 | −3.7 | −14.3 | 2.3 | 7.6 | 2.5 |
| Finland | 5.3 | 4.4 | 5.3 | 0.3 | −8.5 | 3.3 | 2.7 | 0.1 |
| France | 3.7 | 2.5 | 2.3 | −0.1 | −3.1 | 1.7 | 1.7 | 0.2 |
| Germany | 3.1 | 3.7 | 3.3 | 1.1 | −5.1 | 4.2 | 3.0 | 0.8 |
| Greece | 3.5[b] | 5.5[b] | 3.0[b] | −0.2[b] | −3.3[b] | −3.5[b] | −6.9[b] | −6.0 |
| Hungary | 4.2 | 3.9 | 0.1 | 0.9 | −6.8 | 1.3 | 1.6 | −1.2 |
| Ireland | 9.3 | 5.3 | 5.2 | −3.0 | −7.0 | −0.4 | 0.7 | 0.4 |
| Italy | 3.7 | 2.2 | 1.7 | −1.2 | −5.5 | 1.8 | 0.4 | −2.3 |
| Latvia | 5.7 | 11.2 | 9.6 | −3.3 | −17.7 | -0.3 | 5.5 | 4.3 |
| Lithuania | 12.3 | 7.8 | 9.8 | 2.9 | −14.8 | 1.4 | 5.9 | 2.9 |
| Luxembourg | 8.4 | 5.0 | 6.6 | 0.8 | −5.3 | 2.7 | 1.6 | 0.4 |
| Malta | – | 3.1 | 4.4 | 4.1 | −2.6 | 2.5 | 2.1 | 1.0 |
| Netherlands | 3.9 | 3.4 | 3.9 | 1.8 | −3.7 | 1.6 | 1.0 | −0.3 |
| Poland | 4.3 | 6.2 | 6.8 | 5.1 | 1.6 | 3.9 | 4.3 | 2.4 |

**Table 3A.1** *contd*

| Country | 2000 | 2006 | 2007 | 2008 | 2009 | 2010 | 2011 | 2012[a] |
|---|---|---|---|---|---|---|---|---|
| Portugal | 3.9 | 1.4 | 2.4 | 0.0 | −2.9 | 1.4 | −1.6 | −3.0 |
| Romania | 2.4 | 7.9 | 6.3 | 7.3 | −6.6 | −1.6 | 2.5 | 0.8 |
| Slovakia | 1.4 | 8.3 | 10.5 | 5.8 | −4.9 | 4.2 | 3.3 | 2.6 |
| Slovenia | 4.3 | 5.8 | 6.9 | 3.6 | −8.0 | 1.4 | -0.2 | −2.3 |
| Spain | 5.0 | 4.1 | 3.5 | 0.9 | −3.7 | −0.3 | 0.4 | −1.4 |
| Sweden | 4.5 | 4.3 | 3.3 | −0.6 | −5.0 | 6.2 | 3.9 | 1.1 |
| United Kingdom | 4.2 | 2.6 | 3.6 | −1.0 | −4.0 | 1.8 | 0.8 | −0.3 |
| EU27 | 3.9% | 3.3% | 3.2% | 0.3% | −4.4% | 2.1% | 1.5% | −0.3% |

*Source*: European Commission, 2013 (last data update 6 December 2012).

[a]Forecast; [b]Provisional.

**Table 3A.2** *Total expenditure on health, as percentage of GDP, EU27 2000–2011*

| Country | 2000 | 2006 | 2007 | 2008 | 2009 | 2010 | 2011 |
|---|---|---|---|---|---|---|---|
| Austria | 10.0 | 10.2 | 10.3 | 10.5 | 11.2 | 11.0 | – |
| Belgium | 8.1 | 9.6 | 9.6 | 10.0 | 10.7 | 10.5 | – |
| Bulgaria | 6.18 | 6.9 | 6.82 | 6.98 | 7.24 | 6.88 | – |
| Cyprus | 5.78 | 6.28 | 6.06 | 6.04 | 6.14 | 5.98 | – |
| Czech Republic | 6.3 | 6.7 | 6.5 | 6.8 | 8.0 | 7.5 | – |
| Denmark | 8.7 | 9.9 | 10.0 | 10.2 | 11.5 | 11.1 | – |
| Estonia | 5.3 | 5.0 | 5.2 | 6.0 | 7.0 | 6.3 | – |
| Finland | 7.2 | 8.3 | 8.0 | 8.3 | 9.2 | 8.9 | 8.8 |
| France | 10.1 | 11.1 | 11.1 | 11.0 | 11.7 | 11.6 | – |
| Germany | 10.4 | 10.6 | 10.5 | 10.7 | 11.7 | 11.6 | – |
| Greece | 8.0 | 9.7 | 9.8 | 10.1 | 10.6 | 10.2 | – |
| Hungary | 7.2 | 8.3 | 7.7 | 7.5 | 7.7 | 7.8 | – |
| Ireland | 6.1 | 7.6 | 7.8 | 8.9 | 9.9 | 9.2 | – |
| Italy | 8.0 | 9.0 | 8.6 | 8.9 | 9.3 | 9.3 | 9.1 |
| Latvia | 5.96 | 6.78 | 6.98 | 6.6 | 6.6 | 6.68 | – |
| Lithuania | 6.46 | 6.2 | 6.22 | 6.6 | 7.54 | 7.04 | – |
| Luxembourg | 7.5 | 7.7 | 7.1 | 6.8 | 7.9 | – | – |
| Netherlands | 8.0 | 9.7 | 10.8 | 11.0 | 11.9 | 12.0 | – |
| Poland | 5.5 | 6.2 | 6.3 | 6.9 | 7.2 | 7.0 | – |
| Portugal | 9.3 | 10.0 | 10.0 | 10.2 | 10.8 | 10.7 | – |
| Romania[a] | 4.3 | 5.1 | 5.2 | 5.4 | 5.6 | 5.9 | 5.8 |
| Slovakia | 5.5 | 7.3 | 7.8 | 8.0 | 9.2 | 9.0 | – |
| Slovenia | 8.3 | 8.3 | 7.8 | 8.3 | 9.3 | 9.0 | – |
| Spain | 7.2 | 8.3 | 8.5 | 9.0 | 9.6 | – | – |
| Sweden | 8.2 | 8.9 | 8.9 | 9.2 | 9.9 | 9.6 | – |
| United Kingdom | 7.0 | 8.5 | 8.5 | 8.8 | 9.8 | 9.6 | – |
| EU27[a] | 8.06 | 8.95 | 8.89 | 9.19 | 9.93 | 9.88 | – |

*Sources*: OECD 2013; [a]WHO Regional Office for Europe, 2013.

**Table 3A.3** *Annual growth rate of total expenditure on health in real terms, EU27 2000–2010*

| Country[a] | 2000–1 | 2005–6 | 2006–7 | 2007–8 | 2008–9 | 2009–10 |
|---|---|---|---|---|---|---|
| Austria | 1.6 | 1.7 | 4.2 | 3.6 | 2.7 | 0.4 |
| Belgium | 2.9 | −2.5 | 3.2 | 5.0 | 3.7 | 1.1 |
| Czech Republic | 4.9 | 3.3 | 3.0 | 7.8 | 11.7 | −4.1 |
| Denmark | 5.3 | 5.0 | 2.2 | 1.2 | 5.9 | −1.7 |
| Estonia | −2.4 | 10.0 | 10.6 | 12.6 | −0.5 | −7.3 |
| Finland | 5.2 | 3.4 | 1.5 | 3.5 | 1.1 | 0.9 |
| France | 3.1 | 1.9 | 2.1 | −0.9 | 3.3 | 1.3 |
| Germany | 2.6 | 2.0 | 1.7 | 3.2 | 4.1 | 2.6 |
| Greece | 16.4 | 6.4 | 4.0 | 3.0 | 0.9 | −6.5 |
| Hungary | 4.6 | 1.6 | −7.0 | −1.9 | −3.4 | 2.0 |
| Ireland | 15.2 | 4.8 | 8.0 | 11.3 | 3.5 | −7.6 |
| Italy | 3.8 | 3.0 | −2.1 | 1.7 | −1.0 | 1.5 |
| Luxembourg | 1.5 | 2.4 | −1.9 | −3.8 | 10.1 | – |
| Netherlands | 6.3 | 2.3 | 15.7 | 3.6 | 4.1 | 2.5 |
| Poland | 7.4 | 6.0 | 9.1 | 14.3 | 6.5 | 0.6 |
| Portugal | 1.6 | −1.7 | 2.0 | 2.2 | 2.8 | 0.6 |
| Slovakia | 3.6 | 13.0 | 16.6 | 9.4 | 8.5 | 2.6 |
| Slovenia | 6.7 | 4.9 | 1.2 | 9.8 | 2.8 | −1.6 |
| Spain | 4.1 | 4.9 | 5.2 | 6.6 | 2.8 | – |
| Sweden | 9.7 | 3.0 | 3.0 | 2.9 | 2.3 | 2.0 |
| United Kingdom | 6.4 | 5.3 | 3.7 | 2.2 | 7.0 | 0.2 |
| EU27 | – | 2.0% | 3.3% | 3.2% | 0.3% | −4.4% |

*Source*: OECD, 2013.

[a]Data not available for Bulgaria, Cyprus, Latvia, Lithuania, Malta and Romania.

**Table 3A.4** *Public expenditure on health, as a percentage of total expenditure on health, EU27 2000–2011*

| Country | 2000 | 2006 | 2007 | 2008 | 2009 | 2010 | 2011 |
|---|---|---|---|---|---|---|---|
| Austria | 75.6 | 75.7 | 75.8 | 76.3 | 76.4 | 76.2 | – |
| Belgium | 74.6 | 73.6 | 73.2 | 74.7 | 76.1 | 75.6 | – |
| Bulgaria | 60.9 | 56.9 | 58.2 | 58.5 | 55.3 | 54.5 | – |
| Cyprus | 41.6 | 42.4 | 42.6 | 41.5 | 41.5 | 41.5 | – |
| Czech Republic | 90.3 | 86.7 | 85.2 | 82.5 | 84.0 | 83.8 | – |
| Denmark | 83.9 | 84.6 | 84.4 | 84.7 | 85.0 | 85.1 | – |
| Estonia | 77.2 | 73.3 | 75.6 | 77.8 | 75.3 | 78.9 | – |
| Finland | 71.3 | 74.8 | 74.4 | 74.5 | 75.2 | 74.5 | 74.8 |
| France | 79.4 | 78.7 | 78.3 | 76.7 | 76.9 | 77.0 | – |
| Germany | 79.5 | 76.5 | 76.4 | 76.6 | 76.9 | 76.8 | – |
| Greece | 60.0 | 62.0 | 60.3 | 59.9 | 61.7 | 59.4 | – |
| Hungary | 70.7 | 69.8 | 67.3 | 67.1 | 65.7 | 64.8 | – |
| Ireland | 75.1 | 75.1 | 75.5 | 75.1 | 72.0 | 69.5 | – |
| Italy | 72.5 | 76.6 | 76.6 | 78.9 | 79.6 | 79.6 | 79.0 |
| Latvia | 54.4 | 64.1 | 60.7 | 62.4 | 61.6 | 61.1 | – |
| Lithuania | 69.7 | 69.5 | 72.9 | 72.4 | 73.4 | 73.5 | – |

**Table 3A.4**  *contd*

| Country | 2000 | 2006 | 2007 | 2008 | 2009 | 2010 | 2011 |
|---|---|---|---|---|---|---|---|
| Luxembourg | 85.1 | 85.1 | 84.1 | 84.1 | 84.0 | – | – |
| Malta | 72.4 | 69.3 | 66.8 | 64.9 | 64.8 | 65.4 | – |
| Netherlands | 66.4 | 82.4 | 84.1 | 84.8 | 85.4 | 85.7 | 85.7 |
| Poland | 70.0 | 69.9 | 70.4 | 71.8 | 71.6 | 71.7 | – |
| Portugal | 66.6 | 67.0 | 66.7 | 65.3 | 66.5 | 65.8 | – |
| Romania[a] | 81.2 | 79.6 | 82.1 | 82.0 | 78.9 | 80.3 | 80.2 |
| Slovakia | 89.4 | 68.3 | 66.8 | 67.8 | 65.7 | 64.5 | – |
| Slovenia | 74.0 | 72.3 | 71.8 | 73.9 | 73.2 | 72.8 | – |
| Spain | 71.6 | 71.3 | 71.5 | 72.6 | 73.6 | – | – |
| Sweden | 84.9 | 81.1 | 81.4 | 81.5 | 81.5 | 81.0 | – |
| United Kingdom | 78.8 | 81.3 | 81.2 | 82.5 | 83.4 | 83.2 | – |
| EU27[a] | 74.8 | 75.6 | 75.6 | 76.0 | 76.5 | 76.2 | – |

*Sources*: OECD, 2013; [a]WHO Regional Office for Europe, 2013.

**Table 3A.5**  *Physicians per 100 000 population, EU27 2000–2011*

| Country | 2000 | 2006 | 2007 | 2008 | 2009 | 2010 | 2011 |
|---|---|---|---|---|---|---|---|
| Austria | 381 | 444 | 453 | 460 | 468 | 478 | – |
| Belgium | 283 | 289 | 291 | 292 | 292 | 297 | – |
| Bulgaria | 337 | 365 | 364 | 361 | 369 | 371 | – |
| Cyprus | 259 | 253 | 273 | 280 | 286 | 289 | – |
| Czech Republic | 337 | 356 | 357 | 354 | 356 | 358 | – |
| Denmark | 291 | 339 | 340 | 343 | 348 | – | – |
| Estonia | 326 | 319 | 326 | 333 | 327 | 324 | – |
| Finland | 220 | 268 | 269 | 272 | – | – | – |
| France | 330[a] | 370[a] | 350[a] | – | 340[a] | – | 315 |
| Germany | 326 | 345 | 350 | 356 | 364 | 373 | – |
| Greece | 433 | 535 | 556 | 603 | 612 | 610 | – |
| Hungary | 268 | 304 | 280 | 309 | 302 | 287 | – |
| Ireland | 220[a] | 274 | 284 | 294 | 306 | 315 | 327 |
| Italy | 420[a] | 370[a] | – | 420[a] | 350[a] | – | – |
| Latvia | 287 | 294 | 304 | 311 | 299 | 291 | – |
| Lithuania | 363 | 365 | 372 | 370 | 365 | 372 | – |
| Luxembourg | 214 | 258 | 269 | 272 | 271 | 277 | 279 |
| Malta | 265[a] | 390[a] | 340[a] | – | 304 | 307 | 322 |
| Netherlands | 244 | 280 | 279 | 287 | 292 | – | – |
| Poland | 222 | 218 | 219 | 216 | 217 | 218 | – |
| Portugal | 310 | 341 | 350 | 359 | 370 | 383 | – |
| Romania | 192 | 216 | 212 | 221 | 226 | 237 | 238 |
| Slovakia | 323 | 320 | 320 | 340 | 330 | 330 | – |
| Slovenia | 215 | 236 | 239 | 238 | 241 | 243 | – |
| Spain | 331 | 363 | 365 | 350 | 354 | 378 | 397 |
| Sweden | 309 | 360 | 368 | 373 | 380 | – | – |
| United Kingdom | 196 | 245 | 249 | 258 | 267 | 273 | 276 |
| EU | 283 | 312 | 316 | 323 | 329 | 334 | – |

*Sources*: WHO Regional Office for Europe, 2013; [a]World Bank, 2013b.

**Table 3A.6** *Nurses per 100 000 population, EU27 2000–2011*

| Country | 2000 | 2006 | 2007 | 2008 | 2009 | 2010 | 2011 |
|---|---|---|---|---|---|---|---|
| Austria | 721 | 741 | 752 | 767 | 776 | 783 | – |
| Belgium | – | – | – | – | 1 531 | 1 585 | – |
| Bulgaria | 436 | 455 | 465 | 468 | 465 | 465 | – |
| Cyprus | 422 | 440 | 460 | 456 | 474 | 467 | – |
| Czech Republic | 805 | 846 | 843 | 835 | 847 | 848 | – |
| Denmark | 1 261 | 1 474 | 1 456 | 1 501 | 1 573 | – | – |
| Estonia | 632 | 663 | 670 | 670 | 642 | 641 | – |
| Finland | 955 | 970 | 973 | 1 002 | 997 | – | – |
| France | 713 | 831 | 817 | 848 | 883 | 903 | 930 |
| Germany | 978 | 1 056 | 1 071 | 1 094 | 1 126 | 1 151 | – |
| Greece | 293 | 342 | 342 | 345 | 354 | – | – |
| Hungary | 548 | 628 | 628 | 632 | 638 | 639 | – |
| Ireland | – | 1 264 | 1 288 | 1 282 | 1 272 | 1 312 | – |
| Italy | 587 | 633 | 635 | 647 | 658 | 659 | – |
| Latvia | 477 | 566 | 556 | 554 | 485 | 488 | – |
| Lithuania | 802 | 740 | 733 | 739 | 724 | 722 | – |
| Luxembourg | 756 | 1 127 | – | – | – | 1 667 | 1 716 |
| Malta | – | 593 | 621 | 675 | 655 | 682 | 706 |
| Netherlands | – | 834 | 845 | 855 | – | – | – |
| Poland | 553 | 565 | 575 | 578 | 584 | 585 | – |
| Portugal | – | 481 | 510 | 534 | 561 | 587 | – |
| Romania | 530 | 586 | 589 | 577 | 589 | 546 | 551 |
| Slovakia | 748 | 633 | 661 | 657 | 636 | 637 | – |
| Slovenia | – | 763 | 775 | 785 | 806 | 823 | – |
| Spain | 373 | 425 | 453 | 478 | 509 | 504 | – |
| Sweden | – | 1 160[a] | 1 190[a] | – | – | – | – |
| United Kingdom | – | – | 1 014 | 1 019 | 1 036 | 1 020 | 947 |
| EU | 744 | 792 | 797 | 811 | 829 | 834 | – |

*Sources*: WHO Regional Office for Europe, 2013; [a]World Bank, 2013a.

**Table 3A.7**  *Number of physicians employed in the public sector in selected countries, 2006, 2008 and last available year*

| Country | 2006 | 2008 | Last available year | Change 2006 to last available year (%) |
|---|---|---|---|---|
| Portugal | 23 003[a] | 24 659[b] | 20 311[c] (2011) | −2 692 (−13.3%) |
| Italy | 105 860[d] | 106 266[e] | 107 333[f] (2009) | 1 473 (1.8%) |
| Ireland[g] | 7 712 | 8 109 | 8 142 (2011[h]) | 430 (5.3%) |
| Spain[i] | 203 153 | 248 938 | 222 993 (2010) | 19 840 (8.9%) |

*Sources*: [a]Direcção-Geral da Saúde, 2006 (Elementos Estatísticos- Informação Geral/Saúde, http://www.dgs.pt/upload/membro.id/ficheiros/i010517.pdf); [b]Direcção-Geral da Saúde, 2008 (Elementos Estatísticos- Informação Geral/Saúde, http://www.dgs.pt/upload/membro.id/ficheiros/i013685.pdf); [c]ACSS, 2011 (Inventário de Pessoal do Sector da Saúde, http://www.acss.min-saude.pt/Portals/0/Invent%C3%A1rio_vf.pdf); [d]Ministero della Salute, 2006 (Personale delle A.S.L. E Degli Instituti di Cura Pubblici, http://www.salute.gov.it/imgs/C_17_pubblicazioni_840_allegato.pdf); [e]Ministero della Salute, 2008 (Personale delle A.S.L. E Degli Instituti di Cura Pubblici, http://www.salute.gov.it/imgs/C_17_pubblicazioni_1489_allegato.pdf); [f]Ministero della Salute, 2009 (Personale delle A.S.L. E Degli Instituti di Cura Pubblici, http://www.salute.gov.it/imgs/C_17_pubblicazioni_1736_allegato.pdf); [g]Health Service Executive, 2006, 2008 (Health Service Personnel Census at 31 December 2006, 2008, http://www.hse.ie/eng/staff/Resources/Employment_Reports/Census.pdf); [h]2011 data refer to September 2011 employment figures and so caution should be exercised in comparing these data with the previous years' figures for December; [i]Ministerio de Sanidad, 2011 (Indicadores clave del Sistema Nacional de Salud, España, November 2011 (http://www.fmdv.org/Es/Unidades/OSPC/DocumentosOSPC/Indicadores%20clave%20Ministerio%20Sanidad/Indicadores%20clave%20del%20Sistema%20Nacional%20de%20Salud%20%28Espa%C3%B1a.%20Noviembre%20de%202011%29.pdf); numbers calculated by dividing the ratio of physicians and nurses registered in the Professionals Councils per 1 000 population and then multiplying it by the total number of population in the country. (All links accessed 8 October 2013.)

**Table 3A.8**  *Number of nurses employed in the public sector in selected countries, 2006, 2008 and last available year*

| Country | 2006 | 2008 | Last available year | Change 2006 to last available year (%) |
|---|---|---|---|---|
| Portugal | 36 622[a] | 39 018[b] | 41 058[c] (2011) | 4 436/10.8% |
| Italy | 265 444[d] | 261 943[e] | 264 093[f] (2009) | −1 351/−0.5% |
| Ireland[g] | 36 737 | 38 108 | 35 993 (2011[h]) | −744/−2.1% |
| Spain[i] | 233 560 | 248 938 | 262 155 (2010) | 28 595/10.9% |

*Sources*: [a]Direcção-Geral da Saúde, 2006 (Elementos Estatísticos- Informação Geral/Saúde, http://www.dgs.pt/upload/membro.id/ficheiros/i010517.pdf); [b]Direcção-Geral da Saúde 2008 (Elementos Estatísticos- Informação Geral/Saúde, http://www.dgs.pt/upload/membro.id/ficheiros/i013685.pdf); [c]ACSS, 2011 (Inventário de Pessoal do Sector da Saúde, http://www.acss.min-saude.pt/Portals/0/Invent%C3%A1rio_vf.pdf); [d]Ministero della Salute, 2006 (Personale delle A.S.L. E Degli Instituti di Cura Pubblici, http://www.salute.gov.it/imgs/C_17_pubblicazioni_840_allegato.pdf); [e]Ministero della Salute, 2008 (Personale delle A.S.L. E Degli Instituti di Cura Pubblici, http://www.salute.gov.it/imgs/C_17_pubblicazioni_1489_allegato.pdf); [f]Ministero della Salute, 2009 (Personale delle A.S.L. E Degli Instituti di Cura Pubblici, http://www.salute.gov.it/imgs/C_17_pubblicazioni_1736_allegato.pdf); [g]Health Service Executive, 2006, 2008 (Health Service Personnel Census at 31 December 2006, 2008, http://www.hse.ie/eng/staff/Resources/Employment_Reports/Census.pdf); [h]2011 data refer to September 2011 employment figures and so caution should be exercised in comparing these data with the previous years' figures for December; [i]Ministerio de Sanidad, 2011 (Indicadores clave del Sistema Nacional de Salud, España, November 2011 (http://www.fmdv.org/Es/Unidades/OSPC/DocumentosOSPC/Indicadores%20clave%20Ministerio%20Sanidad/Indicadores%20clave%20del%20Sistema%20Nacional%20de%20Salud%20%28Espa%C3%B1a.%20Noviembre%20de%202011%29.pdf); numbers calculated by dividing the ratio of physicians and nurses registered in the Professionals Councils per 1 000 population and then multiplying it by the total number of population in the country. (All links accessed 8 October 2013.)

in terms of volumes, the GDP at current prices are valued in the prices of the previous year and the thus computed volume changes are imposed on the level of a reference year; this is called a chain-linked series. Accordingly, price movements will not inflate the growth rate.

## References

Albreht T (2011). Health workforce in times of financial crisis. *European Journal of Public Health,* 21(1):1–3.

Buchan J, Seccombe I (2012). *Overstretched, under-resourced: the UK nursing labour market review 2012*, London, Royal College of Nursing (http://www.rcn.org.uk/__data/assets/pdf_file/0016/482200/004332.pdf, accessed 5 December 2013).

Buchan J, Seccombe I (2013). The end of growth? Analysing NHS nurse staffing *Journal of Advanced Nursing,* 69(9):2123–2130.

Commission on Social Determinants of Health (2008). *Final report: closing the gap in a generation. Health equity through action on the social determinants of health, 2008.* Geneva, World Health Organization (http://www.who.int/social_determinants/thecommission/finalreport/en/index.html, accessed 2 January 2014).

Dussault G, Perfilieva G, Pethick J (2012). *Implementing the WHO Global Code of Practice on International Recruitment of Health Personnel in the European Region.* Copenhagen, WHO Regional Office for Europe (http://www.euro.who.int/__data/assets/pdf_file/0020/173054/Policy-Brief_HRH_draft-for-RC62-discussion.pdf, accessed 2 January 2014).

*El Correo* (2012). Más de 2.000 estudiantes de Medicina no podrán ejercer especialidad alguna. *El Correo.com* (http://www.elcorreo.com/vizcaya/v/20120602/pvasco-espana/estudiantes-medicina-podran-ejercer-20120602.html, accessed 5 December 2013).

*El Pais* (2012). Salud revisará a la baja los planes de necesidades de profesionales. *El Pais,* 30 September (http://ccaa.elpais.com/ccaa/2012/09/30/andalucia/1349036829_777363.html, accessed 5 December 2013).

European Commission (2012). *Staff working document on an action plan for the EU health workforce. Towards a job-rich recovery.* Strasbourg, European Commission (http://ec.europa.eu/dgs/health_consumer/docs/swd_ap_eu_healthcare_workforce_en.pdf, accessed 2 January 2014).

European Commission (2013). *Eurostat statistical database.* Brussels, Statistical Office of the European Communities (http://epp.eurostat.ec.europa.eu/portal/page/portal/eurostat/home/, accessed 5 August 2013).

European Commission and the Economic Policy Committee (2010). *Joint report on health systems.* Brussels, Directorate-General for Economic and Financial Affairs (Occasional Paper No. 74) (http://ec.europa.eu/economy_finance/publications/occasional_paper/2010/pdf/ocp74_en.pdf, accessed 2 January 2014).

European Federation of Nurses Associations (2012). *Caring in crisis: the impact of the financial crisis on nurses and nursing. A comparative overview of 34 European countries.* Brussels, European Federation of Nurses Associations (http://www.efnweb.be/wp-content/uploads/2012/05/EFN-Report-on-the-Impact-of-the-Financial-Crisis-on-Nurses-and-Nursing-January-20122.pdf, accessed 5 December 2013).

European Hospital and Healthcare Federation (2011). *The crisis, hospitals and healthcare.* Brussels, European Hospital and Healthcare Federation (http://www.epha.org/a/5111, accessed 5 December 2013).

*Expresso* (Lisbon) 15 September 2012.

Gené-Badiaa J et al. (2012). Health reform monitor Spanish health care cuts: penny wise and pound foolish? *Health Policy*, 106:23–28.

Government of Portugal (2012). *Revisão do Regime do Internato Médico: Relatório Final, Maio 2012.* Lisbon, Governo de Portugal Secretário de Estado da Saúde (http://www.fnam.pt/informacao/infromacao_files/RevIntMedico.pdf, accessed 5 December 2013).

Habicht T (2012). Estonia: crisis reforms and the road to recovery, *Eurohealth*, 18(1):10–11.

Howie M (2011). Spanish and Portuguese nurses fill the gaps in the NHS. *The Guardian*, 20 December (http://www.guardian.co.uk/society/2011/dec/20/nurses-spain-portugal-fill-gap-in-nhs, accessed 5 December 2013).

Junta of Andalucia (2012). *Consejeria de Salud. Estudio 201-2039 de las necesidades de profesionales sanitarios en Andalucía. Enero 2012.* Seville, Junta de Andalucia.

Kaitelidou D, Kouli E (2012). Greece: the health system in a time of crisis. *Eurohealth,* 18(1):12–14.

Kuznetsova D (2012). [*Issues and challenges in medical education.*] Sofia, Open Society Institute (http://osi.bg/?cy=10&lang=2&program=1&action=2&news_id=579, accessed 19 December 2013).

*Levante* (2012). Ecuador llama a sus médicos a regresar a sus hospitales. *Levante*, 10 October (http://www.levante-emv.com/comunitat-valenciana/2012/10/10/ecuador-llama-medicos-regresar-hospitales/942835.html, accessed 5 December 2013).

López-Valcárcel BG (2011). La sanidad en tiempos de crisis. *Revista Economistas*, 126 extra, March (http://www.econ.upf.edu/~jimenez/my-public-files/La-sanidad-en-tiempos-de-crisis.pdf, accessed 5 December 2013).

McKee M, Basu S, Stuckler D (2012). Health systems, health and wealth: the argument for investment applies now more than ever. *Social Science and Medicine*, 74(5):684–687.

Mladovsky P et al. (2012). *Health policy responses to the financial crisis in Europe*. Copenhagen, WHO Regional Office for Europe on behalf of the European Observatory on Health Systems and Policies (Policy Summary 5).

Morgan D, Astolfi R (2013). *Health spending growth at zero: which countries, which sectors are most affected?* Paris, Organisation for Economic Co-operation and Development (OECD Health Working Paper No. 60) (http://dx.doi.org/10.1787/5k4dd1st95xv-en, accessed 2 January 2014).

National Audit Office (2012). *Healthcare across the UK: A comparison of the NHS in England, Scotland, Wales and Northern Ireland*. London, National Audit Office:13.

OECD (2011). *Health at a Glance 2011: OECD indicators*. Paris, Organisation for Economic Co-operation and Development.

OECD (2012). *International migration outlook 2012*. Paris, Organisation for Economic Co-operation and Development.

OECD (2013). *Health data: StatExtracts*. Paris, Organisation for Economic Co-operation and Development (http://stats.oecd.org/Index.aspx?DataSetCode=SHA, accessed 9 October 2013).

Pita Barros P, Martins B, Moura A (2012). *A economia da farmácia e o acesso ao medicamento*. Lisbon, Estudo da Nova School of Business & Economics (http://momentoseconomicos.files.wordpress.com/2012/09/estudo-unl_conclusc3b5es_vfinal.pdf, accessed 5 December 2013).

Portuguese Ministry of Finance (2012). *Relatório Orçamento do Estado para 2013*. Lisbon, Ministério das finanças.

Portuguese Observatory on Health Systems (2012). *Crise e Saúde: Um país em Sofrimento. Relatório Primavera, 2012*. Lisbon, Observatório Português dos Sistemas de Saúde (http://www.observaport.org/sites/observaport.org/files/RelatorioPrimavera2012_OPSS_3.pdf, accessed 5 December 2013).

*Radio Renascença* (2012). Bastonário dos Médicos considera essencial diminuir vagas. *Radio Renascença*, 27 January 2012 (http://rr.sapo.pt/informacao_detalhe.aspx?fid=25&did=66054, accessed 5 December 2013).

Ramesh R (2012). NHS figures reveal 5 000 fewer nurses since 2010. *The Guardian*, 21 August (http://www.guardian.co.uk/society/2012/aug/21/nhs-figures-reveal-fewer-nurses?newsfeed=true, accessed 5 December 2013).

*Revista Redaccion Médica* (2012). Aumenta la emigración médica en España ante los recortes. *Revista Redaccion Médica*, 30 July (http://www.redaccionmedica.es/noticia/el-medico-espanol-huye-de-los-recortes-sanitarios-6133, accessed 5 December 2013).

Royal College of Nursing (2011). *Frontline first: November 2011 update*. London, Royal College of Nursing.

Saar P, Habicht J (2011). Migration and attrition: Estonia's health sector and cross-border mobility to its northern neighbour. In Wismar M et al., eds. *Health professional mobility and health systems. Evidence from 17 European countries*. Copenhagen, WHO Regional Office for Europe on behalf of the European Observatory on Health Systems and Policies:339–364.

Sahuquillo MR, Sevillano EG (2012). El éxodo de médicos y enfermeras se duplica por los recortes sanitarios. *El País*, 6 August (http://politica.elpais.com/politica/2012/08/06/actualidad/1344284347_177524.html, accessed 5 December 2013).

Snow T (2012). Decrease in student places poses "significant risk" to care standards. *Nursing Standard*, 26:5.

*Sol* (2012). Enfermeiros portugueses procuram Espanha e Inglaterra. *Sol,* 13 July (http://sol.sapo.pt/inicio/Sociedade/Interior.aspx?content_id=54270, accessed 5 December 2013).

Statistics Portugal (2012). *Database 2012*. Lisbon, Instituto Nacional de Estatística (http://www.ine.pt/xportal/xmain?xpid=INE&xpgid=ine_main, accessed 5 December 2013).

Stuckler DS et al. (2009). The public health effect of economic crises and alternative policy responses in Europe: an empirical analysis. *Lancet*, 374(9686):315–332.

Thomas S, Burke S (2012). Coping with austerity in the Irish health system. *Eurohealth*, 18(1):7–9.

Tjadens F, Weiland C, Eckert J (2012). *Mobility of health professionals. Health, systems, work, conditions and patterns of health workers' mobility in, from and to 25 countries at the crossroads of a major crisis*. Bonn, WIAD (Scientific Institute of the Medical Association of German Doctors) (MoHProf Summary Report) (http://www.mohprof.eu/LIVE/DATA/National_reports/national_report_ Summary.pdf, accessed 2 January 2014).

UCAS (2012). *How have applications for full-time undergraduate higher education in the UK changed in 2012?* Cheltenham, UK, UCAS (Media release, 9 July) (http://www.ucas.com/news-events/news/2013/how-have-applications-full-time-undergraduate-higher-education-uk-changed-2012, accessed 2 January 2014).

WHO (2009). *Financial crisis and global health: report of a high-level consultation.* Geneva, World Health Organization.

WHO (2010). *WHO global code of practice on the international recruitment of health personnel.* Geneva, World Health Organization (Sixty-third World Health Assembly, WHA63.16) (http://www.who.int/hrh/migration/code/ WHO_global_code_of_practice_EN.pdf, accessed 1 October 2013).

WHO Regional Office for Europe (2013). *European Health for All database* [online/offline database]. Copenhagen, WHO Regional Office for Europe (http://data.euro.who.int/hfadb/, accessed 9 October 2013).

Williams D (2012). Trust looks to Portugal for new nursing recruits. *Nursing Times*, 26 July (http://www.nursingtimes.net/nursing-practice/clinical-zones/ management/trust-looks-to-portugal-for-new-nursing-recruits/5047509. article, accessed 5 December 2013).

Wismar M et al., eds. (2011). *Health professional mobility and health systems. Evidence from 17 European countries.* Copenhagen, WHO Regional Office for Europe on behalf of the European Observatory on Health Systems and Policies.

World Bank (2013a). *World development indicators: nurses.* New York, World Bank (http://data.worldbank.org/indicator/SH.MED.NUMW.P3, accessed 9 October 2013).

World Bank (2013b). *World development indicators: physicians.* New York, World Bank.

Zahariev B (2012). [*Discussion on human resources in the Bulgarian health sector.*] Sofia, Open Society Institute (http://www.osf.bg/?cy=10&lang=1&program=1 &action=2&news_id=553, accessed 19 December 2013).

# Chapter 4

# Mobility of health professionals before and after the 2004 and 2007 EU enlargements: evidence from the EU PROMeTHEUS project

*Diana Ognyanova, Claudia B. Maier, Matthias Wismar, Edmond Girasek and Reinhard Busse*

## 4.1 Introduction

The accession of 12 new EU Member States (the EU12)[1], in May 2004 and January 2007 with a total population of over 100 million citizens, expanded the EU labour market considerably and diversified the region culturally and economically[2]. One of the fundamental principles in the EU, the free movement of people, allows health professionals to move across borders and take up employment in other EU Member States. This freedom of movement applies to the EEA, which includes the EU27 and the three European Free Trade Association members, Iceland, Norway and Liechtenstein.[3]

However, the two EU enlargement rounds did not automatically open the labour markets to all EU/EEA countries. Many Member States used the transitional period to introduce labour market restrictions. In 2004, most

---

1 In 2004, Cyprus, Czech Republic, Estonia, Hungary, Latvia, Lithuania, Malta, Poland, Slovakia and Slovenia (EU10); in 2007 Bulgaria and Romania. Please note that the research for this chapter was carried out prior to the accession of Croatia to the EU in July 2013.

2 The material presented here has also been published in http:dx.doi.org/10.1016/j.healthpol, 2012.10.006.

3 Switzerland is a member of the European Free Trade Association but not the European Economic Area; it is bound by a separate bilateral agreement on free movement with the EU.

countries implemented labour market restrictions for nationals of 8 out of the 10 new EU Member States. Countries lifted their restrictions only gradually in the following years (Table 4.1). A similar development happened for nationals of the two 2007 accession states.

**Table 4.1** *Transitional arrangements on the free movement of labour in the EU (as of January 2013)*

|  | Access to EEA labour markets for nationals of EU10 (excluding Malta and Cyprus) in | Access to EEA labour markets for nationals of EU-2 in |
|---|---|---|
| No restrictions implemented | Since 2004: Ireland, Sweden, United Kingdom[a] | Since 2007: Cyprus, Czech Republic, Estonia, Finland, Latvia, Lithuania, Poland, Slovakia, Slovenia, Sweden |
| Restrictions lifted | Since 2006: Finland, Greece, Iceland, Italy, Portugal, Spain<br><br>Since 2007: Luxembourg, Netherlands<br><br>Since 2008: France<br><br>Since 2009: Belgium, Denmark, Norway<br><br>Since 2011: Austria, Germany, Malta, Liechtenstein, Switzerland[b] | Since 2009: Denmark, Greece, Hungary, Portugal, Spain |
| Restrictions in place: |  | up to 31 December 2013: Austria, Belgium, France, Germany, Iceland, Ireland, Italy, Liechtenstein, Luxembourg, Malta, Netherlands, Norway, United Kingdom, Switzerland[c] |

*Sources*: authors' own compilation, based on: http://ec.europa.eu/social/main.jsp?catId=466&langId=en, and https://ec.europa.eu/eures/main.jsp?acro=free.

[a] Free access to labour market but compulsory registration with worker registration scheme; [b] Entitled to restore the restrictions until 31 May 2014; [c] Restrictions extendable until 31 May 2016.

The EU/EEA Member States have since the mid-1970s adopted directives on the mutual recognition of qualifications and certificates of health professionals. The European Commission Directive on the recognition of professional qualifications (European Commission, 2005) covers five health professions: medical doctors, general care nurses, midwives, dentists and pharmacists. It provides for recognition if the minimum requirements of number of hours and theoretical/practical training are met.

For those health professions and specializations not covered by this Directive, the "general system" applies. It requires national competent authorities to assess the qualifications of individuals on a one-by-one basis. In that case, the Member State where the individual has sought employment is not obliged to automatically recognize the qualifications and could impose, as appropriate, compensating measures such as an aptitude test or an adaptation period (Peeters, McKee & Merkur, 2010).

Following the dissolution of the USSR, the health care systems of the Central and Eastern European Member States have undergone major health reforms. In many countries, the crisis in public finance has led to a lack of resources in the health sector. On average, pay and working conditions for health workers in the new EU Member States are still considered to be worse than those of the old Member States. In 2003, the average per capita GDP in purchasing power parity of the accession EU12 countries was roughly half that of the old EU Member States (EU15). By 2009, the average per capita GDP in purchasing power parity of the new EU Member States had increased by 10 percentage points, to approximately 60% of the average in the old EU Member States (European Commission, 2013a).

Because of this income gap, which represents a major migration incentive, many expected a mass migration of health professionals from the new EU Member States (GVG, 2002). Surveys carried out in the then-applicant countries as well as country reports confirmed these expectations (Gál et al., 2003). However, to date, a systematic analysis of the effects of EU enlargement on the mobility of health professionals has been lacking (OECD, 2008). Previous research on this issue is scarce and focused merely on the mobility of one profession (e.g. medical doctors; García-Pérez, Amaya & Otero, 2007), not based on quantitative data (Avgerinos, Koupidis & Filippou, 2004) or only focusing on a limited number of countries (Gerlinger & Schmucker, 2007).

This study aims to assess the scale of mobility of health professionals from the new to the old EU Member States before and after the 2004 and 2007 EU enlargements. It discusses the relevance of the phenomenon for some affected health systems and sheds light on whether the expectations and fears about a mass migration of health professionals hold true. This information could sensitize national and European policy-makers to possible migration flows arising from future EU enlargements.[4]

In view of the emerging workforce challenges, EU Member States, the European Commission and the European Parliament have fostered discussion and collaboration on workforce issues, including mobility of health professionals. Under the Belgian Presidency in 2010, the Member States adopted Council Conclusions on the health workforce that encouraged exchange of good practices, including on the collection of high-quality and comparable data, to better support the development of health workforce policies in Member

---

4 As of Feb 2014, the candidate countries were The former Yugoslav Republic of Macedonia, Montenegro, Turkey and Iceland. Accession negotiations with Croatia were successfully concluded on 30 June 2011. Potential candidates are Serbia, Albania, Bosnia and Herzegovina and Kosovo (in accordance with United Nations Security Council Resolution 1244 (1999)).

States, with particular attention to effective health workforce planning; the development of an action plan providing options to support the development of health workforce policies; the improvement of planning methodologies taking into account identified health needs, CPD and recruitment and retention strategies; and a joint action providing a platform for cooperation between Member States on forecasting health workforce needs and health workforce planning in close cooperation with Eurostat (Statistical Office of the European Communities), OECD and WHO (EU Council, 2010). This was further endorsed by the Hungarian Presidency in 2011, which put mobility of health professionals on the agenda of the Council.

The initiatives of the EU Member States were preceded by a Commission Green Paper and a consultation process on the European Workforce for Health (European Commission, 2008). In parallel, the European Parliament adopted a declaration on the *EU Workforce for Health* (Antonescu et al., 2010). On the international level, the World Health Assembly adopted in 2010 a Code of Practice for the International Recruitment of Health Personnel. The Code provides ethical guidance on international recruitment and discourages recruitment from countries facing workforce shortages (WHO, 2010).

## 4.2 Methodology

This chapter uses the two methodological approaches employed in PROMeTHEUS, the EU-funded project on mobility of health professionals: (1) secondary data collection and (2) in-depth case studies for selected countries.

Secondary data collection provides information on mobility of health professionals from a wide range of data sources: registries of national authorities and professional bodies, labour market statistics, census data, work permit data and other relevant sources. Country coverage includes 28 EEA countries (all EU Member States plus Norway), 5 OECD countries outside the EU (Canada, Australia, New Zealand, the United States, often cited as among the top destination countries, and Turkey) and Ukraine.

Between August 2009 and February 2010, country experts from the European countries covered requested time series data from national authorities and other data holders and filled in a standardized, pilot-tested, data collection sheet covering stock and flow data on medical doctors, nurses and dentists. Furthermore, they provided detailed meta-data information including coverage of data sources, definitions and use of indicators. The three professional groups were chosen by the scientific project leaders because of the importance of the health services provided and data availability considerations. The data collection sheet allowed for additional data on other health professions that the country experts considered important with regard to mobility. The data delivered within the PROMeTHEUS project were complemented whenever necessary by those available from the OECD.

Data were checked against and complemented by the findings of 17 in-depth country case studies on the mobility of health professionals covering 15 EU Member States plus Serbia and Turkey (Wismar et al., 2011). This triangulation was undertaken in order to enhance data validity and completeness and to qualitatively assess the effects of EU enlargement on health workforce mobility. The case studies follow a standardized template, covering the mobility profile of the country, the impact of EU enlargement, personal motivations for migration, the relevance of mobility vis-à-vis other health workforce issues, its impact on the health systems affected, and the policies and instruments used to manage migration.

### 4.2.1 Limitations of the data collected

The data collected are characterized by limitations in terms of country coverage, data sources and the availability of mobility indicators. In particular the datasets on nurses and dentists have significant shortages in terms of country coverage because a number of countries do not record and could not provide data on the migration of these health professionals (see Annex 4.1 and Annex 4.2). The scarce dataset on nurses has inconsistencies: while the data provided by some countries refer to nurses only, the data provided by countries such as Germany and the United Kingdom refer to nurses and midwives.

The available data on immigration (stock of foreign health professionals and annual inflows) refer to three indicators: country of birth, training and nationality. Each of the indicators has its limitations in terms of measuring labour migration. "Foreign-born" includes health professionals who were born abroad but may have been trained in and/or became nationals of the destination country. "Foreign-national" may include health professionals who were born and/or trained in the destination country but never acquired its nationality. "Foreign-trained" may include health professionals who were trained in a different country and then returned to their country of nationality (e.g. study tourism).

As most countries delivered data on only one of the migration indicators, the aggregated data presented in Figs 4.1 and 4.2 (below) refer to different indicators, which poses a further methodological limitation. In the exceptional cases in which countries delivered data on more than one indicator, the preferred indicator used in the aggregated data was country of training (followed by country of nationality and country of birth) as it is deemed to most accurately measure labour migration.

The presented data do not distinguish between short-term and long-term or permanent migration. Other limitations of the database include the availability of data on active versus registered (active plus non-active) health professionals. Furthermore, the data used refer to head counts and not full-time equivalents.

## 4.3 Results

### 4.3.1 Magnitude of health workforce mobility in the EU

Before assessing the effects of migration on mobility of health professionals, the data available were aggregated to provide an overview on the magnitude of health professional migration. The data collected show that in 2007 the vast majority of EU health professionals (92% for medical doctors, 95% for nurses and 95% for dentists) worked in their country of nationality, training or birth (Fig. 4.1).

Regarding foreign EU health professionals, 3–4% of all medical doctors worked in an EU country other than their country of nationality/training or birth. The same applies for dentists. However, only 1–2% of all nurses from the EU worked in an EU country other than their country of nationality/training or birth. In 2007, at least 109 413 medical doctors, nurses and dentists from the EU worked in an EU country other than their country of nationality/training or birth. This figure, however, is an underestimation of the real stock of foreign-trained/foreign-national/foreign-born health professionals as a number of EU Member States did not provide data on the nationality, country of training or birth of their health professionals. A huge number of irregularly employed

**Fig. 4.1** *Stock of health professionals in EU Member States, 2007 (see Annex 1 on data restrictions)*

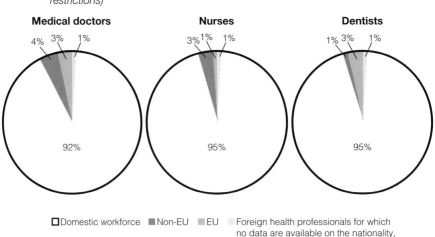

Source: See Annex 4.3.

health professionals, nurses in particular, who are mainly working in the home-based long-term care sector are also excluded.

Compared with overall migration within the EU, mobility of health professionals does not appear to differ by much. According to Eurostat data (European Commission, 2013b), in 2007 about 10.2 million EU citizens were residents in an EU country other than their country of citizenship (around 2% of the total population in the EU). This represents an increase of approximately 30% compared with 2003. In 2010, the total number reached 12.3 million. Migration within the EU (stock of EU citizens who are nationals of a foreign EU country) increased after the 2004 and 2007 EU enlargements, but the highest growth rates compared with the previous year were registered in 2008 (about 11%) and 2007 (9%) (European Commission, 2013b).

Regarding foreign non-EU health professionals, 4% of all medical doctors working in the EU in 2007 were either citizens of, born in or trained in a non-EU country. The corresponding figures were 1% and 3% for dentists and nurses, respectively. The percentage of non-EU citizens among the total population in the EU increased slightly from 3.8% in 2007 to 4% in 2010.

### 4.3.2 EU enlargement reinforcing "east–west" migration

Despite the relatively moderate percentage of EU health professionals working in another country of the EU, the PROMeTHEUS data show that outflows from the new EU Member States towards the western region of the EU increased. Countries are affected by this movement to different extents. Although such an "east–west" trend of health professional mobility existed well before the EU enlargement and can be traced back to the dissolution of the former Soviet Union, the EU enlargement rounds appear to have reinforced these already existing flows. Furthermore, the data suggest that emigration from EU12 peaked around the years 2004 and 2007 rather than a constant, linear rise (Wismar et al., 2011).

The number of medical doctors and dentists from the EU12 clearly increased from 2003 to 2007 in major destination countries of the EU15 for which data were available: Austria, Belgium, Denmark, Finland, Germany, Sweden and the United Kingdom. In absolute (Fig. 4.2 and Tables 4.2–4.4) and relative (Fig. 4.3) terms, the increase in health professionals from the EU12 working in the EU15 is most pronounced for medical doctors and dentists; while the increase in nurses seems marginal, it is based on significantly incomplete data. The percentage of medical doctors from the EU12 among all medical doctors in some EU15 countries more than doubled from 0.7% in 2003 to 1.5% in 2007.

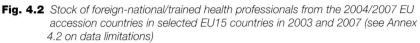

**Fig. 4.2** *Stock of foreign-national/trained health professionals from the 2004/2007 EU accession countries in selected EU15 countries in 2003 and 2007 (see Annex 4.2 on data limitations)*

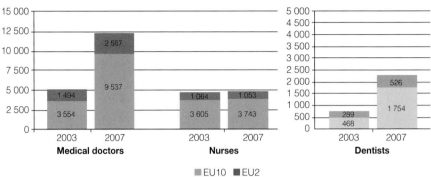

*Source*: See Annex 4.3.

*Notes*: EU10: Cyprus, Czech Republic, Estonia, Hungary, Latvia, Lithuania, Malta, Poland, Slovakia and Slovenia.
EU2: Bulgaria and Romania.

**Fig. 4.3** *Foreign-national/trained health professionals from the 2004/2007 EU accession countries in selected EU15 countries as a percentage in 2003 and 2007 (see Annex 4.2 on data limitations)*

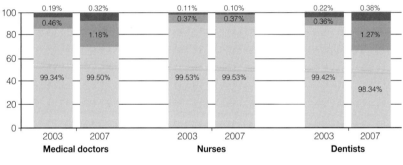

*Source*: See Annex 4.3.

*Notes*: EU10: Cyprus, Czech Republic, Estonia, Hungary, Latvia, Lithuania, Malta, Poland, Slovakia and Slovenia.
EU2: Bulgaria and Romania.

The incomplete data for nurses demonstrate only a minor increase in the stock of foreign-national/foreign-trained nurses, and the percentage of nurses from the EU12 working in EU15 countries remained roughly unchanged at 0.5%. However, the available data have major limitations in terms of country coverage; for example, a major destination country for nurses – the United Kingdom – is not included and data from Germany refer to nurses subject to social insurance contributions and excludes self-employed nurses. Anecdotal evidence suggests that huge numbers of foreign nurses are working irregularly or in a legal grey area, as caregivers or home-helps for the elderly, for example in Germany, Austria and Italy (Bertinato et al., 2011).

With regard to dentists, the absolute numbers of professionals from the EU12 working in EU15 countries appear to be very low. This is mainly because the

**Table 4.2** Stock of foreign national/trained medical doctors from the 2004/2007 EU accession countries in EU15 countries in 2003 and 2007

| | Cyprus | Czech Republic | Estonia | Hungary | Latvia | Lithuania | Malta | Poland | Slovakia | Slovenia | Total EU10 | Bulgaria | Romania | Total EU2 | Total EU12 |
|---|---|---|---|---|---|---|---|---|---|---|---|---|---|---|---|
| **2003** | | | | | | | | | | | | | | | |
| Austria | 7 | 22 | 1 | 87 | 0 | 0 | 1 | 155 | 9 | 4 | 286 | 25 | 67 | 92 | 378 |
| Belgium | 1 | 4 | 0 | 1 | 0 | 0 | 0 | 5 | 1 | 0 | 12 | 0 | 4 | 4 | 16 |
| Denmark | 0 | 3 | 2 | 3 | 3 | 50 | 1 | 46 | 0 | 0 | 108 | 13 | 45 | 58 | 166 |
| Finland | | | 21 | 2 | | 1 | | 4 | | | 28 | 1 | | 1 | 29 |
| France | | | | | | | | | | | | | | | |
| Germany | 42 | 175 | | 248 | 37 | 37 | 4 | 919 | 155 | 11 | 1 628 | 308 | 635 | 943 | 2 571 |
| Greece | | | | | | | | | | | | | | | |
| Ireland | | | | | | | | | | | | | | | |
| Italy | | | | | | | | | | | | | | | |
| Luxembourg | | | | | | | | | | | | | | | |
| Portugal | | | | | | | | | | | | | | | |
| Spain | | | | | | | | | | | | | | | |
| Sweden | | | | 65 | | | | 319 | | | 384 | 58 | | 58 | 442 |
| The Netherlands | | | | | | | | | | | | | | | |
| United Kingdom | 0 | 204 | 6 | 204 | 16 | 8 | 291 | 338 | 33 | 8 | 1 108 | 112 | 226 | 338 | 1 446 |
| **2007** | | | | | | | | | | | | | | | |
| Austria | 9 | 48 | 1 | 130 | 0 | 0 | 1 | 149 | 45 | 10 | 394 | 23 | 62 | 85 | 479 |
| Belgium | 3 | 8 | 0 | 8 | 1 | 5 | 0 | 29 | 8 | 0 | 62 | 7 | 126 | 133 | 195 |
| Denmark | 0 | 5 | 5 | 8 | 6 | 91 | 1 | 106 | 1 | 0 | 223 | 25 | 51 | 76 | 299 |
| Finland | | | 94 | 3 | 6 | 5 | | 1 | 1 | | 110 | 12 | 18 | 30 | 140 |
| France | 1 | 17 | | 17 | 9 | 17 | 1 | 108 | 280 | 2 | 192 | 13 | 156 | 169 | 361 |
| Germany | 52 | 304 | 27 | 359 | 43 | 61 | 5 | 1 332 | 454 | 28 | 2 665 | 462 | 824 | 1 286 | 3 951 |
| Greece | | | | | | | | | | | | | | | |
| Ireland | 1 | 74 | 0 | 104 | 5 | 21 | 23 | 242 | 52 | 3 | 525 | 18 | 65 | 83 | 608 |
| Italy | | 17 | 3 | 75 | | 15 | 20 | | | 28 | 158 | 78 | 564 | 642 | 800 |
| Luxembourg | | | | | | | | | | | | | | | |
| Portugal | | | | | | | | | | | | | | | |
| Spain | | | | | | | | | | | | | | | |
| Sweden | | | | 380 | | | | 827 | | | 1 207 | 126 | | 126 | 1 333 |
| The Netherlands | | | | | | | | | | | | | | | |
| United Kingdom | 0 | 735 | 45 | 971 | 111 | 211 | 396 | 2 075 | 313 | 19 | 4 876 | 284 | 567 | 851 | 5 727 |

*Source:* See Annex 4.3.

*Note:* Empty cells mean no data available.

**Table 4.3** Stock of foreign national/trained nurses from the 2004/2007 EU accession countries in EU15 countries in 2003 and 2007

| | Cyprus | Czech Republic | Estonia | Hungary | Latvia | Lithuania | Malta | Poland | Slovakia | Slovenia | Total EU10 | Bulgaria | Romania | Total EU2 | Total EU12 |
|---|---|---|---|---|---|---|---|---|---|---|---|---|---|---|---|
| **2003** | | | | | | | | | | | | | | | |
| Austria | 4 | 3 | 3 | 6 | 1 | 0 | 0 | 49 | 7 | 0 | 73 | 4 | 217 | 221 | 294 |
| Belgium | 0 | 0 | 9 | 1 | 0 | 0 | 0 | 36 | 0 | 0 | 37 | 0 | 1 | 1 | 38 |
| Denmark | | | | | | | | | | | | | | | |
| Finland | | | | | | | | | | | | | | | |
| France | | | | | | | | | | | | | | | |
| Germany | | 431 | 17 | 291 | 35 | 62 | | 2 325 | 139 | 195 | 3 495 | 249 | 593 | 842 | 4337 |
| Greece | | | | | | | | | | | | | | | |
| Ireland | | | | | | | | | | | | | | | |
| Italy | | | | | | | | | | | | | | | |
| Luxembourg | | | | | | | | | | | | | | | |
| Portugal | | | | | | | | | | | 0 | | | 0 | 0 |
| Spain | | | | | | | | | | | | | | | |
| Sweden | | | | | | | | | | | | | | | |
| The Netherlands | | | | | | | | | | | | | | | |
| United Kingdom | | | | | | | | | | | | | | | |
| **2007** | | | | | | | | | | | | | | | |
| Austria | 0 | 3 | 3 | 6 | 1 | 0 | 0 | 49 | 7 | 0 | 69 | 4 | 217 | 221 | 290 |
| Belgium | 0 | 0 | 1 | 0 | 2 | 4 | 1 | 45 | 0 | 1 | 54 | 1 | 2 | 3 | 57 |
| Denmark | | | | | | | | | | | | | | | |
| Finland | | | | | | | | | | | | | | | |
| France | | | | | | | | | | | | | | | |
| Germany | | 406 | 17 | 308 | 37 | 96 | | 2 335 | 173 | 219 | 3 609 | 233 | 591 | 824 | 4 433 |
| Greece | | | | | | | | | | | | | | | |
| Ireland | | | | | | | | | | | | | | | |
| Italy | | | | | | | | 2 487 | | | 2 487 | 186 | 7 670 | 7 856 | 10 342 |
| Luxembourg | | | 1 | 2 | | | | 8 | | | 11 | 1 | 1 | 5 | 16 |
| Portugal | | | | | | | | | | | | | | | |
| Spain | | | | | | | | | | | | | | | |
| Sweden | | | | | | | | | | | | | | | |
| The Netherlands | | | | | | | | | | | | | | | |
| United Kingdom | | | | | | | | | | | | | | | |

*Source:* See Annex 4.3.

*Note:* Empty cells mean no data available.

**Table 4.4** Stock of foreign national/trained dentists from the 2004/2007 EU accession countries in EU15 countries in 2003 and 2007

| | Cyprus | Czech Republic | Estonia | Hungary | Latvia | Lithuania | Malta | Poland | Slovakia | Slovenia | Total EU10 | Bulgaria | Romania | Total EU2 | Total EU12 |
|---|---|---|---|---|---|---|---|---|---|---|---|---|---|---|---|
| **2003** | | | | | | | | | | | | | | | |
| Austria | 0 | 58 | 0 | 62 | 1 | 1 | 0 | 69 | 27 | 13 | 231 | 12 | 84 | 96 | 327 |
| Belgium | 0 | 0 | 0 | 1 | 0 | 0 | 0 | 2 | 0 | 0 | 3 | 0 | 0 | 0 | 3 |
| Denmark | 0 | 0 | 0 | 0 | 0 | 0 | 0 | 0 | 0 | 0 | 0 | 0 | 0 | 0 | 0 |
| Finland | | | | | | | | | | | | | | | |
| France | | | | | | | | | | | | | | | |
| Germany | 5 | 42 | 1 | 37 | 5 | 0 | 1 | 130 | 0 | 3 | 2 245 | 31 | 162 | 193 | 417 |
| Greece | | | | | | | | | | | | | | | |
| Ireland | | | | | | | | | | | | | | | |
| Italy | | | | | | | | | | | | | | | |
| Luxembourg | | | | | | | | | | | | | | | |
| Portugal | | | | | | | | | | | | | | | 0 |
| Spain | | | | | | | | | | | | | | | |
| Sweden | | | | | | | | | | | | | | | |
| The Netherlands | | | | | | | | | | | | | | | |
| United Kingdom | 0 | 0 | 0 | 0 | 1 | 0 | 9 | 0 | 0 | 0 | 10 | 0 | 0 | 0 | 10 |
| **2007** | | | | | | | | | | | | | | | |
| Austria | 0 | 57 | 0 | 69 | 2 | 1 | 0 | 72 | 27 | 15 | 243 | 17 | 103 | 120 | 363 |
| Belgium | 0 | 1 | 0 | 3 | 0 | 0 | 0 | 3 | 0 | 0 | 7 | 2 | 1 | 3 | 10 |
| Denmark | 0 | 0 | 0 | 1 | 0 | 3 | 0 | 1 | 0 | 0 | 5 | 1 | 2 | 3 | 8 |
| Finland | | | | | | | | | | | | | | | |
| France | | | | | | | | | | | | | | | |
| Germany | 4 | 39 | 1 | 43 | 6 | 3 | 1 | 135 | 2 | 3 | 237 | 43 | 156 | 199 | 436 |
| Greece | | | | | | | | | | | | | | | |
| Ireland | | | | | | | | | | | | | | | |
| Italy | | | | | | | | | 2 | | 2 | | 20 | 20 | 22 |
| Luxembourg | | | | | | | | | | | | | | | |
| Portugal | | | | | | | | | | | | | | | |
| Spain | | | | | | | | | | | | | | | |
| Sweden | | | | | | | | | | | | | | | |
| The Netherlands | | | | | | | | | | | | | | | |
| United Kingdom | 0 | 49 | 17 | 147 | 22 | 105 | 30 | 853 | 39 | 0 | 1 262 | 45 | 156 | 201 | 1 463 |

*Source:* See Annex 4.3.

*Note:* Empty cells mean no data available.

major destination countries did not deliver data. The percentage of dentists from the EU12, however, more than doubled from 0.6% to 1.7% (Fig. 4.3).

### Inflows into the EU15

The stock and annual inflows of health professionals from the EU12 in major destination countries of the EU15 increased following EU enlargement. This section focuses on seven major destination countries (United Kingdom, Germany, Austria, France, Belgium, Spain, Finland) to demonstrate the changes in the scale of mobility of health professionals before and after the 2004 and 2007 EU enlargements.

In the **United Kingdom**, an important destination country with a long-standing tradition of recruiting foreign-trained health professionals, the percentage of foreign medical doctors and nurses is far above the EU average. The number of registered medical doctors (stock) from EU12 countries increased from 1 446 in 2003 to 5 727 in 2007 and 6 029 in 2008. Also the stock of dentists trained in the EU12 seem to have increased significantly between 2003 and 2008 (Table 4.2). The EU15 countries still account for most of the registered EEA health professionals, but numbers from EU12 countries are rapidly catching up. In 2008, the EU15 and the EU12 accounted for 1 166 and 970 new registrant medical doctors, respectively. Among newly registered nurses and midwives in 2008, 932 were from the EU12 and 437 from the EU15.

It is expected that the share of health professionals from EU Member States will grow in importance as numbers from non-EU countries decrease following the 2006 decline in active international recruitment (particularly from developing countries), while EU residents continue to exercise their right to free movement. The largest increases in numbers of EU12 medical doctors and nurses/midwives have come from Poland, but also other countries such as Hungary, the Czech Republic, Romania, Slovakia, Bulgaria and Lithuania have been represented.

While it is impossible to separate out the precise effects of accession per se from the United Kingdom's recruitment activities in certain countries, it is apparent that following the EU enlargements the United Kingdom became a more available destination country. Even with decreased active recruitment abroad,[5] as a result of increased investment in domestic health workforce, the post-2007 increase in health professionals from Bulgaria and Romania is significant in relative terms. For medical doctors and, to some degree, nurses, there are also other European sources outside the EU. These include the Russian Federation, Ukraine, Serbia and Turkey (Young, 2011).

---

5 Active recruitment abroad means the commencement of a search for foreign-trained health professionals once an organization has identified vacancies that cannot be filled by the domestic workforce.

The data collected from **Germany** show that the stock of medical doctors who are nationals of the EU12 countries has increased from 2 571 in 2003 to 3 951 in 2007 and 4 409 in 2008. Individual EU12 Member States are affected by this trend to different degrees. Major source countries are Poland (total number 919 in 2003, 1 332 in 2007, 1 428 in 2008: an increase of 509 in 2008 compared with 2003), Romania (635 in 2003, 824 in 2007, 927 in 2008: increase of 292 in 2008 compared with 2003), Bulgaria (308 in 2003, 462 in 2007, 541 in 2008: increase of 233), Slovakia (155 in 2003, 454 in 2007, 503 in 2008: increase of 348), Hungary (248 in 2003, 359 in 2007, 430 in 2008: increase of 182) and the Czech Republic (175 in 2003, 304 in 2007, 346 in 2008: increase of 171).

The number of foreign medical doctors with EU12 nationality has increased constantly in Germanyy since 2000 but the highest gross annual inflow of medical doctors occurred in 2003, so before the 2004 EU expansion. This occurred at a time when demand for medical doctors was first diagnosed to be high but the restrictive immigration policy for non-EU nationals still applied to these countries. Hence, the restrictive German law on migration did not prevent the migration of health personnel (Fellmer, 2008).

The total number of nurses and midwives coming to Germany from the EU12 and subject to social insurance contributions increased only very slightly from 4 337 in 2003 to 4 433 in 2007 (Table 4.3). However, it is estimated that there has been a greater increase in the number of nurses from EU12 working self-employed or as irregularly employed home-helps or caregivers in Germany, mainly for elderly people and those with disabilities (Ognyanova & Busse, 2011). The stock of dentists from the EU12 has increased only slightly in Germany.

Even though the 2004 EU enlargement has not caused the predicted dramatic rise in health professional mobility to **Austria**, there has been a rise in the numbers of health professionals from the EU12. The stock of medical doctors who are nationals of the EU12 countries increased from 378 in 2003 to 479 in 2007 and the stock of dentists from 327 to 363.

The increase in nurse migration can be approximated by the number of degree validations. In 2004, there were 159 applications in Austria from foreign-trained nurses from the EU10. Numbers rose more than threefold to 530 in 2006, constituting 37.9% of all validations of nursing degrees in that year. However, numbers then decreased to 235 (30.4%) in 2008. In 2000, there were only five registrations of medical doctors who were EU10 nationals; this number increased to 55 in 2006 with a reversing trend afterwards. Hence, the rising trend in the numbers of foreign health professionals in the Austrian labour market after the 2004 EU enlargement stabilized, and inflows were far from dramatic (Offermanns, Malle & Jusic, 2011).

In **France**, the data show that the immigration of health professionals from the EU12 is less significant than anticipated. Immigration has continued to rise over the last few years but has on the whole remained limited. However, immigration from Romania has increased considerably since the country's accession to the EU: in 2007 there were 174 registered Romanian medical doctors, 819 in 2008 and 1 160 as of 1 January 2009. In 2009, Romanians represented 73% of medical doctors from EU12 countries. In the same year, Romanians were the most numerous group among female foreign medical doctors while Belgians remained the most numerous group among male foreign doctors. In 2010, Romanian doctors constituted the largest national group of foreign medical doctors in France (15.4%), outnumbering those from Belgium, Germany and Italy. The number of migrants from other accession countries remains small: a total of 432 in 2009, excluding Romanians (Delamaire & Schweyer, 2011).

In **Belgium**, the stock of medical doctors who are nationals of EU12 countries increased from 16 in 2003 to 195 in 2007, whereas the number of nurses decreased slightly from 294 to 290 and the number of dentists increased from 3 to 10. Romanian medical doctors and nurses are the most numerous group among the health professionals from the EU12. The number of medical doctors from Romania increased significantly from 4 in 2003 to 126 in 2007. This can be partially explained by the activity of private companies recruiting Romanian nurses and specializing medical doctors to work as assistants in Belgian hospitals. However, it is noteworthy that Romanian medical doctors with basic medical training were migrating to Belgium even before Romania's accession to the EU (Safuta & Baete, 2011).

In **Spain**, there have been no significant inflows from the EU12 although flows appear to be increasing. An exception is Polish medical doctors, whose numbers increased significantly in 2007. In 2008, medical doctors from the EU12 acquired recognition of 268 general medical degrees and 202 specialty degrees. These constitute 3.2% and 36.5%, respectively, of all the degrees recognized in 2008. A larger inflow of medical doctors was observed from the Latin American countries. As yet, there have been no similar influxes of dentists and nurses (López-Valcárcel, Pérez & Quintana, 2011).

In **Finland**, the stock of medical doctors trained in the EU12 increased from 29 in 2003 to 140 in 2007. Finland has not been an attractive destination country for EU citizens, except for Estonians. The number of medical doctors in Finland who were trained in Estonia increased from 21 in 2003 to 94 in 2007. The migration of Estonian health professionals to Finland has been facilitated by active recruitment, similar languages, geographical proximity and close ties between medical organizations. Between 2006 and 2008, Finland granted 505 licences to health professionals from Estonia, mostly medical doctors (266).

Migration from Estonia to Finland was limited before implementation of the free movement policy for the new EU Member States (Kuusio et al., 2011).

In addition to the seven major destination countries discussed above, the Scandinavian countries also appear to be important destination countries. In Sweden, the stock of medical doctors trained in the EU12 increased significantly from 442 in 2003 to 1 333 in 2007. A smaller increase in the stock of medical doctors trained in the EU12 was noticeable also in Denmark, from 166 in 2003 to 299 in 2007. The stock of nurses trained in Denmark increased slightly from 38 in 2003 to 57 in 2007, and the number of dentists increased from 0 to 8.

Mobility of health professionals in the EU has changed not only in terms of intensity but also qualitatively through diversification of the types of mobility. There is evidence of increased short-term mobility since the EU expanded: for example weekend work in the United Kingdom; short-term contracts of several weeks/months offered by health care providers in countries such as Finland, Sweden, Norway and Belgium; and increasing mobility in the home care and long-term care sectors (Wismar et al., 2011).

### Demand and active recruitment stimulating mobility

The precise effect of EU enlargement on mobility of health professionals cannot be separated from the effect of other factors such as the recruitment activities of countries, hospitals and private agencies. In fact, labour migration takes place particularly when there is a high demand for health professionals in the destination countries. The United Kingdom has been involved in active international recruitment for a long time. This is one of the major reasons why more than a third of all medical doctors and every tenth nurse in the United Kingdom is internationally trained. In the late 1990s, the British Government began a policy of massive NHS workforce expansion across all health professions, which instigated a period of active international recruitment on an unprecedented scale. At the same time, a number of foreign health professionals were recruited into private sector hospitals, nursing homes and social care (Smith et al., 2006). The policy of active international recruitment was reversed in 2006 and more restrictive immigration rules were introduced as earlier expansion in United Kingdom training numbers came into effect.

In Germany and Austria, a number of agencies emerged that recruited health professionals from Eastern European countries to fill gaps in the hospital and long-term care sectors. Private Belgian companies have been recruiting nurses and specializing medical doctors from Romania. Finnish and Norwegian recruitment companies have been actively operating in Estonia since 2007.

The active recruitment from Estonia to Finland, together with closely related languages, the small distance between Estonia and Finland and close ties between medical organizations, has facilitated the migration of Estonian health professionals. Active measures for recruiting foreign health professionals have increased in Finland over the past few years.

The Continuing Education Centre at the University of Joensuu in Finland is planning a project for recruiting medical doctors from the Russian Federation. The National Institute for Health and Welfare's International Affairs Unit and Helsinki University Central Hospital have launched a pilot project to recruit nurses from other EU Member States. The project aims to develop ethical recruitment among health care personnel. The Finnish Government Migration Policy Programme issued in October 2006 also emphasizes active recruitment of a migrant labour force.

Shortages of health professionals in Spain have led to the emergence of companies that recruit health professionals in the new EU countries, particularly Poland and Romania. Autonomous communities have also embarked on recruiting expeditions, some of which have been led by the head of the regional health service.

Hence recruitment activities of national, regional and private institutions in response to the emerging shortage of health professionals in the destination countries greatly foster migration. Higher remuneration, better working conditions and training opportunities are the main incentives for health professionals to move.

### *Outflows from the EU12*

From the perspective of the EU12, an increase in outflows or requests for recognition of degrees of health professionals became evident around the years of accession. In most source countries, the only data source available to estimate outflows is intention-to-leave data. Intention-to-leave data stem from the EU's mutual recognition of qualifications, which requires certificates of degree recognition or of good standing. These documents are issued by the competent authorities at the request of the health professional seeking recognition of qualification in another EU country. However, intention-to-leave data provide merely a rough estimate of the real migratory outflows as the holders may choose not to leave the country or may leave only on a short-term basis.

In most countries, the highest numbers of certificates of mutual recognition of qualifications were issued directly in the years of accession or one year later, with decreasing tendency afterwards. In Estonia, the numbers of certificates of recognition peaked in 2004, with 283 for medical diplomas, 118 for nursing diplomas and 29 for dental diplomas. Numbers fell in the following years, between three and fourfold, but increased again slightly in 2009 (Saar & Habicht, 2011). Hungary had high numbers of medical doctors and nurses wishing to emigrate in 2004 and 2005, followed by a slightly more contained development in the subsequent years and a new increase in 2009 (Eke, Girasek & Szócska, 2011).

In Poland, data show that the number of certification requests by medical doctors and dentists increased rapidly in the initial phase following accession but slowed from mid-2007 (Kautsch & Czabanowska, 2011). In Slovakia, the number of medical doctors, dentists and nurses asking for confirmation of equivalency of their education in accordance with EU regulations peaked in 2005 but since then has tended to decrease (Beňušová et al., 2011).

In Lithuania, during the first year of EU membership, 2.7% of all medical doctors obtained certificates. That number almost halved to 1.4% in the period 1 May 2005 to 30 April 2006 and fell to 0.9% in 2009. Nurses show a different pattern: 0.4% of all nurses received certificates in 2004–2005, with relative increases to 0.7% in 2005–2006 and 1.1% in 2009 (Padaiga, Pukas & Starkienė, 2011).

Intention-to-leave data from Romania indicate continuing high outflows of medical doctors; more than 300 certificates per month were issued to Romanian medical doctors in 2010. However, intention-to-leave data must be interpreted with care as the reported number of 4 990 medical doctors in 2007 contrasts sharply with the findings of a separate study that concluded that only 1 421 medical doctors actually left the country. Still, the scale of these outflows is a matter of concern, particularly because the most economically deprived region in the north-east of the country was most affected by emigration (Dragomiristeanu, Farcasanu & Galan, 2008).

Hence, in those countries for which data were available, estimated annual outflows based on intention-to-leave data have rarely exceeded 3% of the domestic workforce. In 2004, qualification recognition certificates issued represented roughly 2.7% of all medical doctors in Hungary and Lithuania. In 2005, qualification recognition certificates issued represented roughly 3% of all registered Polish medical doctors, and approximately 2% of the Estonian active medical workforce after 2004 (but 6.5% at the peak of mobility in 2004). Around 3% of all medical doctors left Romania in 2007 (Wismar et al., 2011).

There are two possible explanations for the high number of intentions to leave in the year of or following accession. On the one hand, it may be that interest to leave these countries was most pronounced in that period. On the other hand, these numbers may reflect a culmination of both prospective and retrospective applications – including not only health professionals residing in the country and wishing to leave but also health professionals already living abroad and requesting recognition retrospectively, as was the case in Hungary.

With regard to nurses, the presented very scarce stock data suggest that mobility following the 2004 and 2007 EU enlargements has remained much lower compared with that of medical doctors and dentists. However, it is very likely that the real scale of nurse migration has been extensively underestimated because of the lack of good-quality data in a considerable number of countries.

For the time being, the effect of the increased mobility of health professionals on the health systems in the new EU Member States appear to be of moderate significance. However, some source countries, and particularly economically deprived regions, experience the consequences of increased outflows of health professionals. In the mid or longer term, continuous outflows add to existing staff shortages and risk undermining the sustainability of the workforce for the future. In Romania, the substantial rise in mobility resulting from both EU enlargement and the financial crisis appears to be of critical concern.

As a response to such concerns, some EU12 countries introduced workforce policies, including salary increases and improvement of working conditions, which may have retained considerable numbers of their domestic health professionals. In several countries, including Estonia, Poland and Lithuania, return migration was observed, presumably as a result of policy changes including salary increases or improved working conditions. Such policies may have furthermore contributed to decreasing the incentives to move abroad and retaining the active workforce in the country. In Estonia and Poland, increased levels of salaries coincided with a significant fall in health professionals applying for recognition of qualifications in subsequent years, implying a causal relationship (Kautsch & Czabanowska, 2011; Saar & Habicht, 2011).

### 4.3.3 Labour market restrictions mitigating mobility

Ireland, Sweden and the United Kingdom had opened their labour markets to nationals of the new EU Member States from the beginning of the 2004 EU enlargement, with no restrictions implemented. Data from the United Kingdom show that since the EU enlargement in 2004 the numbers of incoming health professionals from Central and Eastern Europe increased considerably, constituting a new migration source for the United Kingdom. The numbers of health professionals from Poland, particularly of Polish medical doctors, was particularly high. Although it is impossible to single out the precise effect of EU enlargement on mobility of health professionals, the example of the United Kingdom suggests that opening of labour markets, together with the portability of professional qualifications through the mutual recognition of degrees, has had an effect on the numbers of health professionals moving to the United Kingdom (Young, 2011).

Countries that originally implemented labour market restrictions for nationals from eight East European enlargement countries (EU10 excluding Malta and Cyprus), but which subsequently lifted the restrictions, are Belgium, Denmark, Finland, France, Greece, Italy, Luxembourg, the Netherlands, Portugal and Spain, plus the EEA countries Norway and Iceland. Germany, Austria, Malta, Liechtenstein and Switzerland followed on 1 May 2011. In most countries, a work permit was needed for health professionals, which was time consuming, costly and not always granted. For nationals of Romania and Bulgaria, a smaller number of countries (Denmark, Greece, Hungary, Portugal and Spain) chose to lift their labour market restrictions in 2009, but a considerable number of countries (Austria, Belgium, France, Germany, Iceland, Ireland, Italy, Liechtenstein, Luxembourg, Malta, the Netherlands, Norway, United Kingdom, Switzerland) still have restrictions in place (as of July 2011).

In Germany, one of the countries that delayed full labour market access for the longest period possible, the restrictive labour market approach may have been one of the reasons why, against expectations, the migration of health professionals from Eastern Europe did not produce a mass exodus right after the 2004 EU enlargement. The number of foreign medical doctors from the EU12 increased since 2000, but the highest growth rate of medical doctors from the EU12, approximately 21%, was in 2003: before EU enlargement and when the demand for medical doctors was first diagnosed as high. Numbers slowed down after the EU enlargement in 2004 (Ognyanova & Busse, 2011). One possible explanation might be that health professionals from the new EU Member States might have chosen countries such as the United Kingdom that did not limit the freedom of movement of labour in the way that Germany did, indicating that labour market restrictions may have had a role in influencing professionals' choice of destination country. However, the motivation to move to the United Kingdom may also have been influenced by language- and culture-related factors, the characteristics of the health system, salaries and career development possibilities.

Belgium and Finland did not experience substantial numbers of inflows during and after the transitional periods. Yet the most numerous group among medical doctors from the EU12 who migrated to Belgium was the Romanian holders of basic medical training, despite labour market restrictions being in place. The data demonstrate an increase in the recognitions of Romanian basic medicine degrees in 2007 and 2008. The reason lies in a bilateral agreement that the Belgian French-speaking Université catholique de Louvain signed with the Romanian medical university Gr.T. Popa in Iaşi. It allows, on average, 70 Romanian medical doctors annually to spend parts of their specialization in Belgium. Furthermore, migration is facilitated by the activity of private liaison companies recruiting Romanian specializing medical doctors to work as assistants in Belgian hospitals. The latter are mainly working as self-employed, which does not fall under the labour market restrictions (Safuta & Baeten, 2011).

One phenomenon partly triggered by labour market restrictions is the increasing, but legally grey, work of mobile health professionals, primarily in the home-based care sector. Austria, Germany and Italy report a substantial increase in Eastern European nurses and informal care workers working in the long-term care sector. Recruitment agencies in Germany have identified contractual arrangements to circumvent the labour market restrictions by offering foreign health professionals, nurses in particular, contracts with companies in their home countries that work with partner agencies in Germany. The "delegated" carers usually work in Germany for a year, which in exceptional cases can be extended to up to two years. During that time, the carer pays social insurance contributions and taxes in the country of origin. The German families are not employers of these nurses but an ordering party (customer) to the company that employs the nurse. According to the law, the nurses should perform only strictly predefined activities. Practically, however, it is almost impossible not to give the foreign nurse a concrete order, particularly if the nurse lives with the family. Therefore, in practice, the family is the employer, which makes the employment illegal. Working hours are regulated through the law of the country of affiliation; however, it is not possible to monitor if they are kept. The fact that the carer works and lives in the family suggests a constant addressability comparable to ongoing on-call duty.

Another possibility for nurses from the new EU Member States is to register as self-employed in their home country. This allows them to work in Germany if they prove that they are working for more than one client. Practically, however, this is very difficult, particularly when the nurse is living with the family of the elderly or disabled person, which could be a justification for "disguised employment".

In sum, the labour market restrictions appear to have had several consequences for health professional mobility in Europe: they did naturally limit the numbers of incoming health professionals and played a role influencing the geographical directions of mobility in Europe to some extent, as mobile health professionals are likely to have chosen countries without labour market restrictions. Finally, in those countries with restrictions, they contributed to diverting the nature of work of migrant workers from regular employment to semi-regular or irregular work, particularly in the home-based long-term care sector.

## 4.4 Discussion and conclusions

The data collected within the PROMeTHEUS project demonstrate that the 2004 and 2007 EU enlargements have facilitated and reinforced the migration of health professionals from EU12 to the EU15 Member States, although it is difficult to separate precisely the effect of accession from other factors fuelling migration, such as demand for health professionals in some old EU Member States and their recruitment activities. Even though the outflows are relatively moderate and in line with overall migration in the EU, some countries lost a considerable number of health professionals around the years of accession, although numbers often decreased slightly following initial peaks. The negative impacts of outmigration are particularly perceptible in some underserved regions and for some rare specialties, threatening the goal of adequate service delivery.

Before their accession to the EU, the then-applicant countries, as well as the EU Member States, expected a massive east–west migration of health professionals. Several years after the 2004 EU expansion, a number of countries report that actual migration in the health sector has fallen short of predictions. The outflow of health professionals from the new EU Member States was smaller than expected for several reasons. First, the labour market restrictions applied in several EU15 Member States restricted immigration. Second, in some Eastern European countries, salaries were raised and working conditions improved, which may have helped to retain health professionals by reducing incentives to migrate. Third, predictions were often based on the intention/interest to move, which is certainly higher than actual migration.

Hence, in quantitative terms, migration has remained moderate and is only one of the problems the new EU Member States are facing with regard to health care staffing. For example, in some countries, a large number of health professionals shift to other sectors of the economy. Thus, push factors such as poor working conditions and low pay produce not only emigration but also phenomena such as attrition and maldistribution.

Nevertheless, single countries and regions are affected by shortages of health professionals and emigration (between countries, as well as within the country) poses a threat to their health systems objectives. Retention strategies, which include salary increases, improvement in working conditions and facility renovation with new equipment, have proven to be effective in a number of source countries such as Poland, Lithuania and Estonia. The fear that health professionals might emigrate seems to be an important motive for national governments to reform the domestic health care sector (Buchan & Perfilieva, 2006).

However, the free movement of health professionals does not have only disadvantages. In particular, the chances for international education, the intensified exchange of knowledge and skills, the return of more highly qualified professionals and the more rapid implementation of new medical procedures can improve the quality of health care. Until now, little is known about return migration and no data are available as most countries do not record return migration.

Steps should be taken in order to improve monitoring of health professional mobility. Common definitions of the indicators used to measure mobility can increase validity and comparability of data across countries. Workforce planning is another area where exchange between EU Member States can be improved. While the optimal number of health professionals in a country is a political decision, EU-wide cooperation in workforce planning (exchange on data sources and forecasting methodologies) might reduce uncertainties about national forecasts and workforce policies and provide transparency on the planning of the numbers and skill-mix in the health workforce.

## Annex 4.1 Data restrictions for Fig. 4.1

### Medical doctors

The following countries are included in the diagram: Austria, Belgium, Bulgaria, Denmark, Estonia, Finland, France, Germany, Greece (2001), Hungary, Italy, Ireland, Latvia, Luxembourg, Malta, the Netherlands (2006), Poland, Portugal, Romania, Slovakia, Slovenia, Sweden, Spain (2001), United Kingdom.

For Austria, Belgium, France, Germany, Hungary, Italy, Poland, and Slovakia, the PROMeTHEUS database provides detailed data on the number of foreign national medical doctors; for Denmark, Estonia, Finland, Ireland, Latvia, Malta, Portugal, Slovenia, Sweden, United Kingdom - foreign-trained medical doctors; for Bulgaria - foreign born medical doctors.

The PROMeTHEUS database does not provide detailed data on country of nationality, training or birth of foreign medical doctors for Cyprus, Czech Republic, Greece, Lithuania, Luxembourg, the Netherlands, Romania, and Spain. However, it provides the total number of foreign national medical doctors for Luxembourg and of foreign-trained medical doctors for Romania. The data set was complemented by OECD data on foreign national medical doctors for Greece (2001), foreign-trained doctors for the Netherlands (2006) (OECD, 2012), and foreign born medical doctors for Spain (2001) (OECD, 2007). Countries for which no data were available at all - and which were thus excluded from the diagram - are Cyprus, Czech Republic, and Lithuania.

### Nurses

The following countries are included in the diagram: Belgium, Bulgaria, Czech Republic, Cyprus, Denmark, Finland (2006), France (2005), Germany, Greece, Hungary, Italy, Latvia, Luxembourg, Malta, the Netherlands (2005), Portugal, Sweden, Spain, United Kingdom. For Belgium, Germany, Hungary, and Portugal the PROMeTHEUS database provides detailed data on the number of foreign national nurses; for Cyprus, Bulgaria, Denmark, Latvia, Malta, United Kingdom - foreign-trained nurses; Italy - foreign born nurses. The data for the United Kingdom refers to EEA countries instead of EU.

The PROMeTHEUs database does not provide detailed data on country of nationality, training or birth of foreign nurses in Austria, Czech Republic, Estonia, Finland, France, Greece, Ireland, Lithuania, Luxembourg, the Netherlands, Poland, Romania, Slovenia, Slovakia, Sweden, and Spain.

However, it provides total number of foreign-national nurses for Finland (2006) and Luxemburg; foreign-trained - for Czech Republic, Greece and Sweden. Total number of foreign-trained nurses was retrieved from OECD (2011a) for Netherlands (2005) and of foreign national nurses for France (2005). The total number of foreign national nurses for Spain was obtained from López-Valcárcel et al. (2011). The total number of licensed practicing nurses in the Netherlands (2005) were obtained from OECD health data (OECD, 2012a), as they were not available in the PROMeTHEUS data base. Countries for which no data were available at all – and which are thus excluded from the diagram - are Austria, Estonia, Ireland, Lithuania, Poland, Romania, Slovenia, and Slovakia.

### Dentists

The following countries are included in the diagram: Austria, Belgium, Denmark, Finland, Germany, Greece (2006), Italy, Luxembourg, the Netherlands, Portugal, United Kingdom, Bulgaria, Czech Republic, Estonia, Hungary, Latvia, Malta, Poland, Slovakia.

For Austria, Belgium, Germany, Hungary, Italy, Portugal, Poland, Slovakia, the PROMeTHEUS database provides detailed data on the number of foreign national dentists; for Denmark, Estonia, Latvia, United Kingdom - foreign-trained dentists; for Bulgaria - foreign born dentists.

The PROMeTHEUS database does not provide detailed data on country of nationality, training or birth of foreign dentists for Czech Republic, Finland, France, Greece, Ireland, Lithuania, Luxembourg, Netherlands, Romania and Spain. However, it provides total number of foreign national dentists in Finland (2006), Luxemburg, Netherlands, Czech Republic, of foreign-trained dentists for Malta and of foreign born dentists in Greece (2006). Countries for which no data were available at all – and which are thus excluded from the diagram – are Cyprus, France, Ireland, Lithuania, Romania, Slovenia, Spain and Sweden.

## Annex 4.2 Data restrictions for Figs 4.2 and 4.3

### Medical doctors

Included are: Austria, Belgium, Denmark, Finland, Germany, Sweden, and the UK. Data for Austria, Belgium, and Germany refer to nationality; data for Denmark, Finland, Sweden, and the UK refer to foreign-trained medical doctors.

### Nurses

Included are: Belgium, Denmark, Germany, and Portugal. Data for Belgium, Germany, and Portugal refer to nationality. Data for Denmark refer to foreign-trained nurses.

### Dentists

Included are: Austria, Belgium, Denmark, Germany and the United Kingdom. Austria, Belgium and Germany provide data on foreign national dentists. Denmark and the United Kingdom provide data on foreign-trained dentists.

## Annex 4.3

Sources for Fig 4.1

*Sources*: **Medical doctors**, registry data: Austria: Austrian Medical Chamber; Belgium: the Federal Database of Healthcare Professionals; Bulgaria: Registry of Bulgarian Medical Association; Denmark: Labour Register for Health Personnel, The Danish National Board of Health 2009; Estonia: the register of health care professionals; Finland: Statistics Finland employment register; France: Doctors National Order; Germany: Federal Physicians' Chamber, Federal Association of Statutory Health Insurance Physicians, Federal Statistical Office, Federal Employment Agency; Greece: Pan-Hellenic medical association (2001); Hungary: Working Registry of Medical Doctors; Ireland: Registry of the Medical Council; Italy: Italian Federation of Medical Doctors, Dental Surgeons and Dentists; Latvia: Register of medical persons and medical support persons; Luxembourg: professional register of medical doctors; Malta: Medical Council Registers - Medical Practitioners Registers (Principal, Temporary, and Provisional Registers); Poland: Statistic Bulletins of the Ministry of Health 2004-2008, Statistical Yearbook of Poland 1989 - Central Statistical Office; Portugal: Medical Council; Romania: National Registry of Physicians; Slovak Republic: National Register of Health Professionals - National Health Information Centre; Slovenia: Registry of physicians; Spain: Official Councils of Physicians (2001); Sweden: National Planning Support at the Swedish National Board of Health and Welfare; The Netherlands: Healthcare Providers Registration and Information (2006); UK : 1) List of Registered Medical Practitioners, 2) GP Register, and 3) Specialist Register - held by the General Medical Council (GMC). For Greece and the Netherlands, data complemented by (OECD 2010) and for Spain by (OECD 2007). **Nurses**: Belgium: the Federal Database of Healthcare Professionals; Bulgaria: Professional Register of Bulgarian Association of Health Professionals in Nursing; Czech Republic: Registry of non medical health workers; Cyprus: Nursing and Midwifery council of Cyprus; Denmark: Labour Register for Health Personnel, The Danish National Board of Health 2009; Finland: Statistics Finland employment register (2006); France: Direction for research, studies, evaluation and statistics (DREES), Ministry of social affairs and health (2005); Germany: Federal Employment Agency; Greece: Nurses union of Greece; Hungary: Working Registry of Allied Health workers; Italy: National Federation of Professional Nurses, Health Assistants and Childcare workers (IPASVI); Latvia: Register of medical persons and medical support persons; Luxembourg: professional register of Health professionals; Malta: Register of First

Level Nurse; The Netherlands: Healthcare Providers Registration and Information (2005); Portugal: Nursing Council; Spain: Official Nursing Councils; Sweden: National Planning Service at the National Board of Health and Welfare; UK: Nursing and Midwifery Council (NMC) Professional Register. For France, data complemented by (OECD 2011a), for the Netherlands by (OECD 2011a and 2011b), and for Spain by (Lopez-Valcarcel, Perez and Quintana 2011). **Dentists**, registry data: Austria: Austrian Dental Association; Belgium: the Federal Database of Healthcare Professionals; Bulgaria: Registry of Bulgarian Dental Association; Czech Republic: Czech Dental Chamber; Denmark: Labour Register for Health Personnel, The Danish National Board of Health 2009; Estonia: the register of health care professionals; Finland: Statistics Finland employment register; Germany: Federal Statistical Office, Federal Dentists' Chamber; Greece: Hellenic Dental Federation (2006); Hungary: Working Registry of Dentists; Italy: The Italian National Federation of Medical Doctors, Dental Surgeons and Dentists; Latvia: Register of medical persons and medical support persons; Luxembourg: professional register of dentists; Malta: Medical Council Registers - Dental Practitioners - Principal List; The Netherlands: Healthcare Providers Registration and Information; Poland: Statistic Bulletins of the Ministry of Health 2004-2008, Statistical Yearbook of Poland 1989 - Central Statistical Office; Portugal: Portuguese Dental Association; Slovak Republic: National Register of Health Professionals - National Health Information Centre; UK: Dentists Register and Specialists Register, both collated by the General Dental Council (GDC).

## Sources for Fig 4.2 and 4.3

*Sources*: **Medical doctors**, registry data: Austria: Austrian Medical Chamber; Belgium: the Federal Database of Healthcare Professionals; Denmark: Labour Register for Health Personnel, The Danish National Board of Health 2009; Finland: Statistics Finland employment register; Germany: Federal Physicians' Chamber, Federal Association of Statutory Health Insurance Physicians, Federal Statistical Office, Federal Employment Agency; Sweden: National Planning Support at the Swedish National Board of Health and Welfare; UK : 1) List of Registered Medical Practitioners, 2) GP Register, and 3) Specialist Register held by the General Medical Council (GMC). **Nurse**s: Belgium: the Federal Database of Healthcare Professionals; Denmark: Labour Register for Health Personnel, The Danish National Board of Health 2009; Germany: Federal Employment Agency; Portugal: Nursing Council. **Dentist**s: Austria: Austrian Dental Association; Belgium: the Federal Database of Healthcare Professionals; Denmark: Labour Register for Health Personnel, The Danish National Board of Health 2009; Germany: Federal Statistical Office, Federal Dentists' Chamber; Italy: The Italian National Federation of Medical Doctors, Dental Surgeons and Dentists; UK: Dentists Register and Specialists Register, both collated by the General Dental Council (GDC).

## Sources for Table: 4.2

*Sources (registry data)*: Austria: Austrian Medical Chamber; Belgium: the Federal Database of Healthcare Professionals; Denmark: Labour Register for Health Personnel, The Danish National Board of Health 2009; Finland: Statistics Finland employment register; France: Doctors National Order; Germany: Federal Physicians' Chamber, Federal Association of Statutory Health Insurance Physicians, Federal Statistical Office, Federal Employment Agency; Ireland: Registry of the Medical Council; Italy: Italian Federation of Medical Doctors, Dental Surgeons and Dentists; Sweden: National Planning Support at the Swedish National Board of Health and Welfare; UK : 1) List of Registered Medical Practitioners, 2) GP Register, and 3) Specialist Register held by the General Medical Council (GMC). No data available for Greece, Luxembourg, Portugal, Spain, the Netherlands.

## Sources for Table 4.3

*Sources*: Belgium: the Federal Database of Healthcare Professionals; Denmark: Labour Register for Health Personnel, The Danish National Board of Health 2009; Germany: Federal Employment Agency; Italy: National Federation of Professional Nurses, Health Assistants and Childcare workers (IPASVI); Portugal: Nursing Council. No data available for Austria, Finland, France, Greece, Luxembourg, Spain, Sweden, the Netherlands, and United Kingdom.

## Sources for Table 4.4

*Sources (registry data)*: Austria: Austrian Dental Association; Belgium: the Federal Database of Healthcare Professionals; Denmark: Labour Register for Health Personnel, The Danish National Board of Health 2009; Germany: Federal Statistical Office, Federal Dentists' Chamber; Italy: The Italian National Federation of Medical Doctors, Dental Surgeons and Dentists; UK: Dentists Register and Specialists Register, both collated by the General Dental Council (GDC). No data available for Finland, France, Greece, Luxembourg, Portugal, Spain, Sweden, the Netherlands.

## References

Antonescu EO et al. (2010). *Written declaration pursuant to Rule 123 of the Rules of Procedure on the EU Workforce for Health*. Brussels, European Parliament (http://www.europarl.europa.eu/sides/getDoc.do?pubRef=-//EP//NONSGML+WDECL+P7-DCL-2010-0040+0+DOC+PDF+V0//EN&language=EN, accessed 2 January 2014).

Avgerinos ED, Koupidis SA, Filippou DK (2004). Impact of the European Union enlargement on health professionals and health care systems. *Health Policy,* 69:403–408.

Beňušová K et al. (2011). Regaining self-sufficiency: Slovakia and the challenges of health professionals leaving the country. In Wismar M et al., eds. *Health professional mobility and health systems. Evidence from 17 European countries.* Copenhagen, WHO Regional Office for Europe on behalf of the European Observatory on Health Systems and Policies:479–510.

Bertinato L et al. (2011). Oversupplying doctors but seeking carers: Italy's demographic challenges and health professional mobility. In Wismar M et al., eds. *Health professional mobility and health systems. Evidence from 17 European countries.* Copenhagen, WHO Regional Office for Europe on behalf of the European Observatory on Health Systems and Policies:243–262.

Buchan J, Perfilieva G (2006). *Health worker migration in the European Region: country case studies and policy implications*. Copenhagen, WHO Regional Office for Europe.

Delamaire ML, Schweyer FX (2011). Nationally moderate, locally significant: France and health professional mobility from far and near. In Wismar M et al., eds. *Health professional mobility and health systems. Evidence from 17 European countries.* Copenhagen, WHO Regional Office for Europe on behalf of the European Observatory on Health Systems and Policies:181–210.

Dragomiristeanu A, Farcasanu D, Galan A (2008). Migratia medicilor din Romania [The migration of medical doctors from Romania]. *Revista Medica,* 17 March.

Eke E, Girasek E, Szócska M (2011). From melting pot to laboratory of change in central Europe: Hungary and health workforce migration. In Wismar M et al., eds. *Health professional mobility and health systems. Evidence from 17 European countries.* Copenhagen, WHO Regional Office for Europe on behalf of the European Observatory on Health Systems and Policies:365–394.

EU Council (2010). *Council conclusions on investing in Europe's health workforce of tomorrow: scope for innovation and collaboration;*2010. Brussels, Council of the European Union (http://www.consilium.europa.eu/uedocs/cms_data/docs/pressdata/en/lsa/118280.pdf, accessed 2 January 2014).

European Commission (2005). *Directive 2005/36/EC on the recognition of professional qualifications*. Brussels, European Commission (http://ec.europa.eu/internal_market/qualifications/policy_developments/legislation/index_en.htm, accessed 5 August 2013).

European Commission (2008). *Green paper on the European workforce for health*. Brussels, European Commission (COM(2008) 725 final) (http://ec.europa.eu/health/ph_systems/docs/workforce_gp_en.pdf, accessed 2 January 2014).

European Commission (2013a). *Eurostat statistical database* [online database]. Brussels, Statistical Office of the European Communities (http://epp.eurostat.ec.europa.eu/portal/page/portal/eurostat/home/, accessed 5 August 2013).

European Commission (2013b). *Eurostat statistical database: immigration by sex, age group and citizenship* [online database]. Brussels, Statistical Office of the European Communities [http://appsso.eurostat.ec.europa.eu/nui/show.do?dataset=migr_imm1ctz&lang=en, accessed 2 January 2014).

Fellmer S (2008). Germany restricted the freedom of movement for Polish citizens: but does it matter? *EUMAP online* (*Across fading borders: the challenges of east–west migration in the EU*) (http://pdc.ceu.hu/archive/00003936/01/fellmer.pdf, accessed 2 January 2014).

Gál R et al. (2003). *Study on the social protection systems in the 13 applicant countries: Hungary country study 2003*. Cologne, Gesellschaft für Versicherungswissenschaft (http://www.cor-retraites.fr/IMG/pdf/doc-320.pdf, accessed 9 October 2013).

Galan A, Olsavszky V, Vladescu C (2011). Emergent challenge of health professional emigration: Romania's accession to the EU. In Wismar M et al., eds. *Health professional mobility and health systems. Evidence from 17 European countries*. Copenhagen, WHO Regional Office for Europe on behalf of the European Observatory on Health Systems and Policies:449–478.

García-Pérez MA, Amaya C, Otero A (2007). Physicians' migration in Europe: an overview of the current situation. *BMC Health Services Research,* 7:201.

Gerlinger T, Schmucker R (2007). Transnational migration of health professionals in the European Union 2007. *Cadernos de Saúde Pública,* 23(Suppl 2): 184–192.

GVG (2002). *Study on the social protection systems in the 13 applicant countries: synthesis report 2002*. Cologne, Gesellschaft für Versicherungswissenschaft (http://ec.europa.eu/comm/employment_social/news/2003/jan/report_03_en.pdf, accessed 9 October 2013).

Kautsch M, Czabanowska K (2011). When the grass gets greener at home: Poland's changing incentives for health professional mobility. In Wismar M et al., eds. *Health professional mobility and health systems. Evidence from 17 European countries.* Copenhagen, WHO Regional Office for Europe on behalf of the European Observatory on Health Systems and Policies:419–448.

Kuusio H et al. (2011). Changing context and priorities in recruitment and employment: Finland balances inflows and outflows of health professionals. In Wismar M et al., eds. *Health professional mobility and health systems. Evidence from 17 European countries.* Copenhagen, WHO Regional Office for Europe on behalf of the European Observatory on Health Systems and Policies:163–180.

López-Valcárcel BG, Pérez PB, Quintana CDD (2011). Opportunities in an expanding health service: Spain between Latin America and Europe. In Wismar M et al., eds. *Health professional mobility and health systems. Evidence from 17 European countries.* Copenhagen, WHO Regional Office for Europe on behalf of the European Observatory on Health Systems and Policies:263–294.

OECD (2007). Immigrant health workers in OECD countries in the broader context of highly skilled migration. In OECD, ed. *International migration outlook,* 2nd edn. Paris, Organisation for Economic Co-operation and Development.

OECD (2008). *The looming crisis in the health workforce. How can OECD countries respond?* Paris, Organisation for Economic Co-operation and Development (OECD Health Policy Studies) (http://www.who.int/hrh/migration/looming_crisis_health_workforce.pdf, accessed 15 December 2013).

OECD (2011a). *Health at a glance 2011: OECD indicators.* Paris, Organisation for Economic Co-operation and Development (http://www.oecd.org/health/health-systems/49105858.pdf, accessed 1 October 2013).

OECD (2011b). *Health statistics.* Paris, Organisation for Economic Co-operation and Development (http://www.oecd-ilibrary.org/social-issues-migration-health/data/oecd-health-statistics_health-data-en, accessed 10 December 2013).

OECD/WHO (2010). *Policy brief on the international migration of health workforce.* Paris, Organisation for Economic Co-operation and Development (http://www.oecd.org/dataoecd/8/0/44783714.xls, accessed 8 October 2013).

OECD (2012). *International Migration of Health Workers.* (www.oecd.org/dataoecd/8/0/44783714.xls, accessed 05.11.2012)

OECD (2012a). *OECD Health Data 2012* (http://stats.oecd.org/index. aspx?DataSetCode=HEALTH_STAT , accessed 5.11.2012)

Offermanns G, Malle EM, Jusic M (2011). Mobility, language and neighbours: Austria as source and destination country. In Wismar M et al., eds. *Health professional mobility and health systems. Evidence from 17 European countries.* Copenhagen, WHO Regional Office for Europe on behalf of the European Observatory on Health Systems and Policies:89–128.

Ognyanova D, Busse R (2011). A destination and a source: Germany manages regional health workforce disparities with foreign medical doctors. In Wismar M et al., eds. *Health professional mobility and health systems. Evidence from 17 European countries.* Copenhagen, WHO Regional Office for Europe on behalf of the European Observatory on Health Systems and Policies:211–242.

Padaiga Ž, Pukas M, Starkienė L (2011). Awareness, planning and retention: Lithuania's approach to managing health professional mobility. In Wismar M et al., eds. *Health professional mobility and health systems. Evidence from 17 European countries.* Copenhagen, WHO Regional Office for Europe on behalf of the European Observatory on Health Systems and Policies:395–418.

Peeters M, McKee M, Merkur S (2010). EU law and health professionals. In Mossialos E et al., eds. *Health systems governance in Europe: the role of European Union law and policy.* Cambridge, UK, Cambridge University Press:589–634.

Saar P, Habicht J (2011). Migration and attrition: Estonia's health sector and cross-border mobility to its northern neighbour. In Wismar M et al., eds. *Health professional mobility and health systems. Evidence from 17 European countries.* Copenhagen, WHO Regional Office for Europe on behalf of the European Observatory on Health Systems and Policies:339–364.

Safuta A, Baeten R (2011). Of permeable borders: Belgium as both source and host country. In Wismar M et al., eds. *Health professional mobility and health systems. Evidence from 17 European countries.* Copenhagen, WHO Regional Office for Europe on behalf of the European Observatory on Health Systems and Policies:129–162.

Smith PA et al. (2006). *Valuing and recognising the talents of a diverse healthcare workforce.* London, Royal College of Nursing (http://www.rcn.org.uk/__data/ assets/pdf_file/0008/78713/003078.pdf, accessed 2 January 2014).

WHO (2010). *WHO global code of practice on the international recruitment of health personnel.* Geneva, World Health Organization (Sixty-third World Health Assembly, WHA63.16) (http://www.who.int/hrh/migration/code/ WHO_global_code_of_practice_EN.pdf, accessed 1 October 2013).

Wismar M et al., eds. (2011). *Health professional mobility and health systems. Evidence from 17 European countries.* Copenhagen, WHO Regional Office for Europe on behalf of the European Observatory on Health Systems and Policies.

Young R (2011). A major destination country: the United Kingdom and its changing recruitment policies. In Wismar M et al., eds. *Health professional mobility and health systems. Evidence from 17 European countries.* Copenhagen, WHO Regional Office for Europe on behalf of the European Observatory on Health Systems and Policies:295–335.

# Chapter 5

# Monitoring health professional mobility in Europe

*Claudia B. Maier, James Buchan, Matthias Wismar, Diana Ognyanova,*
*Edmond Girasek, Eszter Kovacs and Reinhard Busse*

## 5.1 Introduction

Policy-makers in Europe are being faced with the challenge of ensuring an adequate supply and distribution of their health workforce. Yet often the information base is patchy, of limited quality and outdated. Moreover, there is often a lack of knowledge of what data sources are available and what the limitations are that will need to be taken into consideration in any response to mobility and domestic workforce developments.

In times of crisis, accurate, up-to-date data and intelligence are even more important. The mobility of health professionals has always had a dynamic and changing nature, but most notably this is evident in periods of major economic or geopolitical change, as highlighted in other chapters in this book. The decision to move to and take up employment in another country by medical doctors, dentists or nurses is closely linked to national employment situations, among other factors, and can change rapidly in times of economic downturn and high unemployment rates (see Chapters 1 and 6). Both Europe and the world as a whole are at the conjunction of several critical developments regarding mobility of health professionals: the economic crisis impacts on the direction and magnitude of mobility flows but often is unmeasured in quantitative terms; the reasons for health professionals to move, settle down or return are highly varied within the EU; the health workforce is ageing in line with population ageing, which is likely to increase demand in the future; and countries have committed to ethical recruitment principles by signing the *WHO Global Code of Practice on the International Recruitment of Health Personnel* (WHO, 2010). These factors have the potential to impact considerably on the health workforce and call for a close and timely monitoring of health professional mobility.

This limitation is acknowledged by analysts and policy-makers in Europe (Wismar et al., 2011). However, because of issues related to a lack of capacity, resources and, in some cases, a lack of political will, a thorough overhaul of the national health workforce information systems in many countries has not happened, and this contributes to an incomplete picture at European level. At the global level, the adoption of the *WHO Global Code of Practice on the International Recruitment of Health Personnel* (WHO, 2010) holds some promise as a tool to improve the monitoring of mobility.

This chapter aims to provide an overview of the data currently available on the mobility of health professionals in Europe from a critical, cross-country perspective. It will then highlight the paucity of, and need for, data on *flows* to measure short-term developments in health professional mobility, a crucial but often neglected data requirement for any analysis of rapid sociopolitical or economic changes and their impacts on mobility. Selected data from international databases and the EU PROMeTHEUS study will be presented to illustrate quality issues directly and when interpreting data on mobility. The chapter will also attempt to answer selected policy questions on mobility in the light of the current data before moving on to assess the monitoring requirements of existing codes of practice on international recruitment of health professionals. Finally, it will provide an overview of recent EU-wide and global policy developments to improve the data situation and suggest policy options to improve the monitoring of health workforce mobility in Europe.

## 5.2 Monitoring mobility: data availability and comparability

Timely monitoring of health professional mobility is the stepping stone to taking action. But monitoring the mobility of health professionals is highly complex and requires statistical assessment of the magnitude of various types of mobility when the boundaries between types are often blurred. As highlighted in Chapter 6, there are (at least) six types of mobile health professional: the "livelihood migrant", the "career oriented", the "backpacker", the "commuter" and the "undocumented", who works unofficially in a foreign country. The "returner" migrates back to the country of origin.

Some of these typologies are more desirable from a workforce planning and sustainability perspective than others; for example, the livelihood migrant or career-oriented migrant is more likely to stay and work in a country for a longer time period than the backpacker, who may soon move on to a third country. Some typologies also act as an early warning signal to policy-makers: high numbers of livelihood migrants from a source country demonstrate the economically unsatisfactory situation for these health professionals. However, if monitoring systems do not assess how many health professionals leave or enter their country, and of which typology, they cannot inform policy-making.

### 5.2.1 Definitions and data sources

According to the WHO, monitoring is the *ongoing* process of data collection towards agreed objectives. The overall purpose is to inform decision-makers and stakeholders in a timely and comprehensive manner to take appropriate decisions (Dal Poz et al., 2009). It is not a one-off activity but rather a regular, continuous assessment of the phenomenon. This section will argue that, currently, timely monitoring of mobility in the majority of countries is insufficient or completely lacking, with a few exceptions, for example the United Kingdom (Young, 2011) or Germany (Ognyanova & Busse, 2011) for medical doctors; however, even in these countries, some gaps exist: for example, return migration is not well monitored.

Box 5.1 provides an overview of commonly used concepts of health professional mobility and data types, focusing on stock data, flows and reliance levels (Maier et al., 2011).

At the international and European level, several databases exist on health professionals, some of which also include data on mobility. Table 5.1 provides an overview of existing databases. In general, there is more information on reliance levels on foreign health professionals by countries (stock data) than there is on yearly inflows. Data on outflows are usually even more limited or non-existent.

The *OECD Health data* also covers health workforce data, as of 2010 as part of a joint WHO Regional Office for Europe/OECD/Eurostat endeavour using a joint questionnaire (OECD, 2011a, b). A high number of health professions are covered, by age, gender and selected specializations, as well as meta-data on definitions and background information. However, the database does not include any information on mobility and migration of health professionals.

However, the aggregate nature of data on health professionals (and non-health professionals) available to the public limits its utility.[1] The EU DG MARKT database on the recognition of professional qualifications is the only database with proxy data on outflows, in the absence of EU-wide statistics on *actual* outflows. It shows the (active) intentions of medical doctors, nurses, dentists

1 Data in non-aggregated format can be obtained on special request.

---

**Box 5.1** *Definition of stock and flow data and reliance levels*

*Stock data*

The total number of health professionals in a country/registry/database at a given point in time. Stock data on mobility show the share of foreign health professionals within a country's health workforce, expressed as a percentage of the total stock.

*Flow data*

The number of health professionals who have newly entered a profession's registry or database: often referred to as the newly registered health profession in a given year, allowing for assessing short-term movements across borders.

*Reliance levels*

A qualifying measure of the extent to which a national health workforce relies on foreign health professionals (percentage of foreign among all health professionals). Levels can be:

- negligible to low: <5%

- moderate: 5% to <10%

- high: 10% to <20%

- very high: >20%.

*Source:* Maier et al., 2011.

---

and pharmacists to work in another country (European Commission, 2011) and is publicly available. The data have major limitations in that they do not measure real movements and vary significantly in terms of EU country coverage, country reporting periodicity, reporting procedures and completeness of data. Finally, although covering a variety of indicators on national health workforces in the WHO European Region, the WHO Health for All database (WHO Regional Office for Europe, 2013) does not include information on migration or mobility.

At individual country level, data are usually better understood in terms of strengths and limitations. In most European countries, the best data in terms of availability, coverage and quality come from registry data on medical doctors, followed by that for dentists. For nurses and midwives, the picture in terms of data quality and availability across Europe is mixed. There is a more general paucity of information on mobility for all other health professions, such as pharmacists, physiotherapists and lower-qualified nurses such as nursing assistants or long-term care workers. In addition, different data collection methodologies, coexisting data sources, decentralized data collection systems in some countries, the existence of different indicators on mobility (foreign-trained; foreign-born; foreign-national) and different registration methodologies

**Table 5.1** *International data availability and limitations in measuring health professional mobility, with a focus on Europe*

| Data holder and source | Data on | | | Periodicity | Limitations |
|---|---|---|---|---|---|
| | Reliance on foreign (stock) | Inflows | Loss/ outflows | | |
| OECD project on international migration of health workforce (OECD/ WHO, 2010; data available in two files[a]) | X | X | – | Published with periodicity of 2–3 years, time lag of 3–5 (up to 8) years | Good information base but limited EU country coverage; no routine data collection;[a] limited description of meta-data |
| OECD health data (OECD, 2012b) | - | - | - | Yearly, time lag of 1–4 years | No information on mobility/migration of health professionals, but general information on health workforce in OECD countries |
| EU Labour Force Surveys (European Commission, 2013; microdata available upon written request to Eurostat) | X | – | – | Yearly, time lag 1–2 years | Major limitation is aggregation of different health professions to one category[b] |
| DG MARKT data on recognition of qualifications (European Commission, 2011) | | | (X) proxy of intention to leave | Yearly, time lag 1–5 years | Limited information base; major limiting factors are the indicator of intention to leave and limited EU country coverage |
| WHO Health for All database (WHO Regional Office for Europe, 2013) | – | – | – | Yearly (updates every 6 months); time lag of 1–4 years | No information on mobility/migration, but comprehensive information on health workforce overall in countries of WHO European region |

[a] Online publication of two Excel files on share of foreign-trained/foreign-national medical doctors and nurses, respectively, and inflows in selected countries (http://www.oecd.org/dataoecd/7/63/44783734.xls and http://www.oecd.org/dataoecd/8/0/44783714.xls, accessed 8 October 2013).

[b] Data are aggregated at International Standard Classification of Occupations 3-digit level and so medical doctors, nurses, traditional and complementary medicine professionals, other health professionals, paramedical practitioners and veterinarians are all subsumed into one category, which considerably limits the use of this data source to assess health professional mobility, particularly for individual health professions.

all complicate the picture. Box 5.2 attempts to provide a yardstick for improved monitoring practices on mobility.

Even where this yardstick is applied, it can only provide an approximate picture of the actual mobility flows and trends in Europe. The routine indicators on

**Box 5.2** *Monitoring mobility: a yardstick for improved data quality*

There is no commonly agreed "gold standard" for measuring health professional mobility. However, some overarching suggestions could improve monitoring policies and practices, indicators and accuracy of information and access to data.

*Coverage*
- High coverage of (at least) the most-common health professions (e.g. medical doctors, nurses, midwives, pharmacists, dentists, others) in a country's health system.
- Mandatory, nationwide registration policies for high completeness and accuracy of data.
- Other options are nationwide surveys, such as the EU Labour Force Surveys or census data with representative samples of the health profession.

*Mobility indicators*
*Inflows/stock*. Ideally this should be described by a collection of all three indicators: foreign-trained, foreign-born and foreign-national, or by two indicators of which one is foreign-trained:

- foreign-trained: best quality indicator, closest to the PROMeTHEUS definition of health professional mobility "*any movement across a border by a health professional after graduation with the intention to work, i.e. deliver health-related services in the destination country, including during training periods*"; however, it will include false positives where nationals went abroad for training and returned;
- foreign-born: proxy measure for mobility with a long time lag and risk of many false positives (e.g. health professionals who migrated early and obtained training/naturalization in the destination country); and
- foreign-national: proxy measure for mobility but a risk of bias in cross-country comparisons because of different naturalization practices in countries.

*Outflows*. This can be sourced from either annual nationwide emigration studies (but resource intensive) or routine international exchange of mobility data among national data holders (feeding back statistics on foreign health professions to the monitoring authorities of the countries of origin).

*Timeliness of monitoring*
Compulsory, annual re-registration policies and data on employment/active workforce ensure that data are up to date and cover short-term mobility. It also quantifies the overall loss of the active workforce. De-registration policies, with additional information on future employment, could help to trace back "returners", those working in other sectors, retirees and losses for other reasons.

---

**Box 5.2** *contd*

*Activity levels*

Information on the activity levels of the health workforce is indispensable. In addition to headcounts, data should include full-time-equivalents. Indicators include:

- practising in health care, e.g. inpatient/outpatient, public/private, specialization
- active in health sector but not directly providing health care, e.g. research, teaching
- licensed (currently) to practise
- registered.

*Triangulation of data*

Where several databases/sources exist, triangulation of data on mobility, in light of the quality of methodologies and registry policies, will enable the best informed estimate to be made.

*International collaboration and exchange of data*

A true added value would be international collaboration among data holders to exchange statistics on mobile health professionals and assess outflows, tracing back health professionals to identify returners.

---

mobility cover only selected types of mobile health professional (see Chapter 6) and do not sufficiently capture the increasing diversification of mobile workers. Some of the short-term, returning and undocumented movements would routinely fall through the gaps of this monitoring system. For example, out of the six typologies described in Chapter 6, the first four (livelihood migrants, career oriented, backpackers, commuters) would most probably be covered by up-to-date monitoring systems where mandatory registration and annual re-registration policies are in place; the remaining two, the undocumented and returners, may not be covered or identified as such. To date, to our knowledge, no study has assessed systematically whether and to what extent short-term mobile workers (e.g. the backpacker or commuter) and returners are documented by routine data. No country appears to be able to track returners routinely: those health professionals who practised and gained additional experience abroad and then returned. This "brain drain" could result in "expertise-gain" without countries being aware of the extent of return migration.

Routine data can be an underestimate of mobility (particularly short term and other types), and reflect, in some cases, just the "tip of the iceberg". This implies that some types of mobility may go entirely unnoticed – something not measured/monitored is often assumed not to exist – and could be growing in relative importance. One example is the presence of large numbers of nurses and nursing assistants, mainly from Eastern European countries, working in "legally grey areas" or unofficially in the homes of elderly people, a phenomenon that usually lacks reliable statistics, as reported in Austria, Germany, Italy and France (Bertinato et al., 2011; Delamaire & Schweyer, 2011; Offermanns, Malle & Jusic, 2011; Ognyanova & Busse, 2011).

The following sections aim to provide an overview of the availability of routine data on mobility from a cross-country perspective in Europe, to consider which policy questions they address and will highlight some of the quality issues by using selected data for illustrative purposes.

### 5.2.2 Indispensable as a measure of scale: stock data

The focus of this section is on understanding the magnitude of health professional mobility. There are two guiding policy questions in that context. To what extent does a country's health workforce rely on health professionals from other countries? Does the situation require interventions?

Stock data are usually the starting point in any analysis of migration and mobility. Stock data represent the cumulative mobility over years, measured by one or several indicators of mobility, in relation to the total number of the domestic workforce (Box 5.1). However, while this information is important to set mobility in context, either with other countries or with other professions and sectors within a country, its utility is constrained. Stock data do not capture or represent the short-term rapid changes that are often the dynamic reality of mobility. They do not show if the mobile health professional arrived yesterday or 10 years ago. While stock data are indispensable as a measure of scale or magnitude, flow data are necessary for any analysis on shorter-term changes and past and current fluctuations.

In most countries stock data are the best information available, and, in some countries they are the only information available. However, even these stock data often face a number of limitations in terms of coverage, comparability, limit in scope and depth and timeliness (Diallo, 2004; OECD/WHO, 2010; WHO Regional Office for Europe, 2013).

### Scale of mobility from a cross-country perspective

Whereas at the aggregate European level, the mobility of health professionals does not represent an excessive phenomenon and is in line with overall labour mobility in the EU (Ognyanova et al., 2012; see also Chapter 4), the data at individual country levels show a different and more detailed picture – from very high reliance on foreign health professionals to virtually no reliance.

Most EU Member States require registration of medical doctors in the respective registries as a mandatory requirement for being able to practise (and often annual re-registration), which provides for high completeness of data (Kovacs, Szocska & Schmidt, 2012). Registries are often fully established, have a long tradition and assess at least one indicator of mobility.

Of the EU27 countries covered by the PROMeTHEUS data collection, 23 had stock data on the reliance on foreign medical doctors. This analysis is the most comprehensive in Europe from a country coverage perspective. Data were complemented with selected countries from the WHO European Region, including Norway, Turkey, Ukraine and Switzerland. Selected OECD countries with traditionally high reliance levels such as Australia, Canada, New Zealand and the United States were also added. Reliance was measured as the share of foreign medical doctors of the total workforce (Fig. 5.1). Moreover, the analysis of mobility focuses on the active, hence economically active or practising, workforce. As will be demonstrated later in the chapter, there can be an enormous important difference between the total number of all health professionals covered by registry data and the total number that are currently practising in the profession.

Based on the PROMeTHEUS classification of reliance levels (Maier et al., 2011), 9 of the 31 countries covered showed a *very high* reliance of >20% for foreign medical doctors who are reported active on the registry: Luxembourg, United Kingdom, Sweden, Ireland and Switzerland from within the European region; New Zealand, United States, Australia and Canada from other continents. Countries vary in terms of size of the workforce; for example, Luxembourg, with a small population and territory that facilitates cross-border movements, has a total population of just 512 000 (Grand Duchy of Luxembourg, 2012) and a low average of 271 medical doctors per 100 000 demonstrates that while reliance levels are very high in relative terms (40.7%), the total number of foreign medical doctors is relatively low – 605 foreign-national medical doctors in 2008. By comparison, the United Kingdom showed a lower reliance level of 36.8% but had a total of 91 064 internationally trained medical doctors registered in 2008 (Fig. 5.1).

When examining data on mobility of nurses, the numerically largest health profession in Europe, two important differences from data on medical doctors emerge: first, the much smaller number of countries with data available and, second, those countries that have data consistently show lower reliance levels on foreign nurses than on doctors (Fig. 5.2). Only 21 of the EU27 and five third countries had data available on the stock of foreign nurses. Not all EU Member States require nurses to register; for example, there is no national nursing registry in Germany or Austria (Offermanns, Malle & Jusic, 2011; Ognyanova & Busse, 2011). Proxy measures can be used but their accuracy can be questionable. Where data are available, there are clearly lower reliance levels on foreign nurses than foreign doctors in the majority of countries. A very high reliance of >20% occurred in only four countries: Luxembourg, Ireland, New

**Fig. 5.1** Reliance levels on foreign-trained, foreign-born and foreign-national medical doctors, 2008 or latest year available for countries

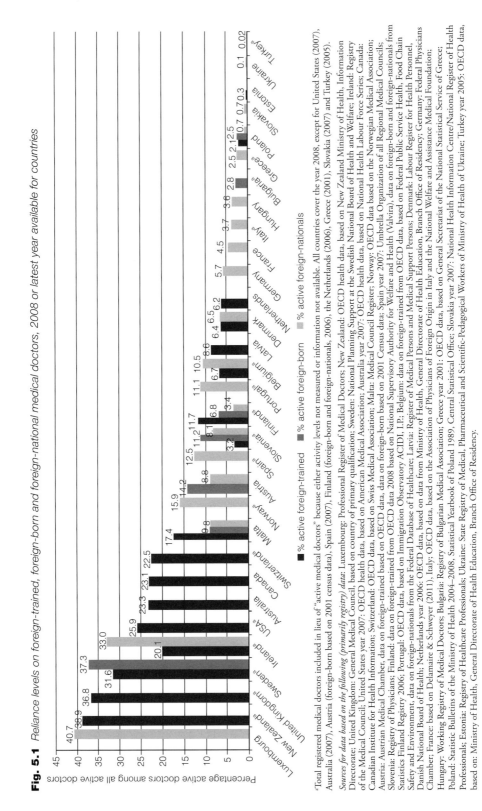

■ % active foreign-trained    ■ % active foreign-born    ▨ % active foreign-nationals

"Total registered medical doctors included in lieu of "active medical doctors" because either activity levels not measured or information not available. All countries cover the year 2008, except for United States (2007), Australia (2007), Austria (foreign-born based on 2001 census data), Spain (2007), Finland (foreign-born and foreign-nationals, 2006), the Netherlands (2006), Greece (2001), Slovakia (2007) and Turkey (2005).

*Sources for data based on the following (primarily registry) data:* Luxembourg: Professional Register of Medical Doctors; New Zealand: OECD health data, based on New Zealand Ministry of Health, Information Directorate; United Kingdom: General Medical Council, based on country of primary qualification; Sweden: National Planning Support at the Swedish National Board of Health and Welfare; Ireland: Registry of the Medical Council; United States year 2007: OECD health data, based on American Medical Association; Australia year 2007: OECD health data, based on National Health Labour Force Series; Canada: Canadian Institute for Health Information; Switzerland: OECD data, based on Swiss Medical Association; Malta: Medical Council Register; Norway: OECD data based on the Norwegian Medical Association; Austria: Austrian Medical Chamber, data on foreign-trained based on OECD data, data on foreign-born based on 2001 Census data; Spain year 2007: Umbrella Organization of all Regional Medical Councils; Slovenia: Registry of Physicians; Finland: data on foreign-trained from OECD data 2008 based on National Supervisory Authority for Welfare and Health (Valvira), data on foreign-born and foreign-nationals from Statistics Finland Registry 2006; Portugal: OECD data, based on foreign-nationals from OECD data, based on Federal Public Service Health, Food Chain Safety and Environment, data on foreign-nationals from the Federal Database of Healthcare; Latvia: Register of Medical Persons and Medical Support Persons; Denmark: Labour Register for Health Personnel, Danish National Board of Health; Netherlands year 2006: OECD data, based on data from Ministry of Health, General Directorate of Health Education, Branch Office of Residency; Germany: Federal Physicians Chamber; France: based on Delamaire & Schweyer (2011), Italy; OECD data, based on the Association of Physicians of Foreign Origin in Italy and the National Welfare and Assistance Medical Foundation; Hungary: Working Registry of Medical Doctors; Bulgaria: Registry of Bulgarian Medical Association; Greece year 2001: OECD data, based on General Secretariat of the National Statistical Service of Greece; Poland: Statistic Bulletins of the Ministry of Health 2004–2008, Statistical Yearbook of Poland 1989, Central Statistical Office; Slovakia year 2007: National Health Information Centre/National Register of Health Professionals; Estonia: Registry of Healthcare Professionals; Ukraine: State Registry of Medical, Pharmaceutical and Scientific-Pedagogical Workers of Ministry of Health of Ukraine; Turkey year 2005: OECD data, based on: Ministry of Health, General Directorate of Health Education, Branch Office of Residency.

**Fig. 5.2** Reliance levels on foreign-trained, foreign-born and foreign-national nurses, 2008 or latest year available for countries

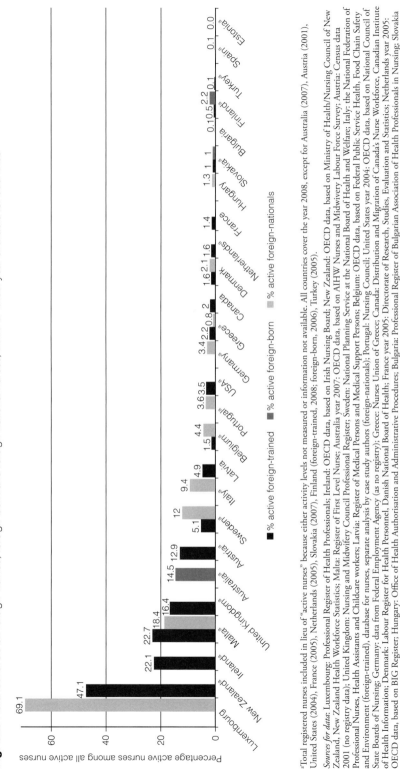

■ % active foreign-trained   ■ % active foreign-born   ▨ % active foreign-nationals

[a]Total registered nurses included in lieu of "active nurses" because either activity levels not measured or information not available. All countries cover the year 2008, except for Australia (2007), Austria (2001), United States (2004), France (2005), Netherlands (2005), Slovakia (2007), Finland (foreign-trained, 2008; foreign-born, 2006), Turkey (2005).

*Sources for data*: Luxembourg: Professional Register of Health Professionals; Ireland: OECD data, based on Irish Nursing Board; New Zealand: OECD data, based on Ministry of Health/Nursing Council of New Zealand, New Zealand Health Workforce Statistics; Malta: Register of First Level Nurse; Australia year 2007: OECD data, based on AIHW Nurses and Midwifery Labour Force Survey; Austria: Census data 2001 (no registry data); United Kingdom: Nursing and Midwifery Council Professional Register; Sweden: National Planning Service at the National Board of Health and Welfare; Italy: the National Federation of Professional Nurses, Health Assistants and Childcare workers; Latvia: Register of Medical Persons and Medical Support Persons; Belgium: OECD data, based on Federal Public Service Health, Food Chain Safety and Environment (foreign-trained), database for nurses, separate analysis by case study authors (foreign-nationals); Portugal: Nursing Council; United States year 2004: OECD data, based on National Council of State Boards of Nursing; Germany: data from Federal Employment Agency (as no registry); Greece: Nurses Union of Greece; Canada: Distribution and Migration of Canada's Nurse Workforce, Canadian Institute of Health Information; Denmark: Labour Register for Health Personnel, Danish National Board of Health; France year 2005: Directorate of Research, Studies, Evaluation and Statistics; Netherlands year 2005: OECD data, based on BIG Register; Hungary: Office of Health Authorisation and Administrative Procedures; Bulgaria: Professional Register of Bulgarian Association of Health Professionals in Nursing; Slovakia year 2007: National Health Information Centre/National Register of Health Professionals; Finland: OECD data (2008 for foreign-trained; 2006 for foreign-born), Statistics Finland; Turkey year 2005: Council of Nurses and Economically Active Population Survey; Spain: Official Nursing Councils; Estonia: Register of Health Care Professionals.

Zealand and Malta (foreign-trained). The majority of countries show reliance levels of <5%. This does not necessarily mean that there are fewer nurses on the move, but, because of the sheer size of the total nursing workforces, the portion of "foreign" (however defined) nurses is smaller in relative terms. However, for individual countries, the data clearly show that their nursing workforces are less reliant on nurses from other countries than is seen for medical doctors.

In measuring mobility, clarity about the type of indicator used and its limitations is crucial. Different indicators will give a different picture of mobility, as is demonstrated for example by Fig. 5.2 on medical doctors. In the majority of countries with more than one indicator (Sweden, Ireland, Malta, Slovenia, Finland, Belgium and Poland) the reliance levels on foreign doctors vary considerably depending on the indicators used. There is a more than 10% point difference in Ireland (20.1% foreign-trained to 33% foreign-national) and more than 5% point difference in Finland (3.4 to 11.7%), Slovenia (3.2 to 11.2%), Malta (8.9 to 17.4%) and Sweden (31.6 to 37.3). These differences can stem from a variety of factors. One reason might be the quality of the different indicators (e.g. voluntary versus mandatory information, self-assessed or drawn from official documentation) or data sources in terms of completeness, representativeness and timeliness. Other reasons may stem from the different naturalization policies in the EU Member States. Reasons need to be analysed in countries' specific health workforce context including the quality and reliability of indicators and data sources.

An additional influencing factor on the accuracy of mobility data is the information available on the total workforce covered, the denominator, for example whether all medical doctors in a registry are covered, all economically active medical doctors or only those practising currently in the profession. At first sight, these may appear to be mere nuances or variations in terminology, but in reality they are decisive to mobility estimates as well as to overall workforce estimates. This dimension is often neglected in data analyses, particularly at international levels. Strikingly, neither data from the OECD/WHO (2010) *Policy Brief on the International Migration of Health Workforce* project nor data from the WHO Health for All database (WHO Regional Office for Europe, 2013) specify what activity levels are exactly covered by the total numbers of national health workforces in their data sets (e.g. registered versus active versus practising). The WHO Health for All database differentiates between head count and full-time equivalents but data on the latter are rare. The annual OECD Health Database does differentiate between levels of activity of the workforce: practising, professionally active and licensed to practise (OECD, 2013) but *not* when it comes to migration estimates, since data from the *Policy Brief on the International Migration of Health Workforce* project were used (OECD/WHO, 2010). Fig. 5.3 illustrates the differences in the total medical workforces in selected EU Member States, comparing the data collected

**Fig. 5.3** *Comparison of international and PROMeTHEUS (national) data on stock of medical doctors (MDs), 2008, selected EU Member States*

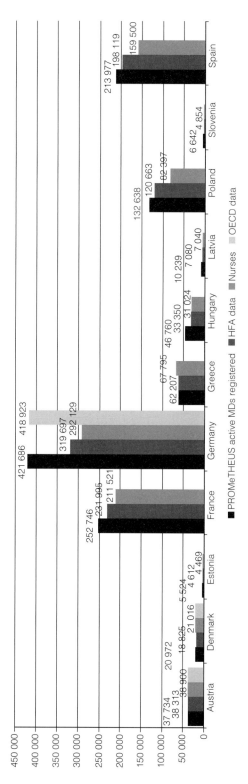

*Sources:* OECD data: OECD/WHO (2010) based on the following (original) sources: Austria 2008: Austrian Medical Chamber/OECD Health Data; Denmark 2008: National Board of Health, Labour Register for Health Personnel; Germany 2008: Federal Physicians Chamber; HFA data: WHO Regional Office for Europe (2013) Health for All database; PROMeTHEUS data collected by country experts, based on the following (primarily registry) data: Austria: Austrian Medical Chamber; Denmark: Labour Register for Health Personnel, Danish National Board of Health; Estonia: Registry of Healthcare Professionals; France (data are for 2007): Doctors National Order (indicator is physician physical persons, no information on data sources or meta-data available); Germany: Federal Physicians Chamber; Greece: Panhellenic Medical Association; Hungary: Working Registry of Medical Doctors; Latvia: Latvian Register of Medical Persons and Medical Support Persons; Poland: Statistic Bulletins of the Ministry of Health 2004–2008, Statistical Yearbook of Poland, Central Statistical Office; Slovenia: Registry of Physicians; Spain: Official Councils of Physicians; WHO Regional Office for Europe (2013) for year 2008; France 2007: indicator is physician physical persons, no information on data sources or meta-data available.

by country experts (as part of the PROMeTHEUS study, see Fig. 5.3 for more details) on total numbers of all medical doctors registered with all "active" medical doctors as per re-registration procedures. These have been compared with the medical workforce statistics provided by the *Policy Brief on the International Migration of Health Workforce* project (OECD/WHO, 2010) and the WHO Health for All database (WHO Regional Office for Europe, 2013).

Several countries, including Germany, Hungary, Latvia, Poland and Slovenia, show that 20% of their total registered medical workforce is *not* active; hence, less than 80% of their medical doctors registered are active in the workforce. In comparing these data with the OECD data on migration of health professionals and Health for All data, such differences can become even more pronounced. Health for All data show lower numbers of the total workforce, even active workforce in France, Germany, Hungary, Poland and Spain, without information on what part of the workforce they actually measure: the total medical workforce registered or active or practising. By contrast, data were quite similar in Austria, Denmark, Estonia, Latvia and Slovenia. OECD data appear to be close(r) to the total number of the registered workforce, yet with substantial differences compared with Health for All data for example; however, again, no information is provided on activity levels.

Such differences in the denominators can lead to heavily biased estimates if data that are not alike are being compared (e.g. all active foreign medical doctors with total medical workforce registered). This may considerably underestimate the real scale of mobility. Workforce planners and decision-makers need to know how many health professionals are actively registered – and even more importantly, how many are actually practising in their profession. Ideally, data would also cover full-time equivalents in addition to head counts, particularly in those professions with a high share of part-time work. This information requirement relates not just to mobility but also to any development of strategic intelligence and service delivery planning.

As demonstrated above, assessing activity levels for a workforce is indispensable in measuring mobility and for informing policy responses. Here registries differ considerably between countries. For example, in Austria, Estonia and Hungary, *active* medical workforce is reflected by registry data, whereas professional bodies in Belgium, France, Poland and United Kingdom cover *total registered* health professionals. Germany and Slovakia have information on both. These differences hamper cross-country comparisons. Moreover, there are other registry specificities that impact on the quality and comparability of data, including mandatory versus voluntary registration, coverage of the private sector, re-registration practices, regional coverage and changes in methodologies over time (Table 5.2).

### 5.2.3 Indispensable for capturing dynamics and short-term movements: monitoring flows

The focus of this section is on understanding the annual movements of health professionals who enter a workforce and compare these movements over time. There are two guiding policy questions in that context. What is the role of current foreign inflows in replenishing the national health workforce and how have they changed over time? What is the extent of annual outflows from the health workforce due to emigration?

Mobility cannot be captured sufficiently by stock data alone. It requires flow data on annual inflows and outflows that are sensitive to short-term and frequent fluctuations. This is particularly relevant in the case of major changes of employment situations, such as those triggered by the recent economic crisis, but also changes in workforce and employment policies, salary negotiations or major EU-wide developments, such as the EU enlargement.

The EU enlargement rounds of 2004 and 2007 demonstrated that mobility is not predictable. There was neither the excessive outmigration from the then acceding states, nor a "swamping" of the destination countries, which contradicted earlier predictions and early warnings (Avgerinos, Koupidis & Filippou, 2004; Buchan & Perfilieva, 2006; Wiskow, 2006; Garcia-Perez, Amaya & Otero, 2007; Ognyanova et al., 2012). The recent financial and economic crisis in Europe is another example demonstrating the need for timely monitoring (Gaál et al., 2011; Fouka et al., 2013; see also Chapter 3).

Timeliness of data, particularly on flows, is perhaps *the* most crucial element in monitoring mobility, but it is also one of its current major limitations. The

**Table 5.2** *Registry methodologies and implications for data quality in selected EU Member States*

| Country | Registration |
| --- | --- |
| Austria | Medical doctors: registration mandatory, only *active* doctors registered, doctors must inform the Medical Chamber about changes regarding employment<br><br>Nurses: no registry with mandatory registration |
| Estonia | No re-registration procedures, hence not all registered health care professionals are still working in the health sector; under a legal change in the registration system, all health professionals had to re-register between 2002 and 2005 |
| Finland | (Valvira) Registry covers all health professionals who have applied for a licence to practise, including health professionals with foreign origin but also a limited number of native Finns who have studied abroad and returned to work in Finland; many of those who have been granted a licence have not actually been employed in the health care sector |
| France | Conseil National de l'Ordre des Médecins: registration not compulsory for all<br><br>Automatisation Des Listes: registration of medical doctors at hospital is not complete |

**Table 5.2** *contd*

| Country | Registration |
|---|---|
| France | Quality of data is better for doctors in private practice than for those working in public hospitals, because of the obligation to register with the National Council when working outside the public sector |
| Germany | Registry data on medical doctors, based on nationality, does not accurately reflect the migrant stocks and inflows of medical doctors in the country; according to micro-census data provided by the Federal Statistical Office, in 2008 approximately 15% of all medical doctors with foreign citizenship were born in Germany, and roughly 57% were estimated to have been trained in Germany (Federal Statistical Office, unpublished data 2010) |
| | Since 2000, the majority of regional physicians' chambers have recorded and can provide data on the outflow of German physicians |
| | Data on return migration is not recorded |
| Poland | Lack of completeness in coverage for medical doctors and nurses |
| | Medical doctors: self-employed doctors are not subject to statistical registration as medical staff working in the public sector; private services are not registered by public statistics |
| | Nurses: accuracy of "denominator" (overestimation) as out of 300 000 registered nurses, estimated that 200 000 work as nurses |
| Slovenia | Medical Chamber of Slovenia: most of the data on "foreign" health professionals fall into the category of foreign-trained, among which there are also some Slovene nationals |
| | Nurses: data on nurses are scarce, but the Nursing Chamber of Slovenia obtained public authorization to keep a nursing and midwifery register in 2008 |
| Spain | Official councils of medical doctors, dentists, nurses and pharmacists (Colegios): registration data of professional councils mostly do not report on citizenship of their members; council registration not required for professionals in the public sector, and in the case of doctors, registration reports only basic medical degree, not specialty degrees |
| | Medical doctors: not all Spanish doctors are registered, but (almost) all recognized foreign doctors register because of professional credibility, leading to overrepresentation of foreign doctors |
| | Nurses: registration figures for nurses are more complete; a strong sense of professional identity encourages nurses to register in great numbers |
| United Kingdom | Lack of comparability across professions: the General Medical Council (GMC) and General Dental Council (GDC) provide data by country of qualification, whereas the Nursing and Midwifery Council (NMC) uses country of qualification (inflows) and domicile (stocks); NMC data prior to 2004 only record EEA not individual countries |
| | Lack of longitudinal data: the GMC has only held the Specialist and General Practice Medical Registers since 1997 and 2006, respectively; the NMC was only set up in 2002; although data exist from previous data holders, it is not computerized |
| | Limited data on outflows: information relates to checks made by EEA/overseas regulators on an individual's intention to leave the United Kingdom, not actual migration |

*Sources*: Albreht, 2011; Delamaire & Schweyer, 2011; López-Valcárcel, Pérez & Quintana, 2011; Kautsch & Czabanowska, 2011; Kuusio et al., 2011; Offermanns, Malle & Jusic, 2011; Ognyanova & Busse, 2011; Saar & Habicht, 2011; Young, 2011.

majority of health profession mobility data currently available at country level are (at least) 12–24 months old. As noted above, at European and international levels, data usually date back at least 3 to 5 years or longer, which also adds to the problem of cross comparisons (OECD/WHO, 2010; WHO Regional Office for Europe, 2013). The remainder of this section looks at the issues surrounding data on inflows and on outflows, and the availability and quality of data.

### Yearly inflows

Usually, data on inflows are more readily available than data on outflows. Good time series data are rare, although with some exceptions. For example, in the United Kingdom, the inflow data on internationally trained medical doctors and nurses and midwives are of reasonably good quality in terms of providing a national assessment of trends in annual international inflow (Young, 2011). United Kingdom data show that there have been major yearly differences in the number of newly registered medical doctors who obtained their first medical qualification abroad. The total number of yearly inflows between 2003 and 2008 decreased more than twofold, particularly among medical doctors trained from outside the EU and EEA (Fig. 5.4).

**Fig. 5.4** *Newly registered foreign-trained doctors in the United Kingdom, 1988, 2003–2008 and major policy developments*

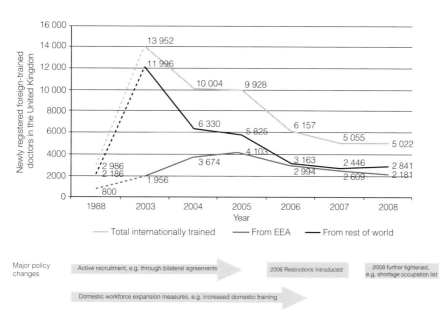

*Source*: General Medical Council unpublished data, cited by Young (2011).

*Note*: New full registrations of doctors with foreign primary medical qualification.

The major policy question that arises is why did numbers decrease so considerably. Fig. 5.4 sets the yearly inflows in context with the timing of major policy initiatives and changes during that period. At the risk of oversimplification, it is interesting to note that yearly inflows of internationally trained medical doctors from overseas and third countries ("rest of world") decreased considerably, even before the 2006 restrictions on active international recruitment were implemented – one reason may be that the growth in United Kingdom domestic medical workforce production came on stream earlier and may have contributed to a decrease in yearly international inflows (Young, 2011; Blacklock et al., 2012). Other reasons may also have contributed and so causality is not clear. This example conveys two main messages: first, yearly flow data are best placed in visualizing short-term changes, which are highly relevant for policy-makers. Second, assessing the reasons that triggered such changes requires careful analysis to assess a causal link. Mobility is a highly complex phenomenon with many influencing factors at the individual, country-specific and international levels. It will require understanding potential drivers and influencing factors such as employment situations or geopolitical events, which may be closely interlinked, but also data methodology issues (e.g. changes in registry methodologies) and it may require the triangulation of different data including qualitative and expert information.

### Data on outflows

Data on yearly outflows are scarce in Europe, not existing in most countries. At best, countries have undertaken one-off studies on outflows, for example Romania for the year 2007 (Galan, Olsavszky & Vladescu, 2011). Most countries rely on proxy measures based on either ad hoc surveys or on routine requests for recognition of qualifications for medical doctors, nurses, midwives, dentists and pharmacists. The exchange of data across borders can improve the accuracy of data. In Belgium, the available data (conformity certificates) were seen as an underestimate of actual outflows as some destination countries (e.g. the Netherlands) do not systematically request these certificates from the holders of Belgian medicine, dentistry and nursing diplomas. Therefore, Belgian data could be supplemented and cross-checked with data from the Ministry of Health, Welfare and Sport in the Netherlands to give a more accurate picture of outflows from Belgium (Safuta & Baeten, 2011).

Fig. 5.5 shows the different data types that can be used in attempting to measure outflows. In terms of rigour of information, a cascade from least to most rigorous can be seen: from self-reported surveys to intention-to-move data (e.g. recognition of diplomas, work permits) to European data on the mutual recognition of diploma emigration studies.

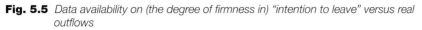

**Fig. 5.5** *Data availability on (the degree of firmness in) "intention to leave" versus real outflows*

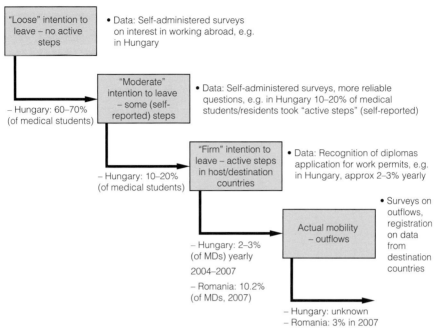

*Sources*: Eke, Girasek & Szócska, 2011 (Hungary); Galan, Olsavszky & Vladescu, 2011 (Romania).
*Notes*: MD, Medical doctors.

The least rigorous is self-reported surveys on (general) interest to work abroad, which has often shown a high level of agreement from survey respondents but a much smaller share of health professionals who actually took active steps and showed a more firm decision to move. Even a "firm" intention to move remains an intention, which subsequently may not translate into actual mobility.

More rigorous are data on intention to move (e.g. recognition of diplomas, work permits or other information), which are available for most countries. However, there are considerable limitations in using these to inform policy. Health professionals may apply for such official documents but decide *not* to move, leading to an overestimate of actual flows. Data from Romania illustrate the discrepancy. In 2007, approximately 10.2% (4 990) of all active medical doctors applied for recognition of diploma, many of whom were already abroad; however, a separate emigration study revealed that 3% (1 421) actually emigrated (Fig. 5.5; Galan, Olsavszky & Vladescu, 2011). Other factors either over- or underestimate mobility. Factors leading to overestimates include health professionals having applied in several countries for recognition of diplomas or having used the recognition scheme to increase (political) pressure in their home countries to improve salaries or working conditions (Saar & Habicht, 2011). Moreover, not all countries systematically request certificates, which can lead to considerable underestimates of flows in both source and destination (Beňušová et al., 2011; Safuta & Baeten, 2011). In some countries, it is reported that health professionals have left without requesting such certificates, for example Polish anaesthesiologists (Kautsch & Czabanowska, 2011).

The European data on the mutual recognition of diplomas (DG MARKT) can be considered as the most close proxy for outflows, hence "firmest" intention-to-leave data in the cascade, since health professionals receive a decision from the destination country on whether their diplomas have been recognized (European Commission, 2011). This provides a rough picture on the firm intention to move across borders for the five health professions covered (European Commission, 2005). The database relies on reporting by national authorities, but in practice not every country reports in a timely manner. In 2007 and 2008, Switzerland and all the EU27 apart from Cyprus submitted data on the decisions regarding the recognition of diplomas of medical doctors by their authorities (European Commission, 2008). In 2009, the number decreased to 23 countries, in 2010 to 18 countries, in 2011 to 14, and in 2012 to just 1, Poland.[2] The limited country coverage over the last two to three years clearly limits the usefulness of the database to assess recent trends. Moreover, the reporting cycles have changed over time, for example from 1999–2000 to 2005–2006, two years seem to be covered (or mid-year coverage levels), followed by full year cycles from 2007 onwards; however, periodicity is not clearly defined in the database. There is limited information on meta-data available; it is unclear on what basis countries submit the data and whether data are being validated. On a positive note, the DG MARKT database, despite the limitations, is the first in the EU that has linked data from source with destination countries, a simple but very effective way to share information (European Commission, 2011).

### 5.2.4 Data on return mobility

Although of high relevance to countries, no routine monitoring of the scale of returners was identified by the countries covered in this chapter. There are small-scale studies on motivations for returning home, based on intentions to leave. For example, a study on foreign nurses in London showed significantly different patterns of intentions from different groups, depending on their source countries: nurses from South Africa were likely to plan to return home; nurses from elsewhere in Africa and from India were planning to stay in the

---

2 2009: Austria, Belgium, Bulgaria, Czech Republic, Denmark, Estonia, Finland, Germany, Greece, Hungary, Ireland, Italy, Lithuania, Malta, Netherlands, Poland, Portugal, Romania, Slovenia, Spain, Sweden, United Kingdom and Switzerland; 2010: Belgium, Bulgaria, Czech Republic, Denmark, Estonia, Finland, Greece, Hungary, Ireland, Italy, Netherlands, Poland, Romania, Slovenia, Spain, Sweden, United Kingdom and Switzerland; 2011: Belgium, Bulgaria, Czech Republic, Denmark, Estonia, Finland, Greece, Hungary, Ireland, Poland, Romania, Slovenia, Sweden and United Kingdom.

United Kingdom, but most nurses from the Philippines were planning to move on to the United States (Buchan et al., 2007). In another survey in Ireland, the Nurse Migration Project showed that 50% of the 337 foreign nurses planned to return "home" and 23% planned to move to a third country for a variety of reasons, including insufficient options in terms of citizenship or family reunification for nurses from non-EU countries (Humphries, Brugha & McGee, 2009). The scale of returners is not known in Europe, despite its significant impacts on the source and destination countries. Particularly for source countries, it is crucial to collect data on return mobility and activity levels: health professionals returning to their "home country" to continue practising in their profession would result in a potential skill-gain for the source country. It is equally important for source countries to assess the underlying reasons for returning: is it for improved employment and working conditions or salary levels, or for other factors that are amenable to policy change, or are the major reasons based on factors that cannot be influenced by policies, such as personal motivation.

The previous two sections have underlined the imperfect data situation in Europe on both stock and particularly yearly in- and outflow data. The key remaining question is what recent developments may influence the situation in the near future. The following section will address this issue.

## 5.3 Policy initiatives and their impacts on monitoring

This section aims to provide an overview of recent policy tools or instruments and their monitoring implications. The guiding question is if recent policy initiatives have triggered improvements in monitoring practices at country level: that is, will policy initiatives get countries closer to the yardstick of good-quality monitoring systems (see Box 5.1). This section will start with an overview at global level, followed by policy initiatives at EU and national levels.

### 5.3.1 Global level

At the global level, there is currently no routine standardized monitoring in place. However, the adoption of the *WHO Global Code of Practice on the International Recruitment of Health Personnel* at the 63rd World Health Assembly in 2010 holds some promise in having an effect on monitoring practices, albeit indirectly and on a voluntary basis (WHO, 2010). It was a landmark policy initiative because of its global reach. For the first time, all WHO Member States committed, on a voluntary basis, to monitoring and sharing information on mobility and health workforce data (WHO, 2010). As discussed in more detail elsewhere in this book (Chapter 13), the *Global Code of Practice* is an important initiative on ethical recruitment and aims to increase global dialogue, share information and improve national workforce intelligence systems. However, because of its voluntary nature, it may risk having limited impact. The *Global Code of Practice* suggests a reporting periodicity of three years, with a first report due at the World Health Assembly in May 2013. Member States were asked to designate a "national authority" responsible for the implementation of the *Global Code of Practice* and for data and information exchange. A "national reporting instrument" has been developed: a self-assessment tool with 15 questions aimed at monitoring first steps of implementation at country levels and providing an overview of the availability of data (WHO, 2011).

There are three critical issues that will determine the success of the *Global Code of Practice* that are directly related to its monitoring function. First, the extent to which countries have the data and intelligence systems in place or show political commitment to develop and improve data over time: any such improvements would be already a success in itself. Second, a determining factor will be how many countries will make (publicly) available their data and monitoring practices every three years: the voluntary nature of the *Global Code of Practice* limits countries' actual reporting practices. By February 2013, 51 countries (of 84 who designated a national authority out of a total of 193 WHO Member States) had reported on their implementation practices. From the WHO European Region, 36 Member States reported (WHO, 2013). From a global perspective, the number of countries that have reported back to date is limited, particularly from regions other than the European region. It remains to be seen how many additional countries will still join the global reporting and to what extent data will be shared and used for cross-country comparisons. The final, equally crucial factor for success will be the extent to which the information will be used by decision-makers and stakeholders to inform policy-making.

Table 5.3 shows the monitoring requirements and practices related to the *Global Code of Practice* and an additional five codes of practice of different scope and reach. Of the two regional codes, the Commonwealth Code of Practice of 2003 does not include any commitment to systematic monitoring, reflecting limited capacity in the Commonwealth Secretariat. The Pacific Code of Practice 2007 highlighted the necessity of monitoring, but in fact there has been no systematic monitoring other than an external review that was commissioned by the WHO Pacific Region but has not been published. Overall, these codes have shown to be weak on improved monitoring, at best suggesting voluntary monitoring as stipulated in the *Global Code of Practice*; ideally, this may change monitoring practices in the future in those countries that are willing to move forward. At worst, some codes do not refer at all to a need for monitoring.

**Table 5.3** *Monitoring requirements and practices of global and regional codes of practice*

| Type of code (year of adoption) | Monitoring requirements (as set out in codes) | (Regular) monitoring practices |
|---|---|---|
| *Global reach* | | |
| WHO Global Code of Practice (WHO, 2010) | Suggests regular reporting every 3 years; first reporting expected in 2013 to World Health Assembly | February 2013: 51 reports by Member States out of 84 countries reporting a designated authority (of 193 WHO Member States adopting the Code) (WHO, 2013) |
| *Regional level* | | |
| Commonwealth Code (Commonwealth Health Ministers, 2003) | No monitoring suggested | No |
| Pacific Code (Ministers of Health for Pacific Island Countries, 2007) | "Should include collection of information on out migration to monitor international recruitment trends including countries targeted and agencies used" | Not systematically; external review was commissioned but not published |
| *European level* | | |
| English Code (Department of Health England, 2004) | NHS Employers responsible for the implementation and managing a list of recruitment agencies with adherence to the Code | "Positive" list: (Regular) update of list of recruitment agencies that comply with Code (NHS Employers, 2013) |
| Scottish Code (Scottish Executive, 2006) | See above | Initially monitored and a 6 monthly report published; now it is covered by NHS Employers "positive" list (see above) |
| *Specific focus (hospitals)* | | |
| EPSU-HOSPEEM (2008) | "By the end of the fourth year" 2012 ... a report on the overall implementation will be published" | n/a |

*Note*: n/a: Not available.

### 5.3.2 European level

At the European level, although a good case can be made for exchange of information and joint monitoring as mobility of health professionals is clearly of cross-border and EU significance, not least through the EU single market, to date there is no systematic or routine monitoring in place. However, the English and Scottish Codes of Practice have had some impact on monitoring in the past, albeit of limited significance on routine monitoring (Department of Health England, 2004; Scottish Executive, 2006). There are two recent policy developments, the *Action Plan for the EU Health Workforce* (European

Commission, 2012) and the joint WHO/OECD/Eurostat data collection (OECD, 2011b, 2012a), which have the potential to include mobility and improve the monitoring of mobility.

### Codes of practice at European level

Among all codes of practice, to date only the England and Scotland Codes of Practice led to the regular "monitoring" of recruitment agency activity but they did not lead to a direct improvement of routine data on health professionals on the move. A positive list has been developed of those recruitment agencies that have agreed to comply with the Codes' principles; non-compliant agencies are not listed. NHS organizations are "urged to only use agencies on this list". While this monitoring practice is clearly the strongest of all codes of practice, with most up-to-date information on implementation (including most recently a summary of the implications of the WHO *Global Code of Practice*), there are limitations. It is mainly linked to the approval of recruitment agencies and to the definition of countries where active recruitment by the NHS is not permitted. It is not based on any systematic monitoring of flow data, which in any case is not available for NHS nurses and some other health professionals (Buchan et al., 2009). Overall, there is no definition of ethical recruitment and no consensus on the significance of harmful recruitment (Connell & Buchan, 2011). The available data do not allow identification of which health professionals have been recruited by the NHS and how many have been recruited by the private sector, by other (non-health) sectors, work illegally or do not work at all (Buchan et al., 2009; Connell & Buchan, 2011). Routine data have not improved with regard to these issues.

The 2008 Code of Conduct produced by the European Federation of Public Service Unions (EPSU) and the European Hospital and Health Care Employers' Association (HOSPEEM) has a more narrow scope, focusing on health professionals working in the hospital sector in the EU (EPSU–HOSPEEM, 2008). It emphasized the need for monitoring and reporting progress. The EU social partner organizations of EPSU and HOSPEEM agreed to implement the Code within a three-year period, up to 2011, with a commitment to yearly monitoring implementation and reporting back to the sectoral social dialogue committee at least once per year. For the end of 2012, a report on the overall implementation was planned (EPSU–HOSPEEM, 2008) but has yet to be published.

### EU Joint Action on Health Workforce Planning and Forecasting

The Joint Action on Health Workforce Planning and Forecasting took up its functions in 2013 (European Commission, 2012). The Joint Action is a form of collaboration between the European Commission and Member States in which both sides enter a contractual agreement and commit resources. Some of the work packages can be delegated to NGOs, including academic institutions or international organizations. Aims of the Joint Action include information sharing of best practices on methodologies, future needs assessments of skills and competences, capacity building, and also providing guidance to the EU on mobility trends and mobility (Lengyel, 2011; Vandenbroele, 2011). Sharing of data is envisaged, particularly updated information on mobility trends; this would clearly have the potential to close some of the knowledge gaps, particularly on outflows and potentially returners in an easier way than if pursued by each Member State alone. However, it remains to be seen to what extent, if at all, the Joint Action will get involved in data sharing or whether it will remain a platform for exchange of knowledge and methodologies.

### Joint WHO EURO/Eurostat/OECD data collection

In 2011, WHO Regional Office for Europe, Eurostat and OECD joined forces on data collection related to health; this is another promising development that could, in theory, include EU-wide data on mobility. However, to date, indicators on mobility are not included. A joint questionnaire on health care statistics was developed that included statistics on the health workforce in Europe with a broad coverage of items, but it missed out indicators on mobility (OECD, 2011b, 2012a).

### 5.3.3 National level

At country level, some recent policy initiatives have been adopted or are in the pipeline with a view to improving monitoring of the workforce, and with it awareness of the mobility of health professionals. Austria, which does not have a mandatory registry for nurses, has been piloting a registry of voluntary nature for those nurses who are members of the major nursing association, the Austrian Association of Nurses (ÖGKV), with plans to implement this registry nationwide (Austrian Association of Nurses, 2011). The English Department of Health is considering a move from voluntary to mandatory registration for public health professionals (Jaques, 2012). In Finland, a specific social security number for each medical doctor from the Finnish Medical Association provides data such as places of residence, ages, genders, specializations, number of graduates and retirement (Matrix Insight, 2012). Similarly, in the United Kingdom, a so-called Electronic Staff Record has been implemented for NHS staff in England and Wales and was reported to have improved the accuracy, timeliness and consistency of data (Matrix Insight, 2012). In France, a so-called directory of health professionals (Répertoire Partagé des Professionnels de

Santé, RPPS) was established in 2009 (Xoual, 2010). It serves as one common platform and database with the aim of covering the major health professions in one single database. As of January 2012, data have been movd to the Répertoire Partagé des Professionnels de Santé for pharmacists, midwives and surgeon-dentists (chirurgiens-dentistes) from the previous registry (ADELI) and for medical doctors from the Conseil National de l'Ordre des Médecins (Sicart, 2012). Each health professional is being registered under a specific number that serves as a single identifier and allows for detailed analyses of data on health professionals, including data on mobility (Xoual, 2010).

The implementation and improvement of registries, and annual mandatory re-registration policies, do not only enhance the regulatory oversight of professions but also substantially improve data availability and data quality if implemented nationwide. Cost implications may pose a challenge as registries are costly and time consuming to set up and maintain; however, in return, policy-makers will have up-to-date data available on the actual size of their overall workforce and can assess the magnitude of mobility in their country-specific context.

The purpose of such data is to inform decision-making adequately and pragmatically. One initial assessment is to determine if a completely new data collection will be necessary because data are either non-existent or of unreliable quality; this must be complemented by improving the data that is collected in such a way that they can support policy action.

## 5.4 Conclusions

This chapter has assessed the quality of data on monitoring health professional mobility in Europe and has underlined the still imperfect data situation, particularly on short-term movements, emigration and return mobility, which are still a "black box" in most European countries. Continuous and up-to-date monitoring is often not feasible at country level, where it is not regarded politically as a priority. Countries hit by the financial and economic crisis are likely to have priorities other than improving their workforce intelligence systems. However, in failing to implement such systems, they may miss out on the impact of mobility on their workforces, with potentially longer-term impacts on health systems and the health of the population. Some of the recent policy developments such as the *WHO Global Code of Practice* hold some promise towards improving the monitoring of health professional mobility; however, because the *WHO Global Code of Practice* is voluntary in nature, it may not live up to its full potential. At the EU level, no EU-wide community action exists to improve health workforce data and intelligence systems. Instead a Joint Action on Workforce Planning was started in 2013, but its impact on countries remains to be seen.

Responding to the sometimes rapid changes in health professional mobility in Europe will require a monitoring system that is up to date and shows reliable data on mobility. Monitoring would need to be embedded in an overall health workforce intelligence system with clear accountability lines, and to be transparent through making the data publicly available. Monitoring and good-quality statistics on the practising workforce will improve workforce planning and forecasting and act as an early warning system on shortages of certain professions or specializations or on regional imbalances that would enable policy-makers to take informed action. Data are not a luxury but a necessity, particularly in times of rapid changes. Yet data collection requires investments, awareness of the need and political commitment, which are not always available.

## References

Albreht T (2011). Addressing shortages: Slovenia's reliance on foreign health professionals, current developments and policy responses. In Wismar M et al., eds. *Health professional mobility and health systems. Evidence from 17 European countries.* Copenhagen, WHO Regional Office for Europe on behalf of the European Observatory on Health Systems and Policies:511–537.

Austrian Association of Nurses (2011). *Registration.* Wien, Austrian Association of Nurses (https://www.oegkv.at/fileadmin/docs/freiwillige_Registrierung/2011_05__Registrierung_Wording.pdf, accessed 2 January 2014).

Avgerinos ED, Koupidis SA, Filippou DK (2004). Impact of the European Union enlargement on health professionals and health care systems. *Health Policy,* 69: 403–408.

Beňušová K et al. (2011). Regaining self-sufficiency: Slovakia and the challenges of health professionals leaving the country. In Wismar M et al., eds. *Health professional mobility and health systems. Evidence from 17 European countries.* Copenhagen, WHO Regional Office for Europe on behalf of the European Observatory on Health Systems and Policies:479–510.

Bertinato L et al. (2011). Oversupplying doctors but seeking carers: Italy's demographic challenges and health professional mobility. In Wismar M et al., eds. *Health professional mobility and health systems. Evidence from 17 European countries.* Copenhagen, WHO Regional Office for Europe on behalf of the European Observatory on Health Systems and Policies:243–262.

Blacklock C et al. (2012). Effect of UK policy on medical migration: a time series analysis of physician registration data. *Human Resources for Health*, 10:35.

Buchan J, Perfilieva G (2006). *Health worker migration in the European Region: country case studies and policy implications*. Copenhagen, WHO Regional Office for Europe.

Buchan J et al. (2007). Internationally recruited nurses in London, a survey of career paths and plans. *Human Resources for Health*, 4:14.

Buchan J et al. (2009). Does a code make a difference: assessing the English code of practice on international recruitment. *Human Resources for Health*, 7:33.

Commonwealth Health Ministers (2003). *The Commonwealth code of practice for the international recruitment of health workers*. Geneva, Commonwealth Health Ministers (Pre-WHA Meeting, 18 May) (http://secretariat.thecommonwealth. org/files/35877/FileName/CommonwealthCodeofPractice.pdf, accessed 2 January 2014).

Connell J, Buchan J (2011). The impossible dream? Codes of practice and the international migration of skilled health workers. *World Medical and Health Policy*, 3(3):1–17.

Dal Poz MR et al., eds. (2009). *Handbook on monitoring and evaluation of human resources for health: with special applications for low- and middle-income countries*. Geneva, World Health Organization.

Delamaire ML, Schweyer FX (2011). Nationally moderate, locally significant: France and health professional mobility from far and near. In Wismar M et al., eds. *Health professional mobility and health systems. Evidence from 17 European countries*. Copenhagen, WHO Regional Office for Europe on behalf of the European Observatory on Health Systems and Policies:181–210.

Department of Health England (2004). *Code of practice for the international recruitment of healthcare professionals*, revised edn. London, DH Publications (http://www.idcsig.org/DoH%20International%20Recruitment.pdf, accessed 2 January 2014).

Diallo K (2004). Data on the migration of health-care workers: sources, uses, and challenges. *Bulletin of the World Health Organization*, 82(8):601–607.

Eke E, Girasek E, Szócska M (2011). From melting pot to laboratory of change in central Europe: Hungary and health workforce migration. In Wismar M et al., eds. *Health professional mobility and health systems. Evidence from 17 European countries*. Copenhagen, WHO Regional Office for Europe on behalf of the European Observatory on Health Systems and Policies:365–394.

EPSU–HOSPEEM (2008). *EPSU–HOSPEEM code of conduct and follow up on ethical cross-border recruitment and retention in the hospital sector.* Brussels, European Federation of Public Service Unions and European Hospital and Healthcare Employers' Association (http://www.epsu.org/a/3715, accessed 2 January 2014).

European Commission (2005). *Directive 2005/36/EC on the recognition of professional qualifications.* Brussels, European Commission (http://ec.europa.eu/internal_market/qualifications/policy_developments/legislation/index_en.htm, accessed 5 August 2013).

European Commission (2008). *Employment in Europe 2008.* Brussels, Directorate-General for Employment, Social Affairs and Equal Opportunities (http://ec.europa.eu/social/main.jsp?langId=en&catId=89&newsId=415, accessed 2 January 2014).

European Commission (2011). *EU single market: regulated professionals database.* Brussels, Eurostat (http://ec.europa.eu/internal_market/qualifications/regprof/index.cfm?action=homepage, accessed 1 October 2013).

European Commission (2012). *Commission staff working document on an action plan for the EU health workforce.* Strasbourg, European Commission (http://ec.europa.eu/dgs/health_consumer/docs/swd_ap_eu_healthcare_workforce_en.pdf, accessed 10 December 2013).

European Commission (2013). *European Union labour force survey.* Brussels, Eurostat (http://epp.eurostat.ec.europa.eu/portal/page/portal/microdata/lfs, accessed 1 October 2013).

Fouka G et al. (2013). The increase in illegal private duty nurses in public Greek hospitals. *Journal of Nursing Management,* 21(4):633–637.

Gaál P et al. (2011). Major challenges ahead for Hungarian healthcare. *British Medical Journal,* 343:d7657.

Galan A, Olsavszky V, Vladescu C (2011). Emergent challenge of health professional emigration: Romania's accession to the EU. In Wismar M et al., eds. *Health professional mobility and health systems. Evidence from 17 European countries.* Copenhagen, WHO Regional Office for Europe on behalf of the European Observatory on Health Systems and Policies:449–478.

Garcia-Perez MA, Amaya C, Otero A (2007). Physicians' migration in Europe: an overview of the current situation. *BMC Health Services Research,* 7:201.

Grand Duchy of Luxembourg (2012). *The first results of the population census July 2012.* Luxembourg City, Grand Duchy of Luxembourg (http://www.

statistiques.public.lu/en/news/population/population/2012/07/20120711/index.html, accessed 2 January 2014).

Humphries N, Brugha R, McGee H (2009). *Retaining migrant nurses in Ireland II. Nurse migration project policy brief 3.* Dublin, Royal College of Surgeons in Ireland.

Jaques H (2012). Government considers statutory regulation of public health professionals. *BMJ Careers* (http://careers.bmj.com/careers/advice/view-article.html?id=20006222, accessed 2 January 2014).

Kautsch M, Czabanowska K (2011). When the grass gets greener at home: Poland's changing incentives for health professional mobility. In Wismar M et al., eds. *Health professional mobility and health systems. Evidence from 17 European countries.* Copenhagen, WHO Regional Office for Europe on behalf of the European Observatory on Health Systems and Policies:419–448.

Kovacs E, Szocska G, Schmidt A (2012). Registration and licensing processes of medical doctors in the European Union. *Conference on Healthcare in Europe; Is the grass always greener on the other side? Mobility of patients, and health- and long-term care professionals to and from Eastern European countries, ECAB session, Ålborg, Denmark, 1 November.*

Kuusio H et al. (2011). Changing context and priorities in recruitment and employment: Finland balances inflows and outflows of health professionals. In Wismar M et al., eds. *Health professional mobility and health systems. Evidence from 17 European countries.* Copenhagen, WHO Regional Office for Europe on behalf of the European Observatory on Health Systems and Policies:163–180.

Lengyel B (2011). Background. *EAHC workshop on joint action on health workforce planning and forecasting, 5–6 December* (http://ec.europa.eu/eahc/documents/news/Workshop_on_JA_5-6_12_2011_Presentations/5_12_2011/JA_2012_SANCO/4_B_Lengyel_JA_workforce.pdf, accessed 2 January 2014).

López-Valcárcel BG, Pérez PB, Quintana CDD (2011). Opportunities in an expanding health service: Spain between Latin America and Europe. In Wismar M et al., eds. *Health professional mobility and health systems. Evidence from 17 European countries.* Copenhagen, WHO Regional Office for Europe on behalf of the European Observatory on Health Systems and Policies:263–294.

Maier CB et al. (2011). Cross-country analysis of health professional mobility in Europe: the results. In Wismar M et al., eds. *Health professional mobility and health systems. Evidence from 17 European countries.* Copenhagen, WHO Regional Office for Europe on behalf of the European Observatory on Health Systems and Policies:23–66.

Matrix Insight (2012). *EU level collaboration on forecasting health workforce needs, workforce planning and health workforce trends: a feasibility study, revised final report.* London, Matrix Insight, Centre for Workforce Intelligence (http://ec.europa.eu/health/workforce/docs/health_workforce_study_2012_report_en.pdf, accessed 2 January 2014).

Ministers of Health for Pacific Island Countries (2007). *Pacific code of practice for recruitment of health workers and compendium.* Manila, Ministers of Health for Pacific Island Countries (endorsed at the Seventh Meeting of Ministers of Health for Pacific Island Countries in Port Vila, Vanuatu) (http://www.wpro.who.int/health_technology/pacific_code_practice_for_recruitment_health_workers.pdf, accessed 2 January 2014).

NHS Employers (2013). *Recruitment agencies. List of recruitment agencies that operate in accordance with the code of practice for the international recruitment of healthcare professionals* (http://www.nhsemployers.org/RecruitmentAndRetention/InternationalRecruitment/Code-of-Practice/agencies/Pages/RecruitersMap.aspx, accessed 8 October 2013).

OECD (2011a). *Health at a glance 2011: OECD indicators.* Paris, Organisation for Economic Co-operation and Development (http://www.oecd.org/health/health-systems/49105858.pdf, accessed 1 October 2013).

OECD (2011b). *Joint questionnaire between OECD, Eurostat and WHO-Europe on non-monetary health care statistics.* Paris, Organisation for Economic Co-operation and Development (Presentation at Meeting of OECD Health Data National Correspondents, October 2011) (http://www.oecd.org/health/health-systems/48831012.pdf, accessed 1 October 2013).

OECD (2012a). *Assessment of results of joint questionnaire between OECD, EUROSTAT and WHO (Europe) on health workforce statistics (with a focus on doctors).* Paris, Directorate for Employment, Labour and Social Affairs, Organisation for Economic Co-operation and Development.

OECD (2012b). *Health data 2012.* Paris, Organisation for Economic Co-operation and Development (http://www.oecd.org/health/health-systems/oecdhealthdata.htm, accessed 1 October 2013).

OECD (2013). *Health data 2013: list of variables.* Paris, Organisation for Economic Co-operation and Development http://www.oecd.org/els/health-systems/oecd-health-data-2013-list-of-variables.htm, accessed 2 October 2013).

OECD/WHO (2010). *Policy brief on the international migration of health workforce.* Paris, Organisation for Economic Co-operation and Development (http://www.oecd.org/migration/mig/44783473.pdf, accessed 8 October 2013).

Offermanns G, Malle EM, Jusic M (2011). Mobility, language and neighbours: Austria as source and destination country. In Wismar M et al., eds. *Health professional mobility and health systems. Evidence from 17 European countries.* Copenhagen, WHO Regional Office for Europe on behalf of the European Observatory on Health Systems and Policies:89–128.

Ognyanova D, Busse R (2011). A destination and a source: Germany manages regional health workforce disparities with foreign medical doctors. In Wismar M et al., eds. *Health professional mobility and health systems. Evidence from 17 European countries.* Copenhagen, WHO Regional Office for Europe on behalf of the European Observatory on Health Systems and Policies:211–242.

Ognyanova D et al. (2012). Mobility of health professionals pre and post 2004 and 2007 EU enlargements: evidence from the EU project PROMeTHEUS. *Health Policy*, 108:122–132.

Saar P, Habicht J (2011). Migration and attrition: Estonia's health sector and cross-border mobility to its northern neighbour. In Wismar M et al., eds. *Health professional mobility and health systems. Evidence from 17 European countries.* Copenhagen, WHO Regional Office for Europe on behalf of the European Observatory on Health Systems and Policies:339–364.

Safuta A, Baeten R (2011). Of permeable borders: Belgium as both source and host country. In Wismar M et al., eds. *Health professional mobility and health systems. Evidence from 17 European countries.* Copenhagen, WHO Regional Office for Europe on behalf of the European Observatory on Health Systems and Policies:129–162.

Scottish Executive (2006). *Code of practice for the international recruitment of healthcare professionals in Scotland.* Edinburgh, Scottish Executive (http://www.scotland.gov.uk/Resource/0041/00412480.pdf, accessed 1 October 2013).

Sicart D (2012). *Les professions de santé au 1er janvier 2012.* Paris, Direction de la recherche, des études, de l'évaluation et des statistiques (Working Document 168) (http://www.drees.sante.gouv.fr/IMG/pdf/seriestat168.pdf, accessed 2 January 2014) [in French].

Vandenbroele H (2011). A proposal in progress. *EAHC workshop on joint action on health workforce planning 5–6 December 2011* (http://ec.europa.eu/eahc/documents/news/Workshop_on_JA_5-6_12_2011_Presentations/5_12_2011/JA_2012_SANCO/4_H_Vandenbroele_JA_HWF.pdf, accessed 2 January 2014).

WHO (2010). *WHO global code of practice on the international recruitment of health personnel.* Geneva, World Health Organization (Sixty-third World

Health Assembly, WHA63.16) (http://www.who.int/hrh/migration/code/WHO_global_code_of_practice_EN.pdf, accessed 1 October 2013).

WHO (2011). Public hearing on the draft guidelines for monitoring the implementation of the WHO Global Code of Practice on the International Recruitment of Health Personnel 21 March to 17 April 2011. ( http://www.who.int/hrh/migration/code/hearing_guidelines_ms/en/index.html , accessed June 2012).

WHO (2013). *The health workforce: advances in responding to shortages and migration, and in preparing for emerging needs.* Geneva, World Health Organization (Report by the Secretariat) (http://apps.who.int/gb/ebwha/pdf_files/WHA66/A66_25-en.pdf, accessed 1 October 2013).

WHO Regional Office for Europe (2013). *European Health for All database* [online/offline database]. Copenhagen, WHO Regional Office for Europe (http://data.euro.who.int/hfadb/, accessed 9 October 2013).

Wiskow C, ed. (2006). *Health worker migration flows in Europe: overview and case studies in selected CEE countries: Romania, Czech Republic, Serbia and Croatia.* Geneva, International Labour Organization (Working Paper 245) (http://www.ilo.org/wcmsp5/groups/public/---ed_dialogue/---sector/documents/publication/wcms_161162.pdf, accessed 14 December 2013).

Wismar M et al., eds. (2011). *Health professional mobility and health systems. Evidence from 17 European countries.* Copenhagen, WHO Regional Office for Europe on behalf of the European Observatory on Health Systems and Policies.

Xoual B (2010). Répertoire partagé des professionnels de santé [Shared directory of health professionals]. *OECD/WHO Technical workshop: monitoring health workforce migration.* Paris, Organisation for Economic Co-operation and Development (http://www.oecd.org/els/health-systems/45491861.pdf, accessed 2 January 2014).

Young R (2011). A major destination country: the United Kingdom and its changing recruitment policies. In Wismar M et al., eds. *Health professional mobility and health systems. Evidence from 17 European countries.* Copenhagen, WHO Regional Office for Europe on behalf of the European Observatory on Health Systems and Policies:295–335.

# Chapter 6

# Health professionals crossing the EU's internal and external borders: a typology of health professional mobility and migration

*Irene A. Glinos and James Buchan*

## 6.1 Introduction

This chapter proposes a twin typology of health professional mobility. The typology is built on two classifications: one of *mobile health professionals* and one of *meanings of borders*[1, 2]. Asking who the mobile health professionals are and what borders they cross unlocks the variety and nuances inherent in health professional mobility. The purpose of the twin typology is to conceptualize and systematize this diversity; it does so by defining six types of mobile health professionals and three categories of borders.

This is not merely a theoretical exercise; it can contribute to better-informed policy. A more accurate conceptualization of health professional mobility serves four purposes: to assess the usefulness of current indicators for measuring flows of mobile health professionals; to spell out how borders determine what is

1 A version of this chapter has been submitted to Policy and Society, Special Issue 'Health, Markets, and the Law' (2014), and appears in the doctoral thesis by Irene A. Glinos *Where border and health care meet: Five studies in movements between health care systems*, Maastricht 2013, ISBN 978 94 6159 256 9.

2 The research leading to this chapter was carried out prior to the adoption of Directive 2013/55/EU of the European Parliament and of the Council of 20 November 2013 amending Directive 2005/36/EC on the recognition of professional qualifications and Regulation (EU) No 1024/2012 on administrative cooperation through the Internal Market Information System ('the IMI Regulation').

mobility and what migration; to develop targeted policies according to the type of mobile health professional leaving or entering a country; and to distinguish health professional mobility from other forms of international migration, in particular by proposing a definition of the phenomenon.

The chapter first explains the relevance of creating a typology. It then considers existing classifications and literature on international migration to draw on the most useful elements for constructing a definition and a typology specific for health professional mobility. The six types of mobile health professional and three meanings of borders are explained in detail before discussing their implications in terms of the usefulness of current indicators, the distinction between mobility and migration and the possibility for policy-makers to better target migration policies.

The starting point for the two classifications is the empirical evidence gathered across Europe and mainly in the EU (Wismar et al., 2011). Given that all EU Member States are confronted with migration to and/or from third countries, any in-depth "European" discussion of health professionals on the move has to be embedded in a global context. The typology reflects the global reality and accentuates the difference between intra- and extra-EU movements. As a conceptual framework for understanding and systematizing health professional mobility, we believe it is also of use for other parts of the world. For the purposes of developing the typology, the chapter considers as "health professional" a person who is qualified and officially authorized to deliver services to patients as a medical doctor, nurse, midwife, dental practitioner, pharmacist, physiotherapist, medical and pharmaceutical technician and nursing and midwifery associate professionals, including during training periods. This approach builds on the professional groups set out by EU Directive 2005/36/EC (European Commission, 2005) and by the International Standard Classification of Occupations (International Labour Organization, 2008).

## 6.2 Rationale for creating a typology

This new approach to conceptualizing health professional mobility serves four purposes. First, the application of a typology for mobile health professionals, devised to be as inclusive as possible in terms of types of mobile health professional, provides a tool to check the validity and comprehensiveness of current migration indicators. In the absence of a commonly accepted definition, the three indicators of "foreign-trained", "foreign-born" and "foreign-national" are used to describe and measure mobility. Yet none of the indicators is perfect. In countries where comparisons between the three are possible, large differences in the quantity of "foreign" health professionals in the total health workforce or in the annual "foreign" inflows are apparent. With no clear definition and no indicator able to capture all facets, our general understanding of health professional mobility is bound to be an approximation – with obvious consequences for data collection, research and policy responses. A merit of the classification is that it allows testing of the usefulness of the three indicators against the six types of mobile health professional identified, and consequently to possibly get closer to a comprehensive definition of health professional mobility.

Second, a typology related to borders demonstrates how such borders are a key determinant of health professional mobility. They symbolize boundaries of legislation that allows (or not) a health professional to move, and by signalling a change of country, borders represent the differences (or similarities) in health systems, culture, language and so on. In this sense, borders determine the opportunities of mobile health professionals. This is particularly true in the context of the EU, which has created a hierarchy of borders par excellence, as intra-EU *mobility* is facilitated by supranational legislation but *migration* between EU Member States and third countries is controlled by national laws (the difference between mobility and migration is discussed below). The importance of borders and their legal value often seems overlooked, perhaps because of a dichotomy in the literature: health professional mobility is approached either from a health systems angle, focusing on the health workforce and the reasons for and consequences of migration and mobility, or from a purely legal perspective in terms of which national and international legal instruments govern movements. The two approaches are rarely bridged but both neglect the spatial dimension inherent in all mobility and migration. Here, the discussion could benefit from the contribution of geographers. A focus on borders captures the legal and cultural nature of movements and can explain why some health professionals have more mobility opportunities than others.

Third, the ability to discern between types of mobile health professional – instead of considering health professional mobility as a monolithic, indistinct mass – is necessary to enable effective policy action to be taken. Very different incentives motivate a junior doctor going abroad to specialize, an experienced nurse emigrating to find better working conditions or a dentist travelling overseas on weekends to increase earnings. Each scenario has specific implications for the home country in terms of loss for the workforce (the types of skills "lost", vacant posts, workload, regional imbalances, etc.) and the likelihood of permanent migration or of return. For the host country, every new foreign entrant will come with a specific set of opportunities and challenges in terms of where they will fit into the workforce and system: matching of skills, expectations, culture and language, duration of stay and so on. To be effective, policy-makers must understand who moves so that they can design policy tools reflecting the variety of in- and outflows and specifically target each group of mobile health professionals with relevant measures.

Finally, the fourth purpose of the typology is to distinguish health professional mobility from other (skilled) migration, for several reasons. One is that of "medical exceptionalism", a position developed by Alkire and Chen (2006, p. 116), who in relation to policy responses and migration argue that "[a]s crucial instruments of health, doctors and nurses should be treated differently for ethical reasons that go far beyond their own well-being". Health and access to health care are recognized as human rights, not least by the Charter of Fundamental Rights of the European Union (Art. 36) (Gekiere, Baeten & Palm, 2010) and by the Universal Declaration of Human Rights (Art. 25(1); United Nations, 1948). In this argument, the vital importance of health services renders health professionals indispensable and their migration too consequential to ignore. Second, health care is unique in that it is a welfare service subject to global market forces. In many parts of Europe, and also elsewhere, the health care sector is considered and governed as a public service and part of the welfare state (despite growing pressures for privatization). As governments have a responsibility to their citizens to provide health care, having the "right" number of health professionals with adequate qualifications and specializations across the national territory becomes a key concern for public authorities. Because of the social and societal importance of the services involved, the mobility of health professionals cannot simply be equated with that of other highly skilled groups such as engineers and accountants; it is more akin to the migration of school teachers and welfare workers. Yet, while the provision of other welfare services is heavily dependent on national curricula and country-specific qualifications, medical education as well as practice standards are increasingly subject to processes of internationalization and so-called market-driven convergence (Cortez, 2009), which facilitate migration. Governments of both source and destination countries can, therefore, have significant policy and electoral interest in managing in/outflows for their health systems but are challenged by the market forces of supply and demand now taking place at global level and in the EU free-mobility zone under a legislative framework that seeks to "liberate" mobility of health professionals as much as possible. Medical doctors were the first professional group for which the European Commission drafted secondary legislation to allow mutual recognition of professional qualifications (in 1969; Zaglmayer & Peeters, 2008). Yet health professional mobility as an issue for health systems and workforce planners has arguably received disproportionately little attention in the EU. Current and forecast health workforce shortages across the world only add to these tensions and to the (ethical) dilemmas between policy-makers "using" foreign inflows to meet their responsibility of providing health care to the population and recruiting from countries that may be facing even worse health workforce problems (Glinos, 2012).

### 6.2.1 Defining health professional mobility and migration

The "exceptionalism" of health care and its professionals does not prevent health professional mobility from sharing some fundamental characteristics with international migration more broadly defined: no consensus on what constitutes "migration" or "a migrant", migratory patterns changing much more rapidly than other population phenomena, and migration being "the only demographic statistic currently produced simultaneously by two different national statistical institutes, one the country of departure and one in the country of arrival" (Thierry et al., 2005). The problems with defining and measuring make it all the more important to have a typology of health professional mobility to draw on existing work in diverse disciplines.

The classification of mobile health professionals takes inspiration from earlier typologies related to migration. An overview of these (Box 6.1) highlights several points:

- the attempt to conceptually systematize migration is no new endeavour; in 1901 the International Statistical Institute at its Budapest Congress stressed the need to differentiate between permanent and temporary emigrants in statistics (Kraly & Gnanasekaran, 1987);

- the many ways in which migration can and has been categorized highlights that it is an unfinished endeavour; diversity in the classification criteria is particularly striking, suggesting none is perfect but also that each has its worth;

- most typologies remain mono-dimensional and only in recent years have scholars started taking a holistic view combining various elements of the migration experience and showing interest in the migrant as individual (e.g. Buchan, Parkin & Sochalski, 2003; Triandafyllidou, 2011); and

- little attention is paid to the legal aspects of migration overall, which is surprising given how laws determine who can enter a country and what employment opportunities they will have; in the EU context, a supranational layer of laws determines if a migrant can enjoy free *mobility* or is subject to *migration* rules depending on the type of border crossed.

Borders embody the formal, legal opportunities of mobile health professionals, just as they embody the informal opportunities in terms of language, culture and geographical proximity. This is why the second classification of the typology

**Box 6.1** *Selected classifications of international migrants, migration and mobility*

*Motivation*
*Iredale (2001).* Five types of motivation: forced exodus, ethical emigration, brain drain, government induced, industry led.

*Cause/migratory force*
*Petersen (1958).* Five types of migratory force: primitive (caused by environment), forced (by authority), impelled (by authority), free (by aspiration), mass (by social momentum).

*Cohen (1997).* Five types of diaspora: victim, labour, trade, imperial, cultural.

*Direction of flows*
*Fairchild (1925).* Flows according to level of civilization: low to high (invasion), high to low (conquest/colonization), same level (immigration). Also discussed by Petersen (1958).

*Iredale (2001).* Flows according to economic development of countries: developing to postindustrialized, postindustrialized to developing, return migration or between postindustrialized.

*European Commission (2005).* Flows according to EU status of migrant and diploma: EU national with EU diploma has free mobility; EU national with non-EU diploma has some restrictions; non-EU national is excluded from free mobility.

*Length of stay*
*United Nations (1998).* Long-term migrant moves for at least 12 months; short-term migrant moves for 3–12 months.

*Iredale (2001).* Length of stay varies for business visitors, skilled transients, temporaries, permanents.

*Buchan, Parkin & Sochalski (2003).* Internationally recruited nurses in the United Kingdom can be permanent (economic migrant, career move, migrant partner) or temporary (working holiday, study tour, student, contract worker).

*European Union (2008),* Treaty on the Functioning of the European Union (TFEU). Free mobility is guaranteed by the freedom of establishment (Art. 49 TFEU) and freedom to provide services (Art. 56 TFEU).

*European Commission (2005).* Mobility to host country is either establishment or service provision of "temporary and occasional nature", assessed in terms of its "duration, frequency, regularity and continuity".

*Mode of integration in host country*
*Iredale (2001).* Integration can be disadvantaged reception, neutral or advantaged incorporation.

> **Box 6.1** *contd*
>
> *Channel/pathway*
>
> *Iredale (2001).* Recruitment channel can be internal labour markets of multinationals, overseas postings, international agencies, local/ethnic networks or via internet.
>
> *Triandafyllidou (2011).* Eight migration pathways: co-ethnicity and returnees, (post) colonial, pre-1989 internal migration, labour-related, asylum-seeking, temporary and seasonal work, "gold-collar", irregular migration.

focuses on the meanings of borders, borrowing some key notions from the disciplines of political and human geography and regional studies.

With a focus on the individual migrant (or mobile individual), we propose the following definition of health professional mobility:

> Any movement across a border by a health professional after graduation with the intention to work, that is, deliver health-related services in the destination country, including during training periods.

The choice of words has the following implications.

*The concept defined.* It should be noted that the definition also applies to (our understanding of) health professional *migration*. The terms mobility and migration overlap conceptually and in common usage. Their difference becomes relevant within the EU where different legal regimes govern intra-EU mobility as opposed to migration between the EU and third countries. As the definition does not specify what kind of border is crossed, it is able to cover mobility as well as migration.

*Movement across a border.* This implies that the health professional changes country to work but without necessarily changing country of residence; this allows for situations of cross-border commuting and working in two countries (i.e. without residing in the country of employment) but clearly excludes movements within a country (e.g. from one region or one sector to another).

*Health professional after graduation.* This implies that certain groups are excluded as they are not officially recognized or authorized to deliver health care: individuals with no previous health-related qualifications who travel abroad to study to become a health professional; individuals with no health-related qualifications although they may provide personal care on a private and/or informal basis (with or without remuneration); as well as health educational and social workers. In terms of the health professionals covered, these include generalist and specialist medical doctors, nurses, assistant nurses, specialized nurses, midwives, dentists, pharmacists, physiotherapists and associated technicians (although terminology varies between countries).

*With the intention to work, that is, deliver health-related services in the destination country.* This has several implications. First, the definition includes health professionals who end up unemployed when abroad but excludes those migrating with no intention to work (the latter being of secondary policy relevance). Work is a broad term covering those employed, self-employed and freelance, whether in the official or informal sector, and whether remunerated (in cash or in kind) or not.

*Health-related services.* This encompasses also activities such as teaching and research by health professionals.

*Including during training periods.* This implies that those who deliver health-related services while receiving specialized training abroad are included in the definition.

### 6.2.2 Developing the twin typology

While most typologies consider migration as a phenomenon of accumulated mass flows and collective behaviour, the classification we propose is built on types of mobile health professional. The approach is not new. Lindberg in his 1930 study on Swedish emigration distinguished three typical migrant profiles corresponding to three distinct periods in the history of emigration to the United States (Petersen, 1958). What is perhaps new is the prominence of the individual's decision to move.

## 6.3 Types of mobile health professional

The typology identifies six types of mobile health professional, taking a variety of elements into account to capture the mobile individual's situation. Each type represents an archetype or model-type of mobile health professional based on motivations for and purpose of migrating, conditions (circumstances) in the home country, conditions in the destination country, personal profile, likely direction of move and likely length of stay abroad. Fundamentally, all migrants seek "something better" abroad but their options for realizing this depend among other things on their skill level, the legal frameworks that govern migration and the labour market in destination countries. This is why "the livelihood migrant" and "the undocumented" are identified as two distinct types: while motivated by much the same incentives, their working conditions and legal situation in the destination are likely to differ substantially. The added value of a holistic approach is that each (arche)type translates into specific advantages and difficulties for data collectors and for policy-makers.

As with all classifications, some degree of overlap and grey areas are unavoidable. A mobile health professional can easily evolve from one type into another; for example, at the moment of leaving the home country he or she might fit the backpacker profile but during the stay abroad come to prefer the foreign system and settle down, becoming a livelihood migrant. Such movements across types only highlight their worth. We also recognize that this fluidity means that the six types are not the only ones possible but are ones we have identified as the most representative and most comprehensive. Although we have sought to cover all the variety of health professional mobility encountered in Wismar et al. (2011), it is impossible to be exhaustive. Finally, the naming of the six types does not follow a strict system as the logic is rather one of highlighting the most prominent characteristic of each type. Some names illustrate the movement undertaken while others focus on the social status or motivation of the mobile health professional.

### 6.3.1 The livelihood migrant

The livelihood migrant moves to earn a (better) living. The classic example is a migrant who leaves the home country for better earnings and better living standards (for the individual but often also for the family). In addition to comparatively low wages, factors in the home country such as unemployment, job insecurity, working below skills level and working conditions in general are likely to encourage the economic migrant. A new variant is the *crisis escapee* from the countries hit hardest by the financial and economic crisis. The purpose of migration can be to settle down abroad, whether permanently or semi-permanently. Because of the strong economic motive, flows within Europe tend to follow clear east-to-west and south-to-north directions, but important flows also come from third countries into the EU. The perception of better earnings and living standards is, of course, relative and depends on home country levels, so Bulgarians work in Romania, Romanians in France and so on (the domino effect of flows).

### 6.3.2 The career-oriented migrant

The career-oriented migrant travels to develop his or her career. The individual may move early on in professional life to receive training and/or education abroad, or in mid-career to (further) specialize or to accelerate professional development. Factors which motivate the ambitious include unfavourable conditions in the home country, such as limited training posts under a numerus clausus; the lack of certain facilities, equipment or specializations; the absence of structured career development plans; a hierarchical and rigid work culture in the health system that hinders career perspectives of (more recently qualified) health professionals; and also curiosity to work in a different system. The stay abroad is likely to be limited in time as the purpose is to obtain qualifications or to gain experience and skills that may boost the career back home, unless the health professional comes to prefer the foreign system and chooses to settle there. The stay may also be limited by legal constraints in the destination country or by the expiration of a guaranteed post in the home country. The direction of flows reflects the available opportunities in terms of training posts, specialized facilities, rewarding jobs and working in a language that opens doors elsewhere. Some systems, for example the United Kingdom, appear to have a certain appeal, including as a stepping stone for those wishing to move further afield, such as to the United States, Australia and New Zealand.

### 6.3.3 The backpacker

The backpacker works to travel. He/she is usually relatively young and independent and is unlikely to have settled down with family ties in the home country. The backpacker sees mobility as an opportunity to experience other countries, (work) cultures and health systems. He/she may try working in several countries and perceive some destinations as stepping stones for the next one. At the moment of leaving, the purpose is not to settle abroad, yet the backpacker may also not have any clear plan as to whether to return home at some point. This will rather depend on the opportunities abroad. As curiosity is a motivator, the direction of flows is less predictable, but the stay in (each) destination country is temporary and rather short. Some flows will be directed by specific national policy instruments, such as the "working holidaymaker" scheme for young nationals from some Commonwealth countries to work in the United Kingdom for limited periods of time.

### 6.3.4 The commuter

The commuting migrant commutes across borders to work. This mobility is characterized by repeated travel at regular and planned intervals. Subvariants exist as some commuters work at just one location while others have work in two countries. One variant is the daily commuter living in one country and working across the border in the neighbouring country. A second is the regular traveller who works part of the week in the home country and on certain days (e.g. weekends) travels to another country to work. This may be in border regions between neighbouring countries where distances are short, but not necessarily. A third variant travels fewer times per year, stays abroad for some weeks or months and may have a residence in both countries. The notions of short- and long-term migration take on a different meaning for this type of mobile health professional since they may commute to work abroad for years, indeed their entire career, but never settle down in the "host" country either temporarily or permanently. Rather, they can be considered as permanent commuters.

### 6.3.5 The undocumented

The undocumented migrant is migrating for work, but unofficially. Similar to the livelihood migrant, the undocumented migrant is motivated by better earnings and a better life in the host country, but works in the informal sector. In most cases, this means being employed by the care-recipient (or the family) and working (and living) in his/her private home. While some intentionally migrate to work as informal carers, others end up in care work and may be providing services below their skills level. Because of the high demand for services in some countries and the often unregulated nature of the sector, getting a job is easy and does not always depend on official qualifications. A distinction should be made between those working in the sector because of their non-regularized status in the destination country and who are more likely to be from non-EU countries, and those with residence permits but whose professional qualifications are not recognized. The work is characterized by a high turnover although the undocumented may live for years in the host country. Reported destination countries include Italy, Germany and Austria. Although some would argue that (home) care services are not *health* care, their inclusion as a distinct type is more than justified by the number of migrants working as carers (easily exceeding a million across Europe; Wismar et al., 2011), the gap in service provision they fill, the significant overlap with health care functions (e.g. nursing for handicapped and/or elderly with chronic conditions) and the challenges for data collection they give rise to.

### 6.3.6 The returner

The returner migrates in reverse. Some intentionally go abroad for a defined length of time or specific goal and simply return home once that is accomplished. Others return from abroad because of a more promising outlook in the home country, for example when salary levels and working conditions (including equipment, infrastructure, etc.) are improved through overall development of the system, or when a downturn in the domestic labour market has been overcome (e.g. the returning *crisis escapee*). Yet others return home due to disappointment as the foreign experience did not match their expectations, they did not find employment, their work permit expired or they became unemployed (e.g. economic difficulties or increased domestic supply in the host country).

## 6.4 Meanings of borders

The classification of borders looks at different meanings (or levels) of borders rather than at distinct types. Unless otherwise stated, we understand "border" as an *external state boundary* (Anderson & O'Dowd, 1999): that is, between two countries. It lies in the nature of borders that their characteristics are not mutually exclusive. The line, whether hypothetical or physical, demarcating a country border may also mark a linguistic border and a cultural one (different traditions, religion, etc.), although this is not necessarily the case (e.g. when neighbouring countries speak the same language).[3] Borders also enclose the outer reach of authority and consequently the limits of any national system, be it the legal system, the health care system, the social protection system, the electoral system or the fiscal system.[4] Paasi (2001) has helpfully described borders as "containers". Ferrera (2005, pp. 23–24) discusses Rokkan's theory on boundary building, which attributes two components to space, namely territory and membership, with the observation that it is relatively easy to cross territorial borders but hard to cross membership (system) boundaries. Membership here should be understood in the broadest sense as encompassing systems such as being part of a country's population, having EU citizenship, speaking a particular dialect or belonging to a community with a distinct history. What counts is that all borders by definition create insiders and outsiders (Rokkan, in Ferrera, 2005). By containing several systems, various characteristics coexist and overlap on a single border giving it different meanings depending on who is trying to cross it and why.

The difference between tourists and migrants is illustrative: while the former often are welcome, the latter are more likely to face obstacles in crossing territorial borders precisely because they intend to also cross the membership border(s) of the destination country (by aspiring to become part of society and the labour market, obtaining citizens' rights, etc.). From the migrant's perspective, borders embody the formal legal opportunities and barriers of the host country but also the informal opportunities in terms of language, culture and geographical proximity. An individual may, for example, be entitled to enter the destination country, settle down and work but experience difficulties in learning the language and integrating; alternatively, a person may face legal entry barriers but have informal advantages in terms of knowing the language

---

3 Language and cultural borders may also run through a country, as in Belgium, Switzerland and Canada.

4 Although the territorial border may be "perforated" to allow expatriated citizens to stay within the system: they may retain electoral rights and vote from abroad, just as they may still have to pay taxes in the home country.

and culture of the country. A border can thus be fluid and easy to cross at some levels, but rigid and difficult to cross in other regards.

Conceiving borders as having many and simultaneous meanings is key to understanding the three categories which follow. While every border we consider is *territorial* in the sense that it occurs between countries (cf. definition of health professional mobility), of interest for the typology is the border's function of delineating membership and systems. The first two categories focus on the legal function(s) of borders that are constructed by states or similar authorities. The third category covers the perceived or informal (i.e. non-binding) meanings of borders: that is, borders which do not depend on legal frameworks and are not created by state powers. While borders may have even more meanings, the three meanings are relevant to understand how health professional mobility and migration are happening within the EU and between the EU and the rest of the world.

### 6.4.1 Free mobility within the EU: the internally removed borders

If health professionals can move freely within the EU, it is in large part thanks to the freedom of movement of persons and of services that form two of the cornerstones of the EU internal market. From these freedoms derive three rights that mobile health professionals benefit from: the rights to free movement of workers, to free provision of services, and to freedom of establishment (Zaglmayer & Peeters, 2008). A series of secondary legislation makes it possible for EU citizens to enjoy these rights in practice by certain guarantees, such as the rights and conditions of residence, equal employment conditions and social security rights for migrating persons and their families.

Of particular importance are the directives on the mutual recognition of professional qualifications, which ensure that the educational requirements of EU Member States are coordinated so that qualified professionals can obtain recognition and exercise their profession elsewhere in the EU. Within this framework is a subgroup of seven professions which enjoy *automatic* diploma recognition thanks to a minimum level of harmonization of educational and training standards. Five are from the health care sector: doctors (with basic training or specialized), nurses responsible for general care, midwives, dental practitioners (specialized or not) and pharmacists. (The other two are veterinary surgeons and architects.) The main health professions thus form a privileged group that host countries may not subject to extra tests or adaption periods if they produce an official diploma (validated by the country of training) as listed in Directive 2005/36/EC (European Commission, 2005).

While mutual recognition is a fundamental measure preventing discrimination between Member States, *automatic* recognition takes free mobility one step further. By removing regulatory and administrative hurdles, it is a key instrument to facilitate freedom of movement (including short-term and temporary moves) as it substantially reduces the time and paperwork needed to work in another Member State. Yet the distinction between "establishment" and "service provision" comes into play as the two have different legal basis in the EU treaties and give rise to different obligations and entitlements (Zaglmayer & Peeters, 2008). Member States retain the right to impose requirements on other EU nationals pursuing a regulated profession provided that such rules apply equally to its own nationals. One example is the obligation to register with a professional body. Directive 2005/36/EC stipulates that such an obligation does *not* apply to health professionals who work temporarily or occasionally in another Member State, that is, they only "provide services".[5] Nor may the host state impose compulsory registration with a public social security body. A light version of requirements thus applies to the temporarily mobile.

It is hard to assess what the direct impact of mutual recognition has been in terms of numbers of health professional mobility in Europe, but the eased procedures and new opportunities to move have most certainly contributed to making mobility a varied phenomenon.

### 6.4.2 National immigration regimes: the externally selective borders

The supranational layer of borders created by the European internal market does not interfere with Member States' legislation on how they deal with migration from third countries. This remains an issue of national competence and the EU does not as yet have a common immigration policy.

Countries may impose any sort of competency tests or entry conditions on nationals from third countries.[6] Labour market tests are a way of favouring the country's workforce (i.e. the insiders) by requiring employers to look for suited employees within the country before offering the job to a migrant. While most EU Member States have rather strict immigration rules, and laws have been tightened as a result of the current global financial crisis, it is not uncommon to apply preferential treatment to immigrants with particular sought-after skills. In this sense, borders can be exceptionally perforated to filter foreign arrivals according to the needs of domestic labour markets, and these filters may change over time in response to changes in identified labour market priorities. As

---

5 Yet a Member State may require "automatic temporary registration with or for pro forma membership of such a professional organization or body, provided that such registration or membership does not delay or complicate in any way the provision of services and does not entail any additional costs for the service provider" (Art. 6a).

6 With the exception of citizens from the EEA countries (Switzerland, Lichtenstein, Norway and Iceland), where EU legislation on recognition of professional qualifications also applies.

numerous countries face considerable staff shortages in the health workforce, foreign health professionals are often among the "privileged outsiders" benefiting from easier access procedures. There are a number of examples: in Italy, nurses have been exempt from national immigration quotas since 2002 when the law was changed in acknowledgement of the severe lack of nurses; Ireland has since 2010 applied a fast-track procedure for non-EEA medical doctors to work in the public health service; Spain has simplified work visas for non-EU nationals in shortage professions such as medical doctors; and many countries have bilateral agreements to facilitate and steer migration. However, many preferential mechanisms follow the dictates of the labour market and only last as long as staff shortages do.

### 6.4.3 The culturally constructed border

Separate from their legal function, borders also have softer attributes that influence how permeable they are. This is what brings scholars to talk about the *anthropology of borders* (Wilson & Donnan, 1998), where language, traditions, religion, the feeling of belonging, cultural values and so on play a role. Here, the issue is not what legal texts stipulate,[7] but "the cultural constructions which give meaning to the boundaries between communities and between nations".

For a mobile health professional, emigrating to (and remaining in) a new country will be (perceived as) easier where there is a shared language, culture or history with the destination country. While legal borders coincide with the territory of the competent authority (be it a country or a formalized group of countries such as the EU), culturally constructed borders, and their memberships, do not necessarily conform to territory. Being part of the same language community, therefore, contributes to thousands of Latin American doctors choosing to go to Spain; perhaps less obviously, to Romanian doctors going to France and Belgium thanks to the common roots of French and Romanian languages; and to the often intense flows between neighbouring European countries (e.g. Germany and Austria, Belgium and France, Belgium and the Netherlands) and in their border regions (e.g. the Russian Federation doctors working in north-eastern Estonia, which is geographically linked to Russia and has a significant Russian-speaking population, or the Dutch University Hospital in Maastricht, 5 km from the Belgian border, where 40% of the nursing workforce is Belgian).

Having formerly been part of the same country or (colonial) empire can lead to enduring cultural bonds, and this plays a role in the Slovak health professionals going to the Czech Republic, the many Indian and Pakistani doctors working in the United Kingdom, and Algerians being the most important group of

---

7 As language skills may be an official requirement in some countries to be allowed to work, language may also function as a legal border.

foreign-trained non-EU doctors in France. Moreover, European history and the redrawing of borders have often left minorities behind across the border. Health professionals of Hungarian origin but living, for example, in Romania, Slovakia and Serbia have been returning to Hungary in two main waves, around 1990 and 2004. The 5 000 foreign-born medical doctors and dentists in Poland may suggest that the country attracts health professionals from the Polish diaspora and particularly the former USSR. Similarly, Finland is home to a considerable group of foreign-trained and foreign-born medical doctors from the Russian Federation, many of whom are Ingrian Finns (of historic Finnish descent). Language, cultural and historic ties can thus be decisive in explaining the direction of mobility and migration as the mobile health professional often will choose to go, and stay, where he/she feels least an "outsider", perhaps because of an already existing migrant community, or where their education curricula is more easily accepted because of previous colonial links.

## 6.5 Consequences for data collectors and policy-makers

Combining the six types of mobile health professional with the three levels of border opens up new ways to understand how the motives of individual health professionals interact with the possibilities that borders allow them. The legal and non-legal functions of borders will affect how permeable the border is and is perceived to be by the mobile health professional. While legal borders determine entitlements and requirements, cultural borders influence the choice of destination. Which function of borders matters more is hard to disentangle; for example, the cultural and symbolic value of the Iron Curtain might arguably have been as important as its legal and physical presence.

### 6.5.1 What the indicators do not tell us

One of the purposes of the typology is to test the usefulness of the migration indicators we currently use. In countries where data on foreign-trained, foreign-national and foreign-born migrants are available, comparisons show just how widely different the measurements are: in Austria the share of foreign-born medical doctors (around 14%) is three times higher than that of foreign-trained (around 4%), with foreign-national somewhere between (around 8%). In 2009, Poland identified 858 foreign-national medical doctors but three times as many foreign-trained (2 868) and four times foreign-born (3 887). It is regrettable how rare intra-indicator comparisons are but the discrepancies should not come as a surprise given the variety the typology has revealed. "Unless all sub-populations are identified, it is not certain that the data covers entirely the populations in question" (Thierry et al., 2005, p. 3). The indicators cannot tell the full story of a mobile health professional's journey to, from and between countries, and different indicators will tell different stories.

The livelihood migrant and the career-oriented migrant types are probably the most straightforward groups to capture for data collectors in destination countries as they have to register with professional bodies (where they exist).

The temporary nature of the backpacker's movements and of the commuter alternating between countries implies that these health professionals benefit from less-strict procedures of registration with the professional body of the host country by virtue of EU law. In countries where professional registries are the main source of information on immigration, this leads to potentially large gaps in data. Moreover, backpackers and commuters often do not deregister in the home country, or in the host country, which leads to inaccuracy in calculations of the total active workforce. In this context, it is noteworthy that EU policy-makers have so far not been able to come to an agreement on the time dimension. While Directive 36/2005/EC explicitly distinguishes "establishment" from "temporary provision of services", it does not explicitly define what is meant by temporary. Efforts by the European Commission to set a limit of 16 weeks per year on what is considered temporary work, during its negotiations on the draft Directive 36/2005/EC with the European Parliament and Member States in 2002, did not succeed.

The undocumented migrant and the returner are least likely to be caught by any measurements at all. The undocumented by definition go uncounted – sometimes both in the home and the host country – but the problem might be exacerbated by the strictness of national immigration laws: the harder it is to obtain work permits and official employment for third-country nationals, the more likely it is that non-EU health professionals resort to working in the informal sector, thus driving up the numbers of the undocumented. Returners who never deregistered when leaving the home country may also go unnoticed, which means that governments have little way of knowing whether health professionals are returning or whether any measures to attract them home are working.

Across the categories, the unique border landscape of Europe further blurs the picture. The fragmented and shifting map (and history) of Europe implies a multitude of neighbouring countries with implications for cross-border mobility: distances are short, transport links widely available, languages often shared and cross-border commuting an established practice. Yet, in a context of geographic, cultural, historical and linguistic proximity, indicators cannot capture if the mobile health professional shares ethnic or linguistic ties with the destination country (thus not really being "foreign"). Where host countries do not require conformity certificates – because they are so accustomed to receiving health professionals from the neighbouring country and trust their qualifications – home countries will not have any insight into outflows. Moreover, the EU has created what is the largest international free movement area in the world (see also the next section). Its sheer scale combined with the above-mentioned issues implies a huge potential for free mobility. Paradoxically, what makes Europe potentially unique from a mobility perspective also complicates the task of data collection.

The added value of the typology is specific as well as general. First, it allows singling out which types of mobile health professional are most likely to escape data collection. Because of the temporary, fluctuating or unofficial nature of their movements, four out of the six types – the backpacker, the commuter working in several countries, the returner and the undocumented – will be particularly difficult to correctly detect and measure with the current indicators. Consequently, consideration of this typology may lead to greater awareness among observers and decision-makers on the variety inherent in health professional mobility. To complement national data and fill the gaps, authorities may have to seek data at the level of health care organizations (particularly hospitals) and work together with the countries where their health professionals are going to or coming from to determine possibilities for common data sets, common measurements and common approaches.

### 6.5.2 EU in the world: mobility versus migration

The removal of legal and regulatory borders for the mobility of health professionals within the EU has created the distinction between those moving *within* the EU and those migrating in or out *across* its external borders. First, in relation to health professional mobility, the EU has created a supranational regime of no-borders between its Member States. To the extent possible, it has eliminated national rules, and thereby national borders, in order to build a unified area of unhindered mobility. While mutual recognition schemes exist elsewhere in the world as bilateral agreements (e.g. between New Zealand and Australia) or involving a limited number of countries (e.g. the North American Free Trade Agreement or the Association of Southeast Asian Nations), the one in the EU is unique by its geographical extent and the number of countries covered. Second, the EU seeks to promote the most-free mobility possible in all its variations. The intention to move should not be burdened by unnecessary paperwork, the logic being that if a health professional is good enough to work in one Member State he or she is good enough for any Member State. It is because of this approach that all EU health professionals, and in particular those moving frequently such as the backpacker, the commuter and the career-oriented migrant, are able to change country and seek work where they wish. To the EU legislator, no mobility is inferior to another; temporary mobility is even encouraged. Third, the freeing up of mobility between Member States has generated the distinction between *mobility* and *migration*. This is not a mere difference of wording (movement and mobility suggesting frequency, ease and reversibility compared with the more heavily charged migration). The EU has created a hierarchy between its internal and external borders, and a system where insiders enjoy legal entitlements to free movement whereas outsiders do not. Outsiders are first and foremost nationals of non-EU countries and they face the immigration laws and border controls of individual Member States.

However, exceptions to the border-free logic can also apply to EU citizens. With the accession of new Member States since the early 2000s, existing Member States have felt the need to protect their labour markets from the potential inflow of inexpensive labour. Transitional restrictions on the free movement of persons were imposed, in the case of Bulgaria and Romania for a maximum of seven years (see also Chapter 4 for details on EU Enlargement), effectively creating "mobility insiders" and temporarily "mobility outsiders". Member States may also invoke a safeguard clause allowing them to reinstate restrictions in case of serious domestic labour market disturbances. The Franco-German letter in April 2012, calling for EU Member State governments to be allowed to suspend the Schengen agreement and reintroduce border controls for a limited period of time (30 days) as a measure of last resort (Volkery, 2012), shows the sensitivity of the issue of the EU's internal and external borders. The treaties refer to third countries as those that are not members of the EU. With the creation of a supranational space of entitlements for its citizens, the EU also created a new marker of outsiderhood (Ferrera, 2005) and a multilevel system of migrants. Non-EU citizens are double outsiders: *foreign* to national authorities, and *third-country nationals* to the EU and its Member States.

Since the EU is shaping the mobility entitlements of all EU citizens, Member States are left with deciding the entitlements of "the rest". With no legal instruments to rein in free-mobility provisions, a Member State wishing to limit immigration can only put up barriers on its external border: towards third-country nationals. There might, therefore, be an inverted correlation between the generosity of intra-EU entitlements and the strictness of national immigration laws, particularly in the context of the financial crisis. As health professionals from third countries necessarily must pass through a Member State to enter the EU, they may select a state with easier immigration laws as their entry point in order to then move on to their intended destination, which is tougher to enter from outside the EU.

### *6.5.3 Developing targeted policies*

Individuals are not fixed over time in one of the six types of mobile health professional. They can easily evolve from one type into another: commuters may choose to settle abroad; backpackers may turn career oriented; the undocumented may be given the possibility to regularize; and livelihood migrants may return. While this fluidity provides policy-makers with a chance to influence mobility and migration, identifying and understanding the various types of mobile health professional are prerequisites to conceiving useful policy tools. As health professionals move for different reasons and different purposes, blanket measures will not be effective.

As always, the perspectives of sending and receiving countries diverge. Considering the backpacker. The challenge for the home country is to know what proportion of recent graduates chooses to travel instead of entering the domestic health workforce, and to ensure good work opportunities for young health professionals to encourage their return. Host countries, by comparison, may develop special schemes based, for example, on age-related entry (e.g. for under 28 years of age) or "working holidays" to attract inflows in the hope that backpackers will then stay in the longer term. With regards to the career oriented, similarly, the challenge is for host countries to retain those who have specialized and gained expertise – and potentially taken up training posts – in the country and for the home country to provide adequate job opportunities and re-integration mechanisms to encourage returns. Livelihood migrants who have settled down in the destination might be less easy to influence, although a clear improvement in the salary, working and living conditions in the home country, compared with the host, might provide the greatest incentive to return. Salary levels are likely to play a bigger role than for backpackers or the career oriented. With regards to the undocumented, host countries can take measures to legalize their situation, which would improve their opportunities of employment and of contributing fully to the host health system. An added advantage would be better data collection on this elusive group, including for the home country.

## 6.6 Conclusions

Mobility and migration have been conceptualized in a multitude of ways. The proposed definition of health professional mobility and the twin typology attempt to bridge the interpretations that approach mobility and migration either from a legal or technical angle (focusing mainly on the time dimension or the status of migrant) or from the viewpoint of migration studies (e.g. looking at causal and motivational factors). It does so by considering mobility and migration not as a mass phenomenon but as composed of mobile individuals moving across country borders and legal spaces. Drawing partly on human geography, the approach recognizes the role of individual decision-making and manages to combine the spatial and legal dimensions that are intrinsic to mobility and migration in the modern world. The result is a twin typology that identifies six types of mobile health professional and three meanings of borders. This conceptual framework can reflect the varied and nuanced nature of health professional mobility and allow policies to be targeted accordingly. It can identify which types of mobile health professional are unlikely to be captured by commonly used mobility indicators, and it can show how borders determine the opportunities of mobile health professionals. The distinction between *free mobility* and *controlled migration* is a result of the hierarchy between the EU's *internal* borders among its members and *external* borders with the rest of the world. The generosity of intra-EU entitlements may influence the strictness of national immigration laws. The decision to move is conditioned by the legal frameworks surrounding the individual. Paradoxically, what makes Europe potentially unique from a mobility perspective – the variety, ease and extent of internal mobility – is also what complicates the task of data collectors and decision-makers dealing with health professional mobility.

## References

Alkire S, Chen L (2006). Medical exceptionalism in international migration: should doctors and nurses be treated differently? In Tamas K, Palme J, eds. *Globalizing migration regimes: new challenges to transnational cooperation.* Farnham, UK, Ashgate (Research in migration and ethnic relations series).

Anderson J, O'Dowd L (1999). Borders, border regions and territoriality: contradictory meanings, changing significance. *Regional Studies*, 33:593–604.

Buchan J, Parkin T, Sochalski J (2003). International nurse mobility: trends and policy implications. Geneva, World Health Organization (http://whqlibdoc. who.int/hq/2003/WHO_EIP_OSD_2003.3.pdf, accessed 2 January 2014).

Cohen R (1997). *Global diasporas: an introduction.* London, UCL Press.

Cortez N (2009). International health care convergence: the benefits and burdens of market-driven standardization. *Wisconsin International Law Journal*, 26(3):646–704.

European Commission (2005). *Directive 2005/36/EC on the recognition of professional qualifications.* Brussels, European Commission (http://ec.europa. eu/internal_market/qualifications/policy_developments/legislation/index_ en.htm, accessed 5 August 2013).

European Union (2008). Consolidated Versions of the Treaty on the Functioning of the European Union, Official Journal of the European Union 09.05.2008, C 115/47

Fairchild HP (1925). *Immigration: a world movement and its American significance.* revised edn. New York, McMillan.

Ferrera M (2005). *The boundaries of welfare: European integration and the new spatial politics of social protection.* Oxford, Oxford University Press.

Gekiere W, Baeten R, Palm W (2010). Free movement of services in the EU and health care. In Mossialos et al., eds. *Health systems governance in Europe: the role of European Union law and policy.* Cambridge, UK: Cambridge University Press:461–508.

Glinos IA (2012). Worrying about the wrong thing: patient mobility versus health care professional mobility. *Journal of Health Services Research and Policy*, 17(4):254–256.

International Labour Organization (2008). *ISCO 08: resolution concerning updating the international standard classification of occupations.* Geneva, International Labour Organization (http://www.ilo.org/public/english/bureau/stat/isco/docs/resol08.pdf, accessed 2 January 2014).

Iredale R (2001). The migration of professionals: theories and typologies. *International Migration*, 39(5, Special Issue 1):7–24.

Kraly EP, Gnanasekaran KS (1987). Efforts to improve international migration statistics: a historical perspective. *International Migration Review*, 21(4, Special Issue):967–995.

Lindberg JS (1930). *An economic and sociological study in the dynamics of migration.* Minneapolis, MN, University of Minnesota Press.

Paasi A (2001). Europe as a social process and discourse: considerations of place, boundaries and identity. *European Urban and Regional Studies*, 8:17–28.

Petersen W (1958). A general typology of migration. *American Sociological Review*, 23(3):256–266.

Thierry X et al. (2005). How the UN recommendations and the forthcoming EU regulation on international migration statistics are fulfilled in the 25 EU countries. *The XXV International Population Conference-UIESP, Tours, 18–23 July.*

Triandafyllidou A (2011). Typologies of migration in Europe. Florence, Robert Schuman Centre for Advanced Studies, European University Institute (Presentation given 7 April).

United Nations (1948). *Universal declaration of human rights*. New York, United Nations.

United Nations (1998). *Recommendations on statistics of international migration*. New York, Department of Economic and Social Affairs, Statistics Division (Statistical Papers Series M, No. 58, Rev. 1).

Volkery C (2012). Franco-German Schengen proposal: a vote of no confidence in Europe. *Spiegel Online*, 20 April (http://www.spiegel.de/international/europe/0,1518,828815,00.html, accessed 2 January 2014).

Wilson TM, Donnan H (1998). *Nation, state and identity at international borders*. In Wilson TM, Donnan H, eds. *Border identities: nation and state at international frontiers*. Cambridge, UK, Cambridge University Press.

Wismar M et al., eds. (2011). *Health professional mobility and health systems. Evidence from 17 European countries*. Copenhagen, WHO Regional Office for Europe on behalf of the European Observatory on Health Systems and Policies.

Zaglmayer B, Peeters M (2008). Recognition of qualifications of health professionals in the EEA. In Mår N, Andenaes B, eds. *Klagenemnder: rettssikkerhet og effektivitet*. Oslo, Fagbokforlaget:321–360.

# Part III
# The mobile individual

# Chapter 7

# Health professional migration in Lithuania: why they leave and what makes them stay

*Žilvinas Padaiga, Martynas Pukas and Liudvika Starkienė*

## 7.1 Introduction

Migrant health professionals are usually faced with a combination of economic, social and psychological factors plus family choices. They consider migration when they expect this move can improve their professional and economic situation. In many studies and publications, low salaries, poor working conditions and lack of professional opportunities were identified as push factors, while demand for health professionals in destination countries in combination with higher pay, better working conditions and professional development opportunities act as pull factors (Buchan, 2007). However, various other factors also impact on individual decision-making. For example, a study in the Netherlands found that personal reasons, including marriage, were the most important factors in the move of 1 500 nurses who had arrived there from other EU and accession countries (de Veer, den Ouden & Francke, 2004). Research on international nurses in the United Kingdom highlighted that professional development and education opportunities for children were also main motivators to move (Buchan et al., 2006).

Although research on health professionals' motivations is limited, a certain consistency is revealed relating to the factors that influence them to make decisions regarding mobility. Mostly, the studies were considering countries outside the EU, such as African or Asian regions, and so lacked a deeper insight and analysis about the objective or subjective motivations for health professional migration within the EEA/EU countries (Dumont & Zurn, 2007). Most efforts to stop the outflow of health professionals from Lithuania were aimed at improving the instigating factors by reforming the health care system (better working conditions, social guarantees and higher salaries). Intentions to leave Lithuania were examined by surveying medical doctors and medical residents in 2002 (Stankūnas, Lovkytė & Padaiga, 2004), pharmacists in 2004 (Šmigelskas, Starkienė & Padaiga, 2007) and nurses in 2007 (Matulevičiūtė, 2007). Table 7.1 summarizes their findings on the main factors influencing the migration intentions of Lithuanian health professionals. However, subjective personal reasons remain a subject for future research and this is why it is essential to update the research on health professional migration not only in Lithuania but also in other countries (Pukas, 2008).

This chapter is based on a qualitative analysis based on interviews with Lithuanian health professionals (medical doctors, nurses and dentists) to examine the influencing factors and motivational reasons to migrate, return or stay and practise in Lithuania.

## 7.2 Study design

### 7.2.1 Aim of the study

Health professional retention is critical for health system performance and a key problem is how best to motivate and retain these professionals in the health system. Lithuania is improving workforce planning infrastructure step by step; however, despite recent major planning efforts, which resulted in gathering comprehensive cross-sectional data on physicians, nurses and midwives, timely information about the inflows and outflows of health professionals

**Table 7.1** Factors influencing mobility of Lithuanian health professionals

| Factor type | Components |
| --- | --- |
| Instigating | Low salaries, long working hours, perceived low prestige, unsatisfactory working conditions |
| Activating | *Personal*: better quality of life, desire for a life change, living experience abroad or relatives abroad |
| | *Job-related*: better professional opportunities, CPD, better working conditions and working environment, professional training abroad, professional and social recognition |
| Facilitating | Very active recruitment agencies (e.g. Norway, United Kingdom), attractive induction schemes (e.g. free language courses, social programmes, fewer barriers to start private practice, less bureaucracy) |
| Mitigating | Separation from family, language skills, settling down with family in a destination country |

*Sources*: Stankūnas, Lovkytė & Padaiga, 2004; Matulevičiūtė, 2007; Šmigelskas, Starkienė & Padaiga, 2007.

remains difficult to gather (Starkienė et al., 2011). Migration management and related policies remain relatively new and still lack political attention, which sometimes leads to non-effective retention policies (Padaiga, Pukas & Starkienė, 2011). This study aimed to improve understanding of migration motivations for Lithuanian health professionals and to provide new insights for further development of retention and recruitment policies.

## 7.2.2 Methodology

The study was conducted in three stages and applied quantitative as well as qualitative research methods. Ethical approval was received from the Lithuanian Bioethics Committee.

### Stage one: quantitative survey

An online survey was conducted (via the Monkey Survey website) based on a questionnaire in Lithuanian. The commonly developed survey questionnaire was designed on the basis of evidence from the 17 PROMeTHEUS case studies and literature review. The primary aim of the survey was to identify health professionals (medical doctors, dentists, nurses, physiotherapists, midwives) who could be further interviewed in focus groups. Notification about the survey was sent out to health professional associations (Lithuanian Doctor Union, Lithuanian Junior Doctors Association, Organization of Lithuanian Nursing Specialists, Lithuanian Dental Chamber and other health professional NGOs), Lithuanian communities in the EEA, via e-mails to personally known medical professionals and through other relevant web discussion forums. The survey was open for two months (October and November 2010) and resulted in a total of 1 130 responses. It took approximately 8–10 minutes for each participant to answer the questions, which were mainly focused on personal factors influencing their migration decisions – motivation to leave Lithuania, to commute between Lithuania and other countries, to return back – or reasons to stay and practise in Lithuania.

The survey also included questions on background demographic characteristics (e.g. age, gender, health profession, country of qualification, nationality). Participants who were willing to be followed up for a further interview were also asked for initial consent and contact details (name, telephone number and e-mail). The only criterion for selection for the interviews was personal and independent agreement of respondents to participate in focus group interviews. All of those who agreed were provided with the telephone numbers and e-mail addresses of the researchers for further information if needed.

### Stage two: focus groups

The aim of the focus groups was to reflect more systematically and subjectively the existing evidence on the migration factors that were raised in the online survey. The focus groups were conducted in January and February 2011. Before the interviews, the research group thoroughly explained the purpose of the research and that the interview would be recorded. In addition, notes were taken during the interviews so that interviewers could avoid any inaccurate interpretations. Participants were free to dismiss any questions that tended to constrain their responses because of internal conflict. A semi-structured methodology was used and participants were asked open-ended questions to get a better understanding of instigating, activating, facilitating and mitigating factors:

Why do they think of moving to another country?

Why do they stay in the country of origin?

Why have they come back to the country of origin?

Why have they left the country of origin?

During the focus group discussions (duration of approximately one hour), some probing questions were also asked in addition to the open-ended questions. This helped the interviewers to gain more knowledge of participants' emotional feelings and to resolve any possible misinterpretations. The aim was to find a balance between the open-ended questions, which could constrain emotional answers, and more direct or probing questions to examine the responses in more detail.

### Stage three: analysis of the collected material

The first step was to decide on the central category, which would represent the main theme of the research. Although this category evolved from research, it should be treated as an abstraction. In this study, the central category was the motivational factors to move to other countries or to stay and practise in Lithuania.

All the audiotaped discussions were transcribed. The findings were analysed thematically using a framework approach, which is a matrix-based method using a thematic framework to organize data according to main themes, concepts and categories. Each individual study is unique and has its own thematic framework, which consists of series of main topics, subdivided by series of related subtopics. The data obtained, which usually amounts to several pages, are then refined through familiarization and labelled (Ritchie & Spencer, 2004). The data were then compiled into the report by the Lithuanian research team.

### 7.2.3 Sample description

Sample sizes in qualitative studies are usually smaller than in quantitative studies. The concept or the experience under study is the unit of analysis; given that an individual person can generate hundreds or thousands of concepts, large samples are not necessarily needed to generate rich data sets. The exact number of individuals needed, and the number of interviews, depends on the goals and purpose of the study. In our case, respondents were chosen according to their availability and willingness to talk (Morse, 2000). However, the quality of a study is not impaired by a low sample size if that sample size is able to provide a full understanding of the topic.

Seven focus groups in total were conducted, six in Lithuania and one in Sweden. Sweden was chosen deliberately because of several personally known Lithuanian medical doctors working in Swedish health care institutions. Purposive sampling, where the sample is chosen on the basis of who the researchers think would be appropriate for the study, used the specialties of health professionals as detailed in Table 7.2.

**Table 7.2** Respondent sampling by medical profession and specialty

| Focus group | Specialization | Number of respondents |
|---|---|---|
| Medical doctors | Neurology, geriatrics, paediatrics, oncology, internal medicine, general practice, neonatology, dermatovenerology, cardiology, endocrinology, psychiatry, ophthalmology, otorhinolaryngology, rheumatology, surgery, maxillofacial surgery, interventional radiology | 29 |
| Nurses | Childcare, general care and mental health care. | 10 |
| Dentists | Prosthetic dentistry, general practice | 4 |

The purposive sampling was done in order to divide the focus groups according to profession, which it was hoped would encourage participants to feel more open and not so rigorous. All health professionals (except dentists, who were self-employed or employed in private clinics) were employed in public institutions – primary health care centres and hospitals.

The seven focus groups contained, respectively, six medical doctors, four nurses, ten medical doctors, four dentists, six nurses, nine medical doctors and four medical doctors. The last was conducted in Sweden. These focus groups (all professions included) represent almost all Lithuanian regions (Fig. 7.1) but it should be noted that the greatest proportion came from the largest Lithuanian cities, Vilnius, Kaunas and Klaipėda (18 medical doctors (75%); 10 nurses (100%), 4 dentists (100%)); one respondent was Lithuanian living

**Fig. 7.1** *Percentage of interviewed health professionals (all) by region*

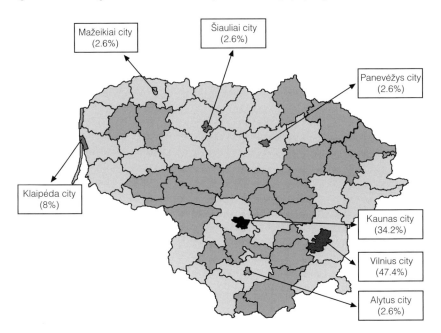

and practising in the United Kingdom (Scarborough region) and four were Lithuanians living and practising in Sweden (Gothenburg region).

Almost 78.6% of interviewed medical doctors (including emigrants) were women and all the nurses; interestingly, male dentists were more active and formed 60% of the dentist respondents. Respondents' ages varied from 35 to 62 years.

### 7.2.4 Limitations

Representativity for the groups was calculated using the statistical programme Statcalc, taking into account that in the year 2011 there were 12 293 medical doctors and 22 843 nurses practising in Lithuania. Even though the response rate to the web survey for medical doctors and nurses was representative (not for dentists), only a small percentage of medical doctors (29 out of 635 responses (4.6%)), nurses (10 out of 398 responses (2.5%)) and dentists (4 out of 45 responses (8.8%)) were positive about having an interview. Interviews were carried out in the two biggest cities (Vilnius and Kaunas) and reimbursement for catering, transportation and living expenses was offered for specialists from other Lithuanian areas. However, the focus groups did consist mainly of health professionals from these two biggest cities.

Research on motivational factors also carries certain methodological constraints. Motivation is an internal state that is difficult to measure, is usually very subjective and is influenced by many factors. To try to avoid these issues, "open" and non-structured questions were asked.

## 7.3 Results

### 7.3.1 Medical doctors

Interviews with medical doctors showed that most of the participants had had previous experience of either working or improving their professional qualifications abroad. Destination countries varied from Scandinavian countries to the United States, and even South American countries. Interview groups were very different and consist of doctors from a wide range of medical specialties (Table 7.2).

### *Instigating and activating factors*

#### *Remuneration*

When asked about the push factors to work abroad, interestingly, financial incentives did not play the major role. Financial incentives were closely interrelated with very human wishes and rights: that is, to have better living conditions. Nevertheless, participants complained that the work they were doing in Lithuania was undervalued and their wages were not proportional to the work they were doing, their qualifications and all the embedded legal requirements:

> …the only field among other sectors is medicine, where financial benefits does not coincide with the work we do. And … Hard to admit but this is tolerated in our country.

Medical doctors felt they were undervalued compared with the financial situation for hospital administration. They named it as "*social injustice*" when hospital directors received five or even ten times bigger salaries and other financial benefits. Respondents also identified very big financial gaps between them and, for example, lawyers for the work they do and for the competencies it requires:

> Could you show us a lawyer that had for example as a surgeon make a decision in 10 minutes or half an hour? … and why their salaries differ so much?

Some participants identified the same problem between medical doctors and medical residents:

> their scholarship is about 1 200 litas (about €350) and plus their salary is 900 litas (about €260). Is it fair that they get more than medical doctor with 30 years experience?

A few, particularly older health professionals, said that they missed the additional incentives that were provided based on professional categories (an earlier scheme where medical doctors had special professional levels according to their competencies and working experience, and received additional pay for this, was abandoned) and did not like unified holidays (holiday terms used to be differentiated according to specialties).

*Perceived low prestige*

Even though the majority of the participants were not only driven by financial incentives, the feeling of depreciation of their profession could be felt in all three interviews. The story of one medical doctor best illustrates it:

> English medical doctors went on strike. They went on strike in order to increase their salaries. But you know what their motive was? To secure prestige of their profession. And what is situation here, if you get a housemaid's salary, you are treated by the public or managers correspondingly.

*Working conditions and working environment*

Another push factor that was strongly stressed by the respondents was working conditions. Some of the respondents also complained about their working environment:

> I don't even have a place to change my clothes, I work and eat and take rest in my cabinet which is just 10 square metres.

Most of the participants indicated that, apart from medical work, the economic crisis had also imposed financial issues such as limitations for prescriptions of reimbursable medicines or expensive tests: "*every quarter we get reports and if we exceed our quotas we can be obliged to pay from our own pocket*". They also complained about the imposition of other functions such as unnecessary paperwork, social work and psychological help. This clearly became another push factor – absence of teamwork. "*Doctors duty is to treat the patients, but for now our profession is totally distorted …*" stated all participants. Interviews revealed that medical doctors also lacked division of work among themselves and with other health professions:

> If I have to treat a patient with stroke, my duty is just to stabilize his condition from i.e. neurological side, but it should not be my duty to take care of his rehabilitation or further nursing services …

Another factor closely interrelated with intentions to leave was heavy workloads. Medical doctors experienced physiological and psychological burnt-out through having multiple jobs (to earn more money) and having large numbers of patients. Such situations create a lot of stress, for health professionals and patients, with patients sometimes not receiving high-quality service because of lack of time:

> ... unfortunately, we have sometimes just ten to fifteen minutes to examine a patient because I need to do paper or other work. Imagine – during six hours I have to examine forty patients ...

All these push factors can be combined into one issue: lack of up-to-date management-based work organization in Lithuania's health system.

*Better professional opportunities*

Lack of diagnostic or treatment standards was also mentioned as a factor enhancing intentions to leave. Most of the medical doctors felt unsafe because choice of treatment is solely based on their judgement and competence, and, of course, treatment results are their responsibility. If a professional mistake or health disorder occurs, the patient's rights are secured by the Law on the Rights of Patients and Compensation for the Damage to their Health (Seimas of the Republic of Lithuania, 1996). In the absence of the standards that are usually adopted individually by each health care institution, a medical doctor does not have any legal tools for defence. One specialist introduced a term that describes very well how this situation is addressed and the effects of it:

> we develop a defensive medical system, we do not do what we are supposed to do, but everything in order to defend ourselves from administration, patient, prosecutor, patient funds, etc.

Some respondents also mentioned that relations between health professionals and patients had also changed, with changes in patients' attitudes, expectations, mentality and behaviour:

> And to work ten or fifteen years ago for me it was significantly easier than now. That is because relations with patients that come for examinations, their attitude to you, to our mentality has changed a lot.

*Continuous professional training*

Continuous educational and professional training was also a definite push factor to go abroad, although this was a very interesting topic with no clear boundaries. One participant clearly stated that the system of health care institutions did not invest in their professionals. It might seem too unbelievable but CPD barriers exist.

> What does Lithuania? Nothing. How can we go and make scientific presentations, if we do not have any conditions for doing research, inordinate

working conditions. Our scientific activities are just re-copying of what has already been found and trialled.

One medical doctor was even more radical and defined this as total "*educational degradation*" because the obligatory training (needed for prolongation of the licence in Lithuania) was led by academics who had lectured the same things for 20 or even more years and were not keen to keep up with new developments. When it was suggested that the participants might choose professional training abroad, the answer was simple and short: "… *my financial status does not allow me to do this*".

*Health care system management*

Interviews also revealed another significant push factor – health care and hospital management systems. Respondents clearly stated that the Lithuanian health care system awarded hospital administrations the right to manage autocratically. Most complained that practically it was impossible to have any constructive dialogue with their administration and expressed a feeling of being neglected:

> I went to my director to ask for higher salary and you know what the outcome was? He instructed a special commission to check my quality of work.

> administration just cares how to secure their posts and they do not want to go into dialogue with you because they just do not care about you …

Respondents were unanimous in saying that professionalism and good management skills are still some kind of taboo in Lithuania and also gave very distinct answers why:

> hospital managers should not be interlinked with political parties and should not have any binding obligations to them …

Interviews disclosed that managers' rotation should and even must be obligatory so that they are not "… *life sentenced in their posts*".

**Corruption**

Last but not least, perceived corruption in the health system was a push factor. Most respondents indicated that this phenomenon existed in all levels – starting from higher education to the highest levels of health system administration. One very perseptive participant disclosed:

> … when I tried to develop a new high technology in Lithuania, I got such a neglective attitude from public institutions taking care of EU funding, that I understood – it is impossible to get in this the so-called monopoly without corruption.

At first glance, it may seem a very significant complaint; however, it was more like a protest against the current health system management:

> I have enough money to eat, but as for today I am ready to close everything I have (business) and emigrate because corruption kills every young person in Lithuania, who are public-spirited and love their country and believe in its future.

### *Mitigating factors*

As we can see, medical doctors have many complaints about the functioning of the Lithuanian health system, its organization and its management, but they also revealed what kept them practising in Lithuania. Most indicated family reasons, social status, career chosen, age, private business, fear of being an "outlander", absence of attractive proposals, insufficient language skills, discomfort of setting up a new life, and finding friends. However, some factors were more surprising. Several disclosed that it would be difficult to get a medical doctor's position abroad (inadequacy with their health system standards) and also to integrate themselves in different systems. Nevertheless, the most touching factor was motherland love:

> … I would better be a small stone, but in my own garden …

> how can I leave my culture, all traditions, all holidays. I do not want to lose this …

### *Core factors keeping medical doctors at home*

Before ending the interviews we asked the participants to recommend three main priorities that would improve the current situation. Even though more than three recommendations were mentioned, the most significant were:

- health reform should be led by professionals, using up-to-date managerial and evidence-based skills but not political party motivations, and ensure:
  - decentralization of health system reform and development of competitive health care services,
  - total removal of any appearance of corruption,
  - time-limited contracts of health system administrators, and
  - increase in health system financing;
- enhance the evidence-based work organization methods through:
  - developing standards that ensure not only duties, but also health professional and, of course, patient rights and quality of health care services,

- legitimating normal workloads and working conditions to ensure health professionals' social economic safety and psychological comfort,

- improving teamwork methodology and reducing the administrative burden for health professionals, and

- enhancing collective agreements, which would lead to normal dialogues and discussions with administration;

• increase health professions' prestige in society; and

• reform the educational system in the way it meets the future demand and supply model.

### 7.3.2 Medical doctors (emigrants)

The group of medical doctors who have been practising abroad was very varied, including doctors who left Lithuania 20 years previously plus doctors who had been practising in Sweden or the United Kingdom for only a few years.

#### Instigating and activating factors

##### Remuneration

According to the participants, the two decades of Lithuanian independence had introduced only minor changes in health system development. Almost all participants disclosed that the main motivational factor to come and work abroad was financial incentives: "*In 1993 it was impossible to 'survive' from my financial benefits*" or "*I have waited 20 years for changes in our health system, but my social position and financial status have not improved*". Participants clearly indicated that social protection (e.g. health insurance, unemployment insurance or pension schemes) for themselves and their families motivated them to work in their foreign country because they were ensured of: "*…safe tomorrow*" or "*First time in my life I have such a good feeling of being happy and satisfied and safe…*"

##### Personal factors

Just one medical doctor disclosed that her motivational factor was family reasons (marriage to a Swedish partner).

##### Health care system management

Interestingly, one participant who had emigrated recently disclosed that her professional life in Lithuania was one of constant conflict, which emerged from (1) constant "neglective" managers' attitude, "*they do hear, but do not listen …*"; (2) constant shortage of medical resources, "*I could not reanimate a patient because we did not have a defibrillator in our department ..."* or *"I cannot perform more diagnostic examinations than indicated by State Patient Fund because it will be not reimbursed"*; (3) psychological stress, knowing that even with all educational abilities it is not possible to provide high-quality health care services, *"I am thankful to this country [host country] because it values me as a medical doctor, I am sure my country (Lithuania) would not do so ..."* or *"health profession in Lithuania is totally distorted ... we cannot use our specialized knowledge because we have to be neurologist, rehabilitologist and etc. at the same time ..."*.

### Profession-related factors

Participants also noted that in Sweden health professionals had not only duties but also rights. They were not so strictly embedded by legal acts on the rights of patients and compensation for damage to their health because the Swedish attitude on medical faults is based not on how to punish the health professional but to how to make sure that this failure would not happen again. However, in Lithuania they felt as if they were acrobats walking on the rope:

> I was always threatened by my boss that they will lay damages from me if a patient sues me for any failure I could make.

### Mitigating factors

However, the emigrant's fate is not that easy. The feeling of being the "outlander" was common for almost all participants: not professionally as many health professionals are emigrants, *"in many hospitals it is a melting pot consisting of Germans, Greeks, Lithuanians, Bulgarians, Indians, etc."* but in daily life with almost all stating *"You have to be Sweden-born if you want to be a member of the club or at least have a Swedish partner"*.

### Facilitating factors

This feeling of being an outlander did not dwarf their willingness to work abroad:

> I think I am like Lithuanian ambassador ... I do proclamate my country ... and I am proud of that, but it would be ideal to work here and live in Lithuania

> you know it was amazing, but when I started working the first thing I was asked if I need any language courses and was introduced to the commune where I got all the necessary legal information for the settlement and ... believe me ... no bureaucracy at all.

### Core factors needed for emigrants to return to Lithuania

Before concluding the interview, participants were asked what needs to be changed in Lithuania in order for them to return. Their key recommendations included:

- to ensure adequate financial incentives and supplant informal patient out-of-pocket payments, accompanied with protectionism;

- to ensure that health system reform develops not only hospital infrastructure but also a public role in health prevention, promotion and overall attitude to health; and

- to change stagnated management systems and enhance a collaboration between health professionals and their managers through teamwork.

### 7.3.3 Nurses

Analysis of the interview revealed that five nurses had only intentions to leave, three had made a definite decision to move abroad and two were returnees who came back to Lithuania for family reasons. Destination countries mainly were the United Kingdom, Germany and Norway.

### Instigating and facilitating factors

*Heavy workloads, lack of teamwork and low financial benefits*

The participants clearly indicated that they were dissatisfied with the heavy and excessive workload that was metaphorically expressed as: "*oppression at work*" or "*majority of nurses suffers from back aches or other physical disabilities after working 20–25 years*". Respondents mentioned that the term teamwork is still uncommon among department or hospital managers and they usually have to perform tasks that definitely could be redistributed among other staff. This included a lot of paper work plus tasks such as catering and cleaning. For this reason they fearlessly complained that their health care services are unable to provide high quality because of the physical load (rather the large number of patients) and work intensity:

> Due to such workload intensiveness, to constant running from one place to another, we provide a health care service, however, it is not somehow finished … not always of high quality.

This factor was, undoubtedly, closely related to financial incentives, mainly relevant payment schemes for the work carried out. All felt financially undervalued, mentioning things such as "*low social guarantees*", "*Quality of life is low here*". One said:

My friend who works abroad laughs at me by saying "hey look, I earn such amount per month and you have to work half a year". I am 55 and I cannot afford to spend my holidays near the Baltic Sea in Curonian Spit[1].

The majority of participants also claimed that nurses desired graduated payment schemes, according to education level, work experience and work results, that could motivate them.

*Poor continuous professional training*

There are no motivations for continuing professional training as this is not reflected by better managerial or financial evaluation for the individual:

Yes, I did finish my master studies in nursing. So what? My salary increased by €20, but I paid for my studies a rather bigger amount. What is my motive?

This was supported by the opinion that many nursing specialists lack career pathways.

*Professional recognition*

Data analysis revealed that the nurses saw a lack of professional status in their daily work. They felt they could be more autonomous, while taking decisions according to their competencies and educational level. They felt they were competent enough to prescribe nursing medical devices or even prolonged prescribed medicines: "*I know that is very common in the Scandinavian countries*". Interestingly, they linked this with the fact that medical doctors were afraid to give away the services, even if those services did not require their competence, because of the loss of informal out-of-pocket payments. It could not be concluded that nurses desired these out-of-pocket payments, but dissatisfaction could be observed:

Why they [medical doctors] can take it and we cannot? It is an inequality in my opinion, why somebody is higher than me, because he/she can do something more than me….

*Irrelevant management*

Another very important motivational factor that was disclosed during the interviews was relations with medical doctors and, of course, their managers. Most of the nurses felt a lack of respect, which presumably comes from the time spent at medical studies:

1 The Curonian Spit is a UNESCO World Natural Heritage Site on the coast of the Baltic. It is a strip of land which separates the sea from the Curonian Lagoon.

> As regards nursing university studies, you do not know how sceptical medical doctors are. My personal experience … we nurses are usually medical doctors' maids.

Nurses having contacts with mental patients also indicated insecurity at work compared with medical doctors. Patients are usually unstable and aggressive and, *"it is not a secret that we are offended by them quite often …"*. When asked if they have complained about this, the answer was very short and simple: *"If you are not satisfied, there is a long queue waiting for your place …"*. Poor management also affected their working conditions, particularly with regard to a lack of medical devices. Disposable medical devices, of course not things like syringes, are sometimes used a few times, which causes health risks for nurses or patients:

> one day we economize this, another day this. Why do I have to use rubber gloves more than once …?

### Mitigating factors

When participants were asked what makes them stay or return (two of the participants were returnees) to work in Lithuania, most responses were similar. They indicated family reasons such as under-age children, ill parents, fear of being "outlanders", ongoing higher education studies (master studies), insufficient language skills, discomfort of settling into new life, finding friends, and so on.

### Facilitating factors

Good career opportunities were clearly a facilitating factor. A few participants clearly declared that there were several very active recruitment agencies offering good working conditions and, of course, remuneration in Lithuania:

> …they offer about €1 200 a month, give free transportation and accommodation, offer language course … you just need to pay a percentage from your salary (did not indicate) to them.

One participant also indicated that some EU countries give direct proposals to nursing students:

> Just imagine, they offer you free studies in universities, pay for language courses and give you an €800 scholarship … how they can resist? Answer is simple – they just leave if get such an opportunity.

### Core factors keeping nurses at home

Before ending the interviews, the participants were asked to recommend three main priorities from the political perspective that could keep them at home. Messages they wanted to send were:

- enhanced professional recognition and professional respect;

- sufficient financial incentives, including sufficient socioeconomic guarantees, relevant workloads, improved working conditions and teamwork; and

- continuous and strategic health system reform, with special attention paid to hospital management, investment in health professionals' education and continuous training.

### 7.3.4 Dentists

The study demonstrated that three of the four dentists had experienced either working or fellowship abroad. The main countries that temporarily received Lithuanian dentists were Sweden and the United Kingdom.

#### *Instigating and activating factors*

*Financial benefits*

One of the factors that impacted dentists' decisions was financial incentives as most of them were self-employed or working in private clinics. A couple of dentists commented on financial security, for example:

> We did not see any perspective (financial revenues), were not sure what will happen tomorrow, after tomorrow or after the week, a year. The same situation is today. But today at least we have more patients what increased our revenues.

The interview clearly revealed that this uncertainty, particularly in terms of the future, intensified the wish to work abroad: "*Whatever you say, financial background is my security guarantee*".

*Management imperfection*

Analysis of interviews also showed that management imperfection, either at the highest level (ministerial) or at a hospital level, was a threat. Interviewed dentists were unanimous in saying that they saw a large communication gap between ordinary health professionals and managers:

> They do not hear. Indeed, managers' goal is to keep the ownership of their posts.

> People that surround them are more managing by the help of moral force, but not according to any kind of agreements between staff, good atmosphere.

The interview data clearly revealed that hospital administration was in a "neglectful position" with regard to staff: "*Disrespect, if you are lower in position, you have to do everything I say*". For dentists working in the public sector, this factor was accompanied by insufficient health system financing and continuous educational training and poor availability of medical resources. Another managerial problem was high workloads, which were usually not reflected in financial bonuses. Professionals working in the public sector have undefined working hours and, as they say, managers find various ways to manipulate this situation.

> My working hours are till 11:30 … But I have to stay longer because a patient was hospitalized at 12:00. I have to spend over hours, otherwise I will get a disciplinary punishment….

*Changing attitude in society*

During the interview, dentists also identified a problem of negative aspects of globalization. It is of course a great challenge, but many core personal and social values are just flattened out: "*Our community is being influenced by commercialized environment, where moral values do not practically play a significant role*". This was mostly not seen as an optional feature for many participants and some were motivated by this to think about moving abroad. Another motivational factor that attracted dentists to working abroad was warm relations between professional and patient:

> I feel satisfied when patients say thank you. They are thankful to you for the services … and you feel even more satisfaction that you are a qualified doctor, but not the one who pump money from the patient funds.

### Mitigating factors

The factors encouraging dentists to stay in Lithuania were the working situation (more stable job contracts in Lithuania) and belief in the country's development vision.

When returners were asked why they have returned to Lithuania, the responses varied. Some respondents said they did not want to keep their families abroad (e.g. United Kingdom) for an understandable reason: "*This is a foreign country and I do not want to keep them as outlanders*". While countries such as Sweden were identified as being ideal for family life as regards socioeconomic guarantees, and this was mentioned as a partial facilitating factor, personal drivers were more important: "What about friends? How to spend my free time? They have something special … attraction". Another factor that motivated return was commitment to a long-term working contract. Dentists did not want to be tied up professionally and personally for one year contracts abroad.

### Core factors keeping dentists at home

Before ending the interviews, the participants were asked to recommend three things from the political perspective that could keep them at home. A very clear, and practically unanimous, message was sent:

- prompt and improved health system management (either at government or hospital level) reform with special attention paid to hospital managers' rotation and decreased administrative burden;

- relevant workloads interconnected with sufficient financial incentives, including other socioeconomic guarantees; and

- enhance investment in health professionals' education and continuous training.

## 7.4 Scope for policy interventions

There were a number of significant findings from this study that provide indications for areas of policy response that would encourage the retention and return of health professionals. Some important factors appeared to be encompassed by a sense of working pride of the health professional. The findings from the focus groups revealed that almost all health professionals have a considerable pride and satisfaction that they are health professionals and use the skills they had learnt daily. Against this positive side, many negative factors influencing their daily and work life were disclosed.

Many health professionals, particularly nurses, cited financial incentives (in terms of relevant salary, "safe and guaranteed tomorrow" or other allowances) that compared with their competences and workload. They expressed a feeling that they were undervalued for their hard and highly skilled work. However, during the interview, almost all agreed that financial incentives alone would not ensure their satisfaction – it should be integrated with other incentives, discussed below.

Health system – and at a lower level hospital – management appeared to be the second largest negative factor, particularly among medical doctors and dentists. Many of them indicated the problems and even "disabilities" of the ongoing Lithuanian health reforms. Some even called it adverse to the daily work of health professionals. Examples provided included not standardized competencies, irrelevant workload and inadequate hospital leadership skills; corruption at all health system levels was not the least complaint. Interestingly, medical doctors were dissatisfied with the implemented legal acts regarding patient safety. They stated that these legal acts empowered only the patients and the people connected with them, and created many constraints for their daily work. Medical doctors indicated that they felt unsafe and infringed because of possible financial penalties in the case of any after-treatment complications or other complaints.

Resource availability was also a considerable motivating factor for medical doctors and nurses (not dentists, perhaps because they work mostly in the private sector). Medical doctors complained that they could not make full use of advanced technologies for diagnostics and treatment. Nurses said that they had to use unsafe medical equipment, such as unprotected syringes. These comments do not mean that Lithuania does not invest in advanced technologies (which is one of the health system reform priorities) or have high-technology medical equipment. It can best be described as a limited amount of services that are reimbursed by the State Patient Fund because of budget cut-offs during the financial crisis.

Personal recognition from managers or hospital directors was also seen as a big motivator for medical doctors and nurses, and for dentists working in the public sector. Interestingly, managerial antagonism was not unusual in most working environments. A lot of managers, according to the participants, would mostly ignore requests for bigger salaries, better resource availability or any other incentives, and would not even start discussions. Some of the nurses felt regret because they did not always feel valued and supported by medical doctors. Last, but not least, those nurses implied that to some extent they were specialists of a "second class" because they do not have equal opportunities with regard to education (mostly colleges not universities) or CPD. Lithuania has made huge investments in infrastructure since 2004 with the help of EU structural funds; however, a lot more is still needed. This was highlighted by all the health professionals working in the public sector.

These motivating factors are ones that can be influenced by politicians, policy-makers at national, regional and district levels, hospital directors and managers and, of course, the medical community themselves. All levels need to collaborate and take part in political or managerial decision-making processes in order to change health professionals' intentions or decisions to work abroad and to take very urgent decisions for elaborating retention and "return" policies.

However, the interviews also revealed several motivational factors that are of a personal nature and therefore cannot be influenced by policy-makers or managers. One promising young medical doctor left Lithuania for family reasons (husband of foreign nationality) and settled in as a highly skilled health professional elsewhere. For others, particularly medical doctors, the reasons to stay were children and, of course, very close ties with family and friends. Some of the respondents could not move abroad because of needing to care for elderly family members. Researchers were also surprised about the expression of participants' strong motherland love as a factor to stay and practise in their home country.

## 7.5 Conclusions

This study has provided new insights into how to develop more efficient retention policies, and this was clearly indicated by the willingness of the focus group participants when they were asked to give recommendations for politicians and other decision-makers.

Investment in health human resources is an essential prerequisite for delivery and implementation of health care services and other related activities. In the light of financial instability it is obvious that a country needs to assess accurately its current health human resources and to address domestic shortages with respect not only to quantitative indicators but also to qualitative ones. With an ageing population, there is a need to expand the spectrum of health care services and, therefore, to have a sufficient number of active specialists. For Lithuania, this is why it is very important to find effective ways to retain our health professionals in our domestic markets and to motivate them to provide high-quality and accessible health care services for all. Motivational factors for health professionals are undoubtedly diverse; however, in Lithuania, financial incentives and management issues are the main factors. It is important to note that financial incentives alone are not sufficient to keep our health professionals in the domestic market. Other factors, such as public recognition, available resources (e.g. advanced technologies) and appropriate infrastructure, can also help to retain health professionals. It should be emphasized that retention strategies should include very clear career models associated with relevant income levels; a proper and convenient working environment, with attention to safety at work; and a proper and bearable workload. Favourable conditions for CPD and systematic changes in health system management will also be very effective.

Motivational factors usually vary over time, and longitudinal research should be conducted to identify these changes. Capturing reality is not easy, although research around the motivational factors for human health resources must remain a priority.

## References

Buchan J (2007). *Health worker migration in Europe: policy issues and options*. London, HLSP Institute (Technical Approach Paper) (http://www.hlsp.org/ LinkClick.aspx?fileticket=SM55vQDY0bA%3D&tabid=1702&mid=3361, accessed 2 January 2014).

Buchan J et al. (2006). Internationally recruited nurses in London: a survey of career paths and plans. *Human Resources for Health*, 4:14.

de Veer A, den Ouden DJ, Francke A (2004). Experiences of foreign European nurses in the Netherlands. *Health Policy*, 68(1):55–61.

Dumont JC, Zurn P (2007). Immigrant health workers in OECD countries in the broader context of highly skilled migration. In OECD, ed. *International migration outlook,* 2nd edn. Paris, Organisation for Economic Co-operation and Development:161–228.

Matulevičiūtė E (2007). *Nurses' intentions to work abroad* [thesis]. Kaunas, Kaunas University of Medicine.

Morse J (2000). Determining sample size. *Qualitative Health Research*, 10(1): 3–5.

Padaiga Ž, Pukas M, Starkienė L (2011). Awareness, planning and retention: Lithuania's approach to managing health professional mobility. In Wismar M et al., eds. *Health professional mobility and health systems. Evidence from 17 European countries.* Copenhagen, WHO Regional Office for Europe on behalf of the European Observatory on Health Systems and Policies:395–418.

Pukas M (2008). *Lithuanian health-care professionals migration study* [thesis]. Kaunas, Kaunas University of Medicine.

Ritchie J, Spencer L (2004). Qualitative data analysis: the call for transparency. *Building Research Capacity*, 7:2–4 (http://www.tlrp.org/rcbn/capacity/Journal/issue7.pdf, accessed 2 January 2014).

Seimas of the Republic of Lithuania (1996). Law on the rights of patients and compensation for the damage to their health. *Official Gazette*, 102-2317, 145-6425 (http://www3.lrs.lt/pls/inter3/dokpaieska.showdoc_l?p_id=384290, accessed 2 January 2014).

Šmigelskas K, Starkienė L, Padaiga Ž (2007). Do Lithuanian pharmacists intend to migrate? *Journal of Ethnic and Migration Studies*, 33(3):501–509.

Stankūnas M, Lovkytė L, Padaiga Ž (2004). The survey of Lithuanian physicians and medical residents regarding possible migration to the European Union. *Medicina (Kaunas)*, 40(1):68–74 [in Lithuanian].

Starkienė L et al. (2011). Collection of data for purposes of human resources for health planning: questions and practical examples. *Sveikatos Politika ir Valdymas*, 568:37–49 [in Lithuanian].

# Chapter 8

# Motivations and experience of health professionals who migrate to the United Kingdom from other EU Member countries

*Ruth Young, Charlotte Humphrey and Anne Marie Rafferty*

## 8.1 Introduction

Within the broad picture of health professional migration, the United Kingdom has been characterized primarily as a destination country, although some have suggested that it may also serve as an intermediate stepping stone to other English-speaking countries, particularly the United States (Young et al., 2003; Ball & Pike, 2004; Travis, 2009). Currently, more than one in three medical doctors, one in ten nurses and midwives and one in four dentists registered in the United Kingdom obtained their initial professional qualifications abroad (Young, Weir & Buchan, 2010b). The vast majority of these have come from world regions outside Europe. In fact, since the 1950s when significant health professional migration to the United Kingdom first began, migration patterns have largely reflected old colonial ties, particularly with South Asia, Africa and Australia/New Zealand (Aiken & Buchan, 2004; Buchan & Rafferty, 2004; Hann, Sibbald & Young, 2008). However, the relatively smaller share of health professionals migrating from Europe – primarily from the EU but also the wider EEA – has grown in recent years. This increase has been fuelled in part by international recruitment campaigns initiated by the British Government between 2000 and 2006, which targeted doctors, nurses and midwives, dentists and pharmacists in several European countries (Young et al., 2008a, 2010a). In the same period, immigrant health professionals were also recruited by health and social care providers in the independent sector[1] (Smith et al., 2006). The EU enlargements in 2004 and 2007 provided a further source of new migration. By 2008 alone, 9% of all medical doctors registered in the United Kingdom and 19% of new medical registrants came from the EEA, principally EU Member States. For nurses and midwives, the equivalent figures were 1% and 6%, respectively, and for dentists it was as much as 15% and 36%, respectively (Young, 2011; General Dental Council, unpublished data, 2009). The EU15 still accounts for most of the EEA-qualified health professionals registered in the United Kingdom, but numbers from the EU12 are rapidly catching up (European Migration Network, 2006; Pollard, Latore & Sriskandarajah, 2008). Among newly registered nurses/midwives in 2008, for example, more than twice as many came from EU12 as from EU15 countries (Young, 2011).

The right to free movement within the EU means that there is less control over this migration than migration from other sources. Consequently, changes in EU-linked migration flows are felt to pose particular challenges for United Kingdom workforce planning. There are also concerns about the potential negative impacts on source countries of losing professionally qualified staff under circumstances that are difficult to predict. From a human resource management view too, there are questions both about how best to support European health professionals to integrate into the United Kingdom health system and how to encourage potential migrants to stay in their countries of origin and/or to return after a period abroad. Against this background of improving information to aid workforce planning and support/development both in receiver and source countries, there is a need to improve understanding of not only the motivations and drivers that lead individual health professionals from EU Member States to move in the first place but also the factors that affect their subsequent decisions to remain, return to their countries of origin or move on elsewhere.

Factors found in previous research to influence decisions to migrate to the United Kingdom are summarized in Table 8.1. It is not clear how significant the various factors are for European health professional migration, as distinct from international migration from further afield, since previous United Kingdom research has generally focused on migrants from outside Europe (e.g. doctors from India, nurses from the Philippines). Those studies that exist of the migration motivations of European health professionals moving

---

1 Independent sector is used in the United Kingdom as an umbrella term for private, voluntary and non-profit-making health and social care organizations.

**Table 8.1** Factors attracting health professionals to the United Kingdom

| Drivers | Factors |
| --- | --- |
| *Macro-level* | National economic and sociopolitical factors that exert influence across all international labour markets and also affect the health system dynamics relevant to health professionals |
| Economic | Prospect of improved standard of living for self/family, means to remit income to country of origin |
| Health system | Un/underemployment amongst health professionals in home country, poor salaries and working conditions in health sector in home country |
| Political | Political instability in home country versus stability in United Kingdom |
| *Meso-level* | Profession-specific factors (e.g. education/training, job conditions) that frame perceived opportunities in a given occupational sector |
| Progression opportunities | Shortage of postgraduate training opportunities and/or posts in particular specialty/profession in home country |
| Additional skills | Experience working in different system rather than learning from theory, learn to use state-of-the-art equipment, broaden knowledge |
| Career development | Professional challenge associated with different ways of working, reputation and status of United Kingdom system, organization or clinical field, opportunities for involvement in research and/or general networking |
| *Micro-level* | Individual circumstances and attitudes through which macro- and meso-level drivers are viewed but which also influence migration decision-making in their own right |
| Family/social network | Perceived better quality of life for family, desire to give children quality education and cultural experience, partner decision to work in the United Kingdom, choices possible within context of social/migrant networks in the United Kingdom |
| Personal fulfilment | Desire for a life change/excitement, stage in career or life cycle (opportunities at a particular point), experience a different culture, accessing a gateway to Europe |
| Language skills | Desire to improve own/family's English language proficiency, opportunity for children to learn/practise English, English first language, so United Kingdom easier country to work in |
| Opportunity window | One-off opportunity provided by the United Kingdom's former policy of active international recruitment |
| United Kingdom policy | Responsive to positive recruitment strategy from United Kingdom Government |
| Recruitment incentives | United Kingdom market position relative to other countries: barriers to/ease of entry, nature of support provided at recruitment stage |
| Migration stepping stone | Work in United Kingdom attractive as potential stage in onward migration, primarily to the United States |

*Source*: Young, 2011.

to the United Kingdom have also largely looked on a single-country basis at particular recruitment campaigns and/or particular professional groups; they have not compared mobile health professionals from Europe as a whole (Pitts et al., 1998; Bellingham, 2001; Ballard, Robinson & Laurence, 2004; Buchan, 2004; Simmgen, 2004; Wang, 2007). Moreover, little is known about how the different factors combine and interact to influence individual decisions about migration. There is some indication that the relative salience and significance of the different factors is likely to vary for different combinations of source country, professional specialty and demographic characteristics, such as gender, age and career stage (Buchan et al., 2006). However, in the absence of detailed direct evidence about the experience of EU health professionals who choose to migrate to the United Kingdom, the nature of this variation remains unclear.

### 8.1.1 Study aim

The exploratory study whose findings are reported here was undertaken as part of the EU-funded project PROMeTHEUS (Wismar et al., 2011). The aim was to gain insights into the initial motivations of health professionals from across the European region who migrated to the United Kingdom and their experiences of the process of migration. This would allow exploration of how these and other factors influenced subsequent decisions to remain, return home or move on elsewhere. More specifically, the study explored how far the macro-, meso- and micro-drivers identified as encouraging health professional migration to the United Kingdom (Table 8.1) are salient to EU-qualified individuals, and how the various factors interact in terms of instigating, activating, facilitating and/or mitigating for or against the migration process in the European context. The analytical categories of instigating, activating, facilitating and mitigating factors were identified as part of an earlier stage of the PROMeTHEUS project. A further aim was to investigate potential similarities/differences in decision-making between professional groups and source countries, for example in the EU15 and EU12.

## 8.2 Methods

### 8.2.1 Overall design

The United Kingdom was selected to represent a major migration destination country within the PROMeTHEUS study because it receives such a large number of health workers from Europe and it was expected to locate professionals from the widest possible variety of source countries. The groups targeted were medical doctors, nurses, midwives, dentists and physiotherapists who migrated to the United Kingdom at any point in the previous 10 years or more. These groups were chosen because they are the professional groups with greatest incidence of migration to the United Kingdom in number terms from countries within Europe (Young et al., 2010a; Young, 2011). The lengthy timescale was in order to capture both individuals recruited as part of the then British Government's policy of international recruitment, from 2000–2006, and those who have since moved to the United Kingdom "under their own steam". As in Germany and Lithuania, an initial survey instrument was used to locate study participants. This was administered online through an established web provider, potential respondents being alerted via the e-mail networks, web discussion forums, internet blogs and newsletters of relevant professional registration bodies, trade unions and country-specific peer support groups for European health professionals in the United Kingdom. Embassies of EU Member States and a small number of NHS Trusts and Medical Deaneries (employer/educational organizations) were also contacted and asked to forward information about the study to relevant individuals.

Given the exploratory nature of the study, the survey was always intended to be used principally as a screening instrument to locate a qualitative interview sample. The survey, therefore, asked for key demographic details (age, gender, health profession, current employment, country of qualification, nationality and birth country), experiences of migration, reasons why respondents left the country where they originally qualified and why they moved to the United Kingdom. This design was based on evidence of key factors influencing migration decision-making gained from literature reviews undertaken for the earlier, case study phase of the PROMeTHEUS project (Wismar et al., 2011). The survey answers were then used to select an interview sample stratified in order that similarities and differences across the various groups could be explored in more detail. Specifically, the interview sample was stratified to cover the range of target professional groups, demographic characteristics, origin countries, experience of and motivations for migration.

### 8.2.2 Interview sample

The survey elicited 236 responses, from which 42 were interviewed either face to face or by telephone between January and April 2011. The interview sample comprised 16 medical doctors (from Germany, Italy, the Netherlands, Poland, Portugal and Spain), 13 nurses (from Austria, Bulgaria, Croatia, Cyprus, Finland, France, Germany, Greece and Romania), six dentists (from Italy, Portugal, Romania and Sweden), four physiotherapists (from Germany, the Netherlands and Malta), and three midwives (from Latvia, Lithuania and Poland). Twenty-eight of the sample were from EU15 countries, 12 were from EU12 countries and one from an EU candidate country. One-third of the respondents had been in the United Kingdom for less than five years, one-third between five and ten years, and one-third for ten years or more. Some were working in the NHS, some in the private or voluntary health sector and some had academic posts in universities. A few had not found health professional employment in the United Kingdom. Four people were interviewed by telephone in their countries of origin, having temporarily or permanently returned home, but the great majority of respondents were still in the United Kingdom at the time of interview and either intending to stay or were uncertain about their future plans. A limitation of the study is, therefore, that we were able to find out relatively little about the views and experiences of health professionals who migrate to the United Kingdom and then choose not to remain.

### 8.2.3 Data collection and analysis

The interviews were semi-structured, focusing on the motivations and drivers that led individual health professionals to move to the United Kingdom, and on the factors that had affected their subsequent decisions to remain, return to their countries of origin or move on elsewhere. The topic guide allowed for an exploration of the influence of the sorts of macro-, meso- and micro-level migration factors identified in Table 8.1, plus how those actually work in terms of influencing an individual migrant's thinking at the different (instigating, activating, facilitating, mitigating) stages of the migration decision-making process. All of the interviews were recorded and transcribed in full, the transcripts being analysed using the framework approach (Ritchie & Spencer, 1994).

The findings for each respondent were grouped by stage of migration: first, the process of leaving their country of origin and moving to the United Kingdom and, second, their experiences since arriving in the United Kingdom and future plans. Decisions at the first stage were examined in terms of instigating factors (macro-, meso- and micro-level reasons for wanting to leave the country of origin and/or reasons to favour the United Kingdom as a destination) and activating and facilitating factors (macro-, meso- and micro-level) that had precipitated the actual decision to move or enabled the initial process of migration. Experiences after arrival were analysed in terms of factors that helped or hampered the process of getting established professionally and personally in the United Kingdom and factors that influenced plans to stay or return. Throughout the analysis, we looked out for variation between different groups of respondents in terms of profession, country of origin, life stage and other demographic factors. Where there were evident differences between particular groups, these are described below.

## 8.3 Results

### 8.3.1 Reasons and process of leaving

*Instigating factors*

Almost all the factors identified from the wider international migration literature (Table 8.1) as relevant to instigating migration decision-making were also found in this specifically European sample. As has been noted elsewhere, there was great variety in the intensity, balance and combination of push and pull factors (Larsen et al., 2005; Winkelmann-Gleed, 2006; Young et al., 2003, 2008b). Some respondents had strong grounds for leaving their countries of origin while others had simply no compelling reasons to stay. For some, the United Kingdom had been a quite specific choice, while for others it was an almost arbitrary destination. Very few respondents explained their decision to migrate in terms of one single reason.

*Macro-level drivers*

Previous literature has suggested that economic motivations were the most significant underlying drivers for EU-qualified health professionals, albeit more for those from the Central and Eastern European countries than the richer EU15 (Ast, 2004; Krieger, 2004; Simmgen, 2004; Galan, 2006; Smigelskas, Starkienė & Padaiga, 2007; Young et al., 2008a). For a lot of the respondents in this study, mainly but not only those from EU15 countries and higher paid professions (medicine and dentistry), the move to the United Kingdom was not particularly financially beneficial, but this was not perceived as an issue because earning more money was not a key consideration. For others from some of the EU12 countries who simply could not earn enough to live at home, and for particular professions in some countries for whom there were no jobs available at home, the opportunity to earn a reasonable living was clearly more significant. However, as has been observed in other studies (Young et al., 2008b), few even of those respondents cited financial considerations as the main or only reason why they had moved.

> The salary was not the important thing. For me, my main ambition is my academic career more than the economic career. For me it came after my academic ambition, and after my personal ambitions as well – to be with my husband. (Doctor 8, Italy)

> The crude reason was the availability of a job and a salary, something that wasn't there in Italy. But it's not only that, it's the whole system and the whole environment [in the United Kingdom] that is very supportive for academics and research in biomedicine. (Dentist 40, Italy)

> I was happy working and the job was satisfying [in Bulgaria] until I reached the point where I was just working, and couldn't go on holiday, couldn't buy my children new clothes or shoes when they needed them, couldn't provide anything else. I mean I was just working and nothing else. My husband was on and off from work and changing from one to another job and it was very difficult. (Nurse 30, Bulgaria)

> Well, finance was one reason. And then I was quite fascinated about the mix of cultures [and] people you find here which I never came across in my place. In the Capital there you will find maybe a mixture, but it's nothing compared with what you will see here. The patients and even my colleagues are from all over the world. (Nurse 26, Romania)

With regard to political drivers, none of the respondents in our sample mentioned concerns about political stability on a level that threatened their security. Where problems were mentioned, these were to do with economic stagnation, structural problems within the health systems or perceived corruption and professional nepotism – all factors that in one way or another constrained the opportunities for professional progression. Some had, therefore, moved to the United Kingdom in search of better working conditions; finding more, or more rewarding, work to do; or being able to consolidate their activities within a single role rather than having to tout around for work.

> The main reason, I struggle to summarize it in a word, but when you see that the system is not trustable, it's not reliable, it's not fair. Whether it's a matter of career progression, business, driving, or whatever. You mash your face a few times and eventually you decide that this is not a fair system and you want to move somewhere else. I wanted to achieve my freedom. I quite fancy stronger, muscular competition. I hate stabbing from the back basically. (Doctor 1, Italy)

> The NHS system [in Sweden] was going through quite big changes and it was to the worse for dentists. It's not just moneywise, it was the whole system was very difficult to claim and to treat patients, so it felt like we were stuck and it was time maybe to try to do something different. (Dentist 15, Sweden)

> The job opportunities were quite a big factor. In Spain 10 years ago there were no job opportunities to work as a nurse or GP, so people were just surviving doing some out-of-hours or going to little villages maybe two hours from home. That was one of the times that a lot of Spanish doctors went to Portugal, to UK and to Sweden. And it was easy to come here. (Doctor 5, Spain)

*Meso-level drivers*

It has been suggested elsewhere that professional and personal development opportunities are likely to be important motivating factors for migration within Europe, just as they are for international health professionals (Burgermeister, 2004; Mareckova, 2004; Young et al., 2010a). In the study described here, specific opportunities for professional development through postgraduate education were mentioned by some respondents in all professional groups as a key reason why they had made the move to the United Kingdom. The specialist qualifications or research careers they wanted to pursue were either simply unavailable in their countries of origin or excessively competitive to get into. By comparison, the United Kingdom was attractive both because of the variety and accessibility of the courses and research opportunities available, and their perceived quality in terms of the style and culture of learning, because of the high calibre of potential mentors and the chance to study or work with colleagues at the cutting edge in a particular field.

> Choosing the UK [to do a PhD] was because my boss here was like the best thing I could ever choose – this was the best guy in Europe that I could work with, so I chose him. (Doctor 11, Portugal)

> I had a vague idea that it would be interesting to work in another country, good experience. But actually this job was the incentive, at the university here. The research was quite interesting, and I wanted to do interesting research. [In Poland] we don't really have like, research opportunities. So it's much easier to have a career here and also there is more money invested in research, so you can do better research. (Doctor 7, Poland)

> I was clear that at least for some time I would like to go abroad because of the way the [training] system was run in Germany, which I wasn't very happy about – very impersonal, very mechanistic. The way it was set up [in the UK] was very much you get in there and learn while you are doing it and people take you along with them quite happily and that is how you are expected to learn. Of course you still have to do all the reading but it is very experiential and very practically orientated, which is what you actually need. And the culture, this learning culture, which was I felt very encouraging. (Doctor 42, Germany)

> In Austria with nursing not being an academic profession, the training system is an apprenticeship style which delivers a very good basic training. You come out of training with a lot of practical skills actually, fully able to do the work, but the disadvantage is that not having much in terms of specialized pathways you then hit a bit of a ceiling. (Nurse 25, Austria)

> In Germany a physiotherapist works less independently and you have here much more choices and development opportunities. I had to move because there are only a few places where you can do MSc as a physiotherapist in Germany. (Physiotherapist 38, Germany)

> I cannot specialize back home, the island is too small to be able to cater for that. There is definitely a need but they do not allow you to specialize; there is no programme. To put in context how small the island is, we only train 15 physios a year, whereas in the UK you train hundreds. It's very competitive to get into the course, it's more competitive than medicine at times. (Physiotherapist 37, Malta)

*Micro-level drivers*

Apart from the professional opportunities available, the English language was the most frequently mentioned factor behind choosing to move specifically to the United Kingdom. Almost all the respondents already knew some English before migrating and its pervasive presence as a world language in the media and popular culture made the United Kingdom seem more accessible and familiar than many other European countries. At the same time, the fact that it was still in Europe and relatively close to home made it significantly more attractive than other English-speaking countries such as the United States or Australia. In contrast to findings from other studies of international health professionals from outside Europe (Young et al., 2003; Ball & Pike, 2004; Travis, 2009), the United Kingdom was not perceived in this study as a stepping stone for migration further afield. For those for whom improving their own English, or enabling their children to do so, was the key objective, knowing that they could relatively easily find work as a health professional in the United Kingdom had facilitated the decision to move, but the scope or nature of the work potentially available was not a primary consideration.

> The main reason was that I have children, they were at this point seven and eight and I just thought it would be quite good to go to school in England. In the beginning it was just to come for three years, and they could get better language and we will see what is next. (Dentist 16, Sweden)

> It was for the challenge. Discovering a country I always wanted to live in and being bilingual for the benefit of the children. (Physiotherapist 36, Germany)

> Basically it was just like a challenge for me. I was not bored, but I needed something else. So I said, oh well, why not? I don't think it's such a big deal to learn. Basically English is such an international thing. You will easily learn it even if you are watching TV and listening to music. So I thought it's manageable. And another reason was that it's quite close. I was thinking to go to America, but that's just too far. Here it's like only 2.5 hours flight from home, it's basically just round the corner. (Nurse 26, Romania)

> I wouldn't have moved to the US where the commute was jet lag and hours of airplane. While here it's two hours. I can go any time, even for the day. I can look after my family in Italy. That's very relevant. That's major. (Doctor 2, Italy)

### Activating and facilitating factors

There were three main types of factor that precipitated the actual decision to move to the United Kingdom at a particular point in time. The first of these related to very specific personal circumstances (i.e. micro-level drivers), such as a partner living in or moving to the United Kingdom, the chance for a child to receive medical treatment here and specific life events or particular life stages that had prompted respondents to ask themselves questions of the "if not now, when?" variety. For some individuals, the initial decision appeared to have been quite a casual one, prompted by a chance encounter or suggestion.

> My reason was a very good family friend died, and she was only 51 and she kept on saying that she was going to wait until her kids grow up before she does anything. I saw the advert to come and I just thought "I'm going". I was in a dead-end relationship, so I had actually nothing to lose. (Nurse 22, Germany)

> After working a few years, we thought "why not go and try for a year or six months?" Mainly because, if we are going to do something abroad, it's a chance now. At that time we didn't have any mortgage for a house or a flat. We didn't have any child or dog or anything to think about, so it felt at that time quite a good chance to go. (Dentist 15, Sweden)

> My plan was not even leaving Portugal. The only reason I came was because a friend told me he was coming and at the time I thought "Yes, that might be a good opportunity for me". (Dentist 18, Portugal)

A number of respondents also described how micro-level factors provided the particular practical or emotional support necessary to encourage them to take the migration plunge. Mostly this was linked to the presence of friends or family members already in the United Kingdom. For others, the decision "to take the plunge" was facilitated at the professional, or meso-level. In these cases, the assistance provided by a recruiting agency or the certainty of having a specific job or course to come to had been crucial. A few respondents also mentioned the influence of macro-level factors associated with EU enlargement, both in terms of greater opportunities for work or study and a simpler and easier process of migration.

> We came here for four days and the bosses were amazing, organizing everything. Over four days we found a house to rent, schools for the children, we done GDC registration and we looked around the city. It was very intense and probably this helped us in deciding just here on the spot, yes. Because I believe that if I went home and thought about it again I would never do this. But everything looked so amazing and so good, so I thought, why not? (Dentist 16, Sweden)

> I am that type of person that I want at least a little bit of reassurance. I am not a very brave person. I wouldn't have come on my own to the UK and start looking for work. I relied on a professional agency. Having the reassurance from professional bodies as well was encouraging. I didn't feel like I come here and take someone's job. (Dentist 17, Poland)

I had never been to the UK so I didn't know anything about it except what I saw on TV. There was nothing in particular that made me want to come here. It was just this opportunity – they were looking for dentists. When I heard about it on TV it didn't seem real. I thought, "why would they be looking for dentists in other countries, because they should have their own?" They talked about these salaries, and they seemed quite big salaries. I just started to look for information and it was quite quick. I went to interview and they told me I was a suitable candidate, and then I came here. (Dentist 19, Romania)

When I came to the UK to study, Cyprus had already entered the EU so I didn't need a visa, I didn't have any problems with travel or passports or anything, which was a really big push actually. Because when I visited the UK before it was a really different experience. It meant going through customs and "Why are you here? How long are you staying?" It's strange how when they have the lanes to check your passport, how different it feels to go into the "UK/EU" as opposed to the "Other". It's that welcoming feeling, if you like, of knowing I'm not an "Other." (Nurse 32, Cyprus)

### 8.3.2 Experiences after arrival in the United Kingdom

Individual circumstances and experiences after arrival in the United Kingdom varied greatly. Not surprisingly, respondents who came to take up jobs or courses organized and agreed before they arrived had generally been much better supported than those who did not have anything arranged beforehand. While the former group had often received help from their employers in finding accommodation and opening bank accounts as well as advice about working in the United Kingdom health system, others who were fending for themselves were much more reliant on help from friends or chance acquaintances, particularly in the first few months.

Some respondents in all health professional groups had faced particular challenges associated with lack of recognition of their training or qualifications by United Kingdom professional regulatory bodies, lack of clarity about what evidence they needed to provide to obtain registration or problems with supplying that evidence. Those who experienced the least difficulties with migration in professional terms tended to be young people, relatively early in their careers, moving to prearranged postgraduate courses or locum jobs, most often from EU15 countries and working in medicine and dentistry. The group that had encountered the biggest problems were the older nurses and midwives from EU12 countries who had come to the United Kingdom without plans for work already in place, and whose professional backgrounds were least compatible with or familiar to the United Kingdom system.

I had an interview with a locum agency in Holland and they arranged everything really, also to get registered with the GMC [UK General Medical Council]. It was easy, it was no problem. I didn't have to do an exam or language tests. They also organized a bank account for me and [dealt with] the Medical Defence Union. When I arrived, all the junior doctors lived in the hospital, so you didn't have to look for a room. My brother just put all the things in his car and drove me there, unloaded, and that was it. (Doctor 10, Netherlands)

I contacted somebody here in the [university] department and he was interested in the research I did for my PhD. One of the professors here said it would be nice to have a chat, and then after this chat he asked me if I would like to come for two months … and then they offered me a post. (Doctor 7, Poland)

In two months after I first sent my query that I would like to register in the UK, I had my registration. And getting a job was amazingly easy. What I did, I sent e-mails [before coming to UK]. I asked my colleagues which hospitals they would recommend. Then I sent e-mails to unit managers with my CV. Everyone said OK, we have jobs available, apply online. I got three job offers in one go and it was like, I don't even know where to choose. (Nurse 28, Finland)

In the UK you are familiar with Indian education and Indian nurses, you are familiar with Philippine nurses, but nobody knew about Bulgaria. I mean, I have been asked so many silly questions – where is Bulgaria, and is it in Asia and what language are you speaking? Nobody knew it. I'm proving myself everyday, just to prove I am competent to work on an equal basis with others. (Nurse 30, Bulgaria)

In February 2006 I received … permission to work in your country and then I start applying for a job. I was sending about five or six applications every month, and for over two years I didn't receive any answer, any invitation for interview, anything. In the meantime I was working in a kitchen washing dishes. But I was lucky, my manager was midwife before. She just direct me start applying for other jobs, just to put your first foot in the NHS. So I did it and after 18 months I got a job in a walk-in centre as a health care assistant. Again I was very lucky, my boss was very helpful and just push me to apply for midwifery only. And after about 18 months I got a job as midwife again – 4.5 years after first applying. (Midwife 34, Poland)

Every time I apply for cleaner job, housekeeper job, but without result. They said me, "if you midwife you can't work this cleaner or housekeeper job". So I change my CV. I lie about cleaner job 20 years. Now I apply for domestic assistant job. (Midwife 33, Latvia)

Beyond finding work, almost all the respondents had found the wider experience of living and working in a new country challenging in one way or another, at least at first. There were issues to do with unfamiliar processes and systems, cultural expectations and coping with English. In this respect, several people observed that the exceptional linguistic and cultural diversity in the United Kingdom population was both a challenge and a benefit. While colleagues and patients from other countries were often hardest to understand, such colleagues were seen as a particular source of help and support, because of their common experience of migration.

> Everything is challenge because despite help from friends or colleagues or advisers you are just dealing with daily life on your own. I mean every different contact, in the banks and the shops and the post office. With accommodation and estate agents, all this moving from one rented house to another, you just have to deal with it and yes, it's difficult to learn all the rules, because many things are different. (Nurse 30, Bulgaria)

> I thought I was quite good in English but it was quite difficult, especially in London, because people come from different parts of the world and the accents are different. So I kept quite quiet for a long time. Nurses from different countries who were also foreigners here, they made it so much easier because we could share the experiences, how it is and how things are done. (Nurse 28, Finland)

> The first six months was awful. The way you nurse, it's completely different here, so that's been difficult. And the problem with different nurses – Filipino nurses and Indian nurses – it is very, very difficult trying to understand what they are saying. You feel embarrassed to ask them to repeat and you feel stupid. And when you come in a different culture and you don't have any friends, any family, you feel more alone than you've ever been in your life. (Nurse 31, France)

By the time of our interviews, having found their feet in the United Kingdom and become more familiar with both the challenges and opportunities of living and working in this country, many of the respondents had moved on from the jobs and locations to which they had come at first, having identified places to live or work settings that better suited their particular needs, skills and preferences. Reflecting this, some of the respondents had developed quite specific niche roles reflecting their migrant status, such as providing health services for embassy staff or working for international organizations providing advice and support to other migrants.

### 8.3.3 Plans to stay or return

At the point where they first came to the United Kingdom, few of the respondents had definite plans to remain in the longer term. Most perceived their initial decision to move here as a short- to medium-term choice, an open-ended adventure or a means to fulfil a specific, focused goal such as completing a degree. Some were on leave from jobs in their country of origin, to which they were expected to return. Others had already been and returned on several occasions, sometimes over a period of several years, before arriving and staying for a longer period. However, by the time of our interviews, the perspective had changed considerably.

Most respondents thought they were quite likely to stay in the United Kingdom at least until after retirement. Very few had definite intentions to leave unless something significant changed back home, such as being needed to care for elderly parents or unexpectedly being headhunted for their ideal job (in the case of one returner we interviewed abroad, this was just what had happened). Listening to their accounts, it became clear that migration was not a matter of a single decision at a particular point in time but rather a process that had happened by degrees. Many of these respondents were now long-term migrants but had only realized this in retrospect.

> It was first six months. Then another six months. Then they said do you want to do your rotations, so I knew it would be another two years. That was the nice thing. I was independent, no children, no sort of boyfriend, and there was nothing really for me to go back to Holland for. (Doctor 10, Netherlands)

> When I first came, if you asked me in the first three months, probably I would say give my money back, my contract back and go back to Poland, because it wasn't a very good time. But then I started thinking here is a place I want to live, it's a really good environment, I think I can enjoy life here. And I decided to stay here as long as possible, to make it my permanent country. (Dentist 17, Poland)

> It's a kind of domino effect I think. I arrived here because it seemed the right country to go to considering that I spoke a little bit of English. And while I was here I became more acquainted with the culture and professional development opportunities. I did a lot of courses. So the option of going home didn't appeal at all. When I look back and see how much I achieved here in my career and personal and professional development, I would not be able to do even a tiny bit of that back in Croatia. And I never thought about going anywhere else to be honest, because I wanted to work on the things I started, rather than go off and start from the beginning somewhere else. (Nurse 20, Croatia)

> I expected to stay one year. That was my original plan. My expectations and my goals changed because of the support I got here. You expect to get a job as a nurse and gain that professional satisfaction working as a nurse in a good country with a good sort of history. But then when you enter you find out so many other possibilities and options that you can actually get, so plans can

change. Every time I make plans they change. My plan now is to finish with my studies, and I have a job here now, so again it's to develop as much as I can. (Nurse 32, Cyprus)

I still have my job in France. It's kept for 10 years. So if tomorrow I say, "I'm fed up, I want to go home" I just call my manager and say I want to come back. When I went back last time she asked me, "When you come back?" And I said, "I don't think I will come back". And she was, "Are you sure you don't want to change your mind?" For now I'm not going back. (Nurse 31, France)

A few respondents had arrived with clear plans and taken active steps to obtain citizenship and become permanent United Kingdom residents. For most, however, their repositioning as long-term migrants had been less conscious or deliberate. Instead it reflected a gradual accretion of social and emotional ties, practical commitments, professional networks and career investment in the United Kingdom system. In terms of personal biography, some who had moved at earlier stages, because they felt free to do so and sought adventure, now had established careers, partners and/or English-speaking children in secondary education. Consequently, they felt less inclined or able to move again. For some, the experience of living outside their countries of origin and the time spent away had simply changed their views about where they felt they belonged.

Now I am here I probably would not be moving at all from this country because for the first I am tired to move from country to country, and for the second, my children are used to being here. (Dentist 16, Sweden)

When the moment came for choosing a school we had the choice, would they go to a standard English local school or to an international school. We chose [the English school] because we decided that we wanted them to belong somewhere. I know a lot of families that have children who went to international schools and these children are citizens of the world, they are multilingual, but they don't know where they belong. (Doctor 4, Italy)

I am just one in my family and my parents are dead. Nothing, just graves I left. My children just speak English now. We live in an area where there are not Lithuanian people, just English, and friends are English. We have child minder, she is English. I try to do everything as British people. Food and my style of life. I changed everything. Where you live, you should do this. (Midwife 35, Lithuania)

London is a wonderful city, it offers so much. Italy is a big town, it's very closed. And nothing changes, everything's the same. Which is both positive and negative. But once you have lived in London you'd feel a bit claustrophobic living all the time in Italy. (Doctor 2, Italy)

> Back home I was like, oh my God, I don't think I will ever get to see France, or Italy or whatever. Whereas here I go like a weekend break. I say, well I work hard, so I deserve it. So the standards are changing as well. (Nurse 26, Romania)

In addition, a number of respondents felt they would be unable to get appropriate work back in their countries of origin. Either they would not find a job at all or would not find one at a level of seniority commensurate with what they had achieved in the United Kingdom. Several nurses and physiotherapists also commented that they would no longer be able to tolerate the more restricted roles and hierarchical relationships that still prevailed in their countries of origin.

> It would be almost impossible for me to go back and get a job in the [Italian] health service because now people are ahead of me, people are trained after me. My professor is not powerful any more. (Doctor 2, Italy)

> In Germany in principle they have a lack of doctors. But the problem is I haven't worked in Germany for five years now, and I am not the youngest any more. And its like everywhere after a specific age. They might not be interested to take you. (Doctor 13, Germany)

> The people I worked with back home ask me, "when are you coming back?" And then they say "Well you can't expect to come back and swan your way into a senior job, because you have been away and we have been working away at it doing our rotations". You have people there who have been physios for 20 years, have not done any CPD, but purely on the basis that they have 20 years experience, irrespective of the fact that maybe what they do is 20 years old and is not evidence based, they get the senior posts. My main battle is that if I go home I have to start off as a junior, and I find that unacceptable because I refuse to do the same job as someone who has just left university. (Physiotherapist 37, Malta)

> I definitely won't go back, not working as a nurse. Because now I am too adapted to … especially in my current job, where I am practising fairly autonomously. I can't go back to the level of being an underdog to the doctors. It's just not going to happen. (Nurse 25, Austria)

A few respondents had much more actively maintained and cultivated cultural, professional or personal links with their communities and countries of origin in order to keep their options firmly open. One, for example, had sent her children to Saturday school to ensure they learnt about the history and culture of Poland. Another commuted one week each month to work in Italy, taking her children with her to ensure she maintained her professional connections there and that they remained bilingual. The small minority who indicated definite intentions to return home also mentioned strong personal or cultural ties, moral obligations or, in some cases, unhappiness and dissatisfaction with their experiences in the United Kingdom. It should be reiterated that definite returners are likely to be underrepresented in our study, because our sample was necessarily largely drawn from those still in the country.

> It's highly likely that I will go back, though it's not 100%. First, the agreement I have with my hospital that they allowed me to come expecting me to go back. Then, subjective things. I had this idea that people have an obligation to give something back to their society and this would be my contribution to that, help the health care and research in my field to improve and the patients in my group to improve. And then of course, personal reasons. I quite like the city I grew up in, and I have friends and family there. (Doctor 11, Portugal)

> We made a decision to go back this year. After all that experience [in the UK] I know money is not enough. Here we are quite lonely, so we are very homesick. The culture [in the UK] is a little bit shock for me, because we are more religious people and I just can't understand many behaviour here. It's just not what I want for my children to grow up. I know the standard of life will drop dramatically again, but I do have a hope we will manage, together with the love and support of family and friends. (Midwife 34, Poland)

## 8.4 Policy implications

Some have argued that United Kingdom bodies do not need information on European health professionals because their numbers are relatively fewer than from countries outside Europe. This is a short-sighted view because European sources have, in recent years, started to become much more important – at least in relative terms – and, as our study shows, the incentives (economic, professional and personal) for health professionals to move to the United Kingdom from all parts of Europe continue to be significant. Moreover, the relative trend away from migration from non-EU/EEA countries towards more EU/EEA migrants seems likely to continue given that EU-resident professionals can carry on exercising their rights to free movement while work permit regulations for others have changed significantly (Young, 2011). Another point in this context is that the EU itself is significantly raising its profile in respect of Europe's health workforce and is continuing to legislate in a variety of areas to remove further the barriers to professional mobility/migration. Perhaps most significantly, the sheer variety of countries (31 in the EEA alone at the time of writing) and professional cultures represented makes workforce integration equally, if not more, challenging than for other ostensibly more significant movements from single-country sources such as India and the Philippines.

For some in the United Kingdom, the question of language standards is a key concern arising from this increasing migration of European health professionals, particularly those from EEA countries. At issue is the fact that a test of competence in English is not a prerequisite for professional registration for these migrants (Alliance of UK Health Regulators on Europe, 2005; Healthcare Professions Crossing Borders, 2007; Nursing and Midwifery Council, 2005). As the experience of our interviewees illustrated, migrants can be familiar with and feel competent in general with the English language but that does not mean that they automatically have "the right" English to work effectively in the health service. In addition, the United Kingdom, like other EU/EEA States, has its own particular ethos and system of health care delivery that has emerged from cultural and historical factors, which are often intangible and difficult to quantify. Recognition and management of potential difficulties within these areas is vital for three reasons: first, to ensure the individual patient experience is safe and of high quality; second, to enable NHS organizations to get maximum value from employing EU/EEA migrants; and third, to assist individual health professionals to gain positive benefits from moving to work in the United Kingdom. Although dedicated support has been in place, it has often been in the context of particular recruitment campaigns (Ballard & Laurence, 2004; Porter & Powell, 2005). What is needed, then, is a better infrastructure for NHS organizations (and others) to share experience about how best to ensure language competency and to deliver both language training and professional/clinical induction and support.

Another concern from the United Kingdom's viewpoint relates to the exchange of regulatory information between countries across Europe. Although the professional and regulatory bodies have been working to address the challenges involved (Alliance of UK Health Regulators on Europe, 2005; Healthcare Professions Crossing Borders, 2007), the reported view of United Kingdom stakeholders is that assurances of quality are currently inadequate (Young, Weir & Buchan, 2010b). The issue has gained further significance because of certain high-profile cases of medical errors associated, rightly or wrongly, with health professionals moving to the United Kingdom under EU free movement regulations (Meikle, 2009; Meikle & Connolly, 2009). Having the infrastructures in place to support NHS organizations in their induction/support activities is likely, therefore, to become all the more important. It will also be important for the EU as a whole to support all Member States to develop the systems and infrastructures and improve the quality and usefulness of the information they provide to underpin mobility. The view is that if such mechanisms can be developed this would assist both the United Kingdom and Europe as a whole – in the context of professional regulation, quality safeguards and also workforce planning (see also EU Health Policy Forum, 2003).

The evidence is mixed in relation to potential benefits and prospects of return migration: the gains that might be brought back to the home country in terms of additional skills, competencies and experiences, embodied in human capital (Bach, 2003; Krieger, 2004; Blitz, 2005). At a general level, just as the NHS potentially benefits from the challenge of different ways of thinking from abroad, so too can source countries benefit, particularly when returning staff go into professional leadership and/or teaching positions. Equally, however, the United Kingdom experience is not always relevant, and where health professionals develop specialisms in the United Kingdom, the experience and additional qualifications obtained are not always adequately recognized in their countries of origin. For example, in the study of Young et al. (2008a), such problems were reported to be equally applicable to countries in Europe (e.g. Spain, Greece, Czech Republic) as to others elsewhere (see also Blitz (2005) in relation to Spanish doctors). Another issue reported in the same study was the continued un- or underemployment of health professionals in some countries (e.g. Greece), which can mean that more experienced (i.e. more expensive) returning staff are less likely to be employed. Such issues were also highlighted by our interviewees, but more important than factors in countries of origin that restrict opportunities for return migration were the factors that kept them much longer than they had initially expected (if not permanently) in the United Kingdom. Though the United Kingdom clearly has a responsibility not to recruit health professionals from countries that cannot afford to lose them, it seems that countries losing their health professionals also need to do more to encourage them to stay in the first place. In fact, the key finding from this United Kingdom element of the PROMeTHEUS study is how much more difficult it appears to be for countries of origin to encourage return migration – hence the conclusion that the emphasis may need to be on redressing the balance of push–pull factors in the first place between migration sources and destination countries such as the United Kingdom. On the basis of this study, it appears that relevant actions might focus particularly on seeking to ensure the availability of appropriate and attractive employment opportunities for health professionals in their countries of origin and on improving local opportunities for career development and further specialization after initial qualification.

In this context, there is also potentially a development role for the United Kingdom. Codes of practice and ethical policy stances around migration/ recruitment, although essential, can only achieve so much to protect vulnerable countries – including those in Europe – against losing migrant health professionals (Buchan et al., 2009). Again this is a complex debate and one that cannot be given justice here. The key point, however, is that if the United Kingdom really wishes to help to influence the balance of "buyer power" of health professional labour in favour of migration sources, it needs to take proactive action. The literature provides several examples of such "developmental approaches" in the context of the health workforce: bilateral agreements, institutional collaborations, exchange programmes and so on. However, "there is clear scope to increase the effectiveness and strategic impact of this work", including within Europe (Crisp, 2007).

Overall, as one of the largest destinations for migrating health professionals within Europe – and given the added experience of the large-scale recruitment drives of recent years – the United Kingdom is an ideal crucible in which to research this European mobility perspective. From the viewpoint of the United Kingdom, recognizing the potential to make better use of more easily available human resources for health from within Europe may also be a better workforce strategy than having to compete globally with other "bigger players" (e.g. the United States). Being part of a Europe of free-moving workers is then as much an opportunity as it is a challenge to United Kingdom health care. Of course, consideration of source country viewpoints demands that the United Kingdom also gives more thought to developmental approaches and the extent to which recruitment/migration can potentially be linked to real availability of supplies.

In the final analysis, no one driver or constraint to health professional mobility (to and from the United Kingdom) can be singled out as key, for individual migrants, particular professions or source countries. Inflows and outflows are linked and movements to and from different countries change as the balance of drivers versus constraints alters over time. How to capitalize upon the different migration drivers and address constraints in ways that are of benefit to all (receiver and source countries, and individual migrants) is a clear topic for continued Europe-wide debate.

## References

Aiken L, Buchan J (2004). Trends in international nurse migration. *Health Affairs*, 23(3):69.

Alliance of UK Health Regulators on Europe (2005). *Healthcare professions crossing borders. UK Presidency patient safety initiative*. London, Alliance of UK Health Regulators on Europe and Department of Health.

Ast J (2004). A first-hand personal account of the thinking of young Polish doctors. *BMJ Online* (http://www.bmj.com/rapid-response/2011/10/30/first-hand-personal-account-thinking-young-polish-doctors, accessed 2 January 2014).

Bach S (2003). *International migration of health workers: labour and social issues*. Geneva, International Labour Office (Sectoral Activities Programme Working Paper 209).

Ball J, Pike G (2004). *Stepping stones: results from the RCN membership survey 2003.* London, Royal College of Nursing.

Ballard K, Laurence P (2004). An induction programme for European GPs coming to work in England: development and evaluation. *Education for Primary Care*, 15:584–595.

Ballard K, Robinson S, Laurence P (2004). Why do general practitioners from France choose to work in London? A qualitative study. *British Journal of General Practice*, 54:747–752.

Bellingham C (2001). Facing the recruitment and retention crisis in pharmacy: looking abroad. *Pharmaceutical Journal,* 267(7156):45–46.

Blitz B (2005). "Brain circulation": the Spanish medical profession and international medical recruitment in the UK. *Journal of European Social Policy*, 15(4):363–369.

Buchan J (2004). Commentary: nurse workforce planning in the UK. Policies and impact. *Journal of Nursing Management,* 12(6):388–392.

Buchan J, Rafferty AM (2004). Not from our backyard? The United Kingdom, Europe and international recruitment of nurses. In McKee M, MacLehose L, Nolte E, eds. *Health policy and European Union enlargement.* Buckingham, UK, Open University Press:143–156.

Buchan J et al. (2006). Internationally recruited nurses in London: a survey of career paths and plans. *Human Resources for Health*, 4:14.

Buchan J et al. (2009). Does a code make a difference? Assessing the English code of practice on international recruitment. *Human Resources for Health*, 7:33.

Burgermeister J (2004). Exodus of Polish doctors could threaten health system. *British Medical Journal*, 328(7451):1280.

Crisp N (2007). *Global health partnerships: the UK contribution to health in developing countries.* London, Department for International Development (http://www.wales.nhs.uk/documents/DH_083510.pdf, accessed 2 January 2014).

EU Health Policy Forum (2003). *Recommendations on mobility of health professionals.* Brussels, EU Health Policy Forum.

European Migration Network (2006). *Small scale study II: managed migration and the labour market – the health sector 2006.* Brussels, European Migration Network.

Galan A (2006). Romania. In Wiscow C, ed. *Health worker migration flows in Europe: overview and case studies in selected CEE countries – Romania, Czech Republic, Serbia and Croatia.* Geneva, International Labour Organization:37–53.

Hann M, Sibbald B, Young R (2008). Workforce participation among international medical graduates in the National Health Service of England: a retrospective longitudinal analysis. *Human Resources for Health*, 6:9.

Healthcare Professions Crossing Borders (2007). *Healthcare professions crossing borders: Portugal agreement.* London, Healthcare Professions Crossing Borders.

Krieger H (2004). *Quality of life in Europe: migration trends in an enlarged Europe.* Luxembourg, European Foundation for the Improvement of Living and Working Conditions for the European Commission.

Larsen J et al. (2005). Overseas nurses' motivations for working in the UK: globalisation and life politics. *Work, Employment and Society*, 19(2):349–368.

Mareckova M (2004). Exodus of Czech doctors leaves gaps in health care. Hospital officials draw up crisis plans to prepare for May 1 easing of migration restrictions. *Lancet*, 363(9419):1443–1446.

Meikle J (2009). Rules on EU doctors leave patients at risk, say BMA. *The Guardian*, 24 August, p. 6.

Meikle J, Connolly K (2009). German GP who accidentally killed patient advised to "go home". *The Guardian*, 24 August, p. 7.

Nursing and Midwifery Council (2005). *EU language position a "dangerous farce" says NMC President.* London, Nursing and Midwifery Council (Press Release 44/2005).

Pitts J et al. (1998). Experiences and career intentions of general practice registrars from the Netherlands. *Medical Education*, 32:613–621.

Pollard N, Latore M, Sriskandarajah D (2008). *Floodgates or turnstiles? Post-EU enlargement migration flows to (and from) the UK 2008.* London, Institute for Public Policy Research.

Porter E, Powell G (2005). Recruitment of European Union general practitioners: developing a process for the analysis of English language training needs. *Education for Primary Care*, 16:31–35.

Ritchie J, Spencer L (1994). Qualitative data analysis for applied policy research. In Bryman A, Burgess RG, eds. *Analysing qualitative data.* London, Taylor & Francis:173–194.

Simmgen M (2004). Why German doctors enjoy British medicine. *Clinical Medicine,* 4(1):57–59.

Smigelskas K, Starkienė L, Padaiga Z (2007). Do Lithuanian pharmacists intend to migrate? *Journal of Ethnic and Migration Studies,* 33(3):501–509.

Smith PA et al. (2006). *Valuing and recognizing the talents of a diverse healthcare workforce.* London, Royal College of Nursing (http://www.rcn.org.uk/__data/assets/pdf_file/0008/78713/003078.pdf, accessed 2 January 2014).

Travis A (2009). Here today, gone tomorrow: new breed of migrants finds greener grass overseas. *The Guardian,* 6 August (http://www.guardian.co.uk/uk/2009/aug/06/britain-losing-highly-skilled-migrants/print, accessed 2 January 2014).

Wang L (2007). Eastern European pharmacists in the UK. *Pharmaceutical Journal,* 278:7–8.

Winkelmann-Gleed A (2006). *Migrant nurses: motivation, integration and contribution.* Oxford, Radcliffe Press.

Wismar M et al., eds. (2011). *Health professional mobility and health systems. Evidence from 17 European countries.* Copenhagen, WHO Regional Office for Europe on behalf of the European Observatory on Health Systems and Policies.

Young R (2011). A major destination country: the United Kingdom and its changing recruitment policies. In Wismar M et al., eds. *Health professional mobility and health systems. Evidence from 17 European countries.* Copenhagen, WHO Regional Office for Europe on behalf of the European Observatory on Health Systems and Policies:295–335.

Young R et al. (2003). *The international market for medical doctors: perspectives on positioning of the UK.* Manchester, MCHM and NPCRDC, University of Manchester (Report submitted to the Department of Health).

Young R et al. (2008a). Case study reports. In *International recruitment into the NHS: evaluation of initiatives for hospital doctors, general practitioners, nurses, midwives and allied health professionals.* London, Florence Nightingale School of Nursing and Midwifery, King's College London, with Open University Centre for Education in Medicine, Manchester Business School and NPCRDC, University of Manchester (Report submitted to the Department of Health).

Young R et al. (2008b). *International recruitment into the NHS: evaluation of initiatives for hospital doctors, general practitioners, nurses, midwives and allied health professionals.* London, Florence Nightingale School of Nursing and Midwifery, King's College London, with Open University Centre for Education in Medicine, Manchester Business School and NPCRDC, University of Manchester (Report submitted to the Department of Health).

Young R et al. (2010a). Evaluation of international recruitment of health professionals in England. *Journal of Health Services Research and Policy*, 15(4):195–203.

Young R, Weir H, Buchan J (2010b). *Health professional mobility in Europe and the UK: a scoping study of issues and evidence.* Southampton, UK, National Institute for Health Research (Research Report for the Service Delivery and Organisation Programme).

# Chapter 9

# Why do health professionals leave Germany and what attracts foreigners? A qualitative study

*Diana Ognyanova, Ruth Young, Claudia B. Maier and Reinhard Busse*

## 9.1 Introduction

The migration of health professionals has increased globally and within the EU over the last decades, in line with the increased labour mobility facilitated by globalization (Wismar et al., 2011; Ognyanova et al., 2012). Migration patterns are increasingly circular, with people moving back and forth between countries of origin, transit and destination; returning home; and then often migrating again. The patterns are highly complex and change rapidly (Haour-Knipe & Davies, 2008).

The mobility of health professionals affects the performance of health systems by changing the size and composition of the health workforce in both sending and receiving countries and aggravating or alleviating workforce shortages and regional maldistributions (Wismar et al., 2011). In order to respond to current and emergent health workforce challenges and to steer the migration flows of health professionals, policy-makers need up-to-date information on the factors causing migration. In view of the looming demand for nurses in countries with ageing populations, up-to-date research on the migration motivations of nurses is vital.

Germany is both a destination and a source country for mobile health professionals. So far, the mobility of health professionals to and from Germany is not a huge and unmanageable phenomenon, but the inflow of medical doctors, as well as of nurses working in the home-care sector, is increasing, while at the same time German health professionals leave the country for better employment opportunities abroad (Ognyanova & Busse, 2011). Hence research on the migration motivations of medical doctors and nurses could help policy-makers to devise proper retention, recruitment and integration policies.

As part of the EU-funded PROMeTHEUS project, a qualitative study on the motivations for migration of nurses and medical doctors was conducted with health professionals who:

- have migrated to Germany

- have returned to Germany after having worked abroad

- intend to leave the country to work abroad.

While migration is often determined by personal factors, the study strives to highlight health system relevant factors for migration and to show how they differ for medical doctors and nurses, and, for immigrants, emigrants and returners; as well as using the findings of previous research on the migration motivations of health professionals. Furthermore, the study aims to illustrate some of the challenges arising once migration has taken place.

## 9.2 Literature review

The existing research on migration of health professionals often relates to the push–pull theory and reveals a certain degree of consistency relating to the factors that influence health professionals to leave their country of origin (Buchan, 2007). Health workers consider migration when they expect this move can improve their professional and economic situation. The most cited push and pull factors are summarized in Table 9.1.

In her book, Kingma (2006) discussed the various migration motivations of nurses and classified migrant nurses into several, mutually non-exclusive categories: economic migrant, quality-of-life migrant, career move migrant, survival migrant, partner migrant, adventurer, holiday worker and contract worker.

Research on the migration motivations of health professionals to and from Germany is scarce and outdated. Some studies explore the reasons for dissatisfaction among health professionals in Germany or the intentions to leave the particular health profession, but the focus on migration is marginal or non-existent. No research has been carried out on return migration of health professionals. No study compares the migration motivations of different professionals groups for three migrant types.

**Table 9.1** Main push and pull factors in international migration of health workers

| Push | Pull |
|---|---|
| Low pay (absolute and/or relative) | Higher pay (and opportunities for remittances) |
| Poor working conditions | Better working conditions |
| Lack of resources to work effectively | Better resourced health system |
| Limited career opportunities | Career opportunities |
| Limited educational opportunities | Provision of post-basic education |
| Impact of HIV/AIDS | Aid work |
| Unstable work environment | Political stability |
| Economic instability | Travel opportunities |

*Source*: Buchan, 2007.

Research on the migration motivations of nurses to and from Germany is extremely limited. Although some studies have explored the reasons for dissatisfaction among nurses in Germany or for the intention to leave the nursing profession, there has been little or no focus on migration. One study found that the instigating determinants of nurses' decisions to leave their profession include dissatisfaction with working conditions, the work content and work organization; low esteem; a marked effort–reward imbalance; and perceived low pay (Hasselhorn, Müller & Tackenberg, 2005).

With regard to immigration, Hasselhorn, Müller and Tackenberg (2005) stated that there was an upward trend in the inflow of foreign nurses to European countries (including Germany). Possible push factors mentioned in that study include low pay, poor employment, and economic, safety and working conditions. As pull factors facilitated migration within EU countries, active recruitment and the mutual recognition of diplomas in the EU were noted. No detailed research, however, has been conducted on the specific motivational factors and experiences of foreign nurses moving to Germany.

With regard to medical doctors, one of the biggest surveys was conducted by Ramboll Management (2004) and indicated three main instigating factors for ceasing to practise curative medicine or emigrating: (1) the level of remuneration, with medical doctors considering this to be inadequate for the services they provide; (2) the workload and the poor work–life balance; and (3) the increasing bureaucracy and administrative burden faced by medical practitioners. Further factors cited were the hierarchical structure and leadership style in German hospitals, as well as poor mentoring. Ranking of these factors did differ slightly according to gender and career phase.

A study by Janus et al. (2007) suggested that non-monetary factors were important determinants of physicians' job satisfaction, possibly more important than monetary incentives. Factor analysis revealed that decision-making and recognition, continuous education and job security, administrative tasks and collegial relationships were highly significant; specialized technology and patient contact were moderately significant; while research and teaching and international exchange were not significant in contributing to job satisfaction.

A study by Fellmer (2008), based on interviews conducted in 2005 with 20 Polish medical doctors working in Germany, found that both the higher wages and the better working conditions in Germany played a significant role in the decision to migrate for most of the medical doctors who were interviewed. However, the results suggest two further findings: unemployment levels in Poland played only a modest role in the decision to leave but the lack of training opportunities in Poland was a dominant migration motivation for about half of the respondents. A factor discouraging migration at that time was the recognition of their professional qualifications in Germany. If their qualifications were not (or not fully) recognized, this may have resulted in a lower level of income. The study found that leaving family back in Poland was a factor discouraging emigration, but only to a lesser degree.

## 9.3 Methodology

The study described in this chapter follows a three-stage approach. First, an online survey based on an elaborate questionnaire was conducted. While not intended to be a representative study, the primary goal of the survey was to identify health professionals who could be interviewed in a second stage in focus groups and telephone interviews. The online questionnaire built on existing theories from various disciplines of science (synthesized in Massey et al., 1993; Bijak, 2006; di Mattia & Cassan, 2009; Lowell, 2009) and the findings of recent studies on the migration motivations of health professionals. The online questionnaire was sent in electronic form to health professional bodies (Regional Chamber of Physicians Berlin, Regional Chamber of Physicians Brandenburg, German Nursing Association, German Nursing Council), health care providers and personally known health professionals. By means of a Likert scale, approximately 200 survey participants scaled the importance of a number of identified migration factors.

Survey participants who expressed interest in taking part in the follow-up qualitative study were invited to participate in focus groups, which took place at the Berlin University of Technology's Department of Health Care Management. Those health professionals who were interested in the study but could not attend the focus groups were interviewed by telephone. Before the start of the study, approval by the ethical board at the Berlin University of Technology was obtained, confirming that the study adhered to the established ethical guidelines.

The aim of the focus groups and the telephone interviews was to reflect in-depth on the factors causing migration. The online questionnaire served as a preparation to the focus groups as it gave health professionals the possibility to reflect on a wide range of migration motivations and to identify those which were most relevant for their personal situation.

The focus groups were carried out in November 2010 (medical doctors) and January 2011 (nurses) and lasted 1.5 hours each. The focus groups were organized according to profession in order to encourage the discussion of profession-related issues and avoid possible hierarchical interaction patterns in the discussion.

The focus groups and telephone interviews consisted of open and semi-structured questions on the motivations for immigration, emigration and return migration, as well as the hurdles and the facilitating factors. While personal and family factors often played a key role in the decision to migrate, the focus group moderator encouraged a discussion on the health system-related factors that policy-makers are able to influence, the experience of health professionals with different health systems and on the problems arising once migration has taken place. Finally, participants were asked about their future plans and intentions and the conditions under which future movements could potentially happen were discussed.

The total number of health professionals who participated in focus groups and telephone interviews was 52: 27 medical doctors and 25 nurses. Two focus groups, with eight participants each, were held and in addition 36 individual telephone interviews were conducted. Table 9.2 gives an overview on the sample size and composition.

In addition to the focus groups and the telephone interviews with health professionals, the researchers conducted expert interviews with representatives of four private recruitment agencies specializing in the recruitment of health professionals moving to and leaving Germany. Furthermore, an expert interview was conducted with a representative of the Federal Employment Agency, which is involved in the recruitment of Croatian nurses. Although the recruitment agencies were not willing to convey the contact details of the people they had recruited, the information retrieved from the interviews complemented the personal reports of health professionals by giving an aggregated picture of migration motivations to either leave or move to Germany.

**Table 9.2** Sample size and composition

|  | **Medical doctors** | **Nurses** |
|---|---|---|
| *Total* | 27 | 25 |
| *Focus group* | | |
| Total | 8 | 8 |
| Immigrant | 5 | 4 |
| Returner | 2 | 3 |
| Potential emigrant | 1 | 1 |
| *Telephone interviews* | | |
| Total | 19 | 17 |
| Immigrant | 13 | 6 |
| Returner | 4 | 6 |
| Potential emigrant | 2 | 4 |
| Emigrant working abroad | – | 1 |
| *Characteristics* | | |
| Females:males (%) | 58:42 | 84:16 |
| Age range (years) | 28–55 | 23–56 |
| Specializations | Anaesthesiology, gynaecology, general medicine, internal medicine, diabetology, surgery, neurology, radiology, paediatrics, psychiatry, orthopaedics | Psychiatry, geriatric care, paediatric care, nephrology, oncology, surgery, anaesthetics |
| *Movement* | | |
| Federal state | Berlin, Brandenburg, Bavaria, Saxony-Anhalt | Berlin, Bavaria, Baden-Württemberg |
| Countries of origin | Austria, Bulgaria, India, Iraq, Kazakhstan, Latvia, Lithuania, Mongolia, Romania, the Russian Federation, Syria, Ukraine, Vietnam | Australia, Bulgaria, Iraq, Kenya, Poland, the Russian Federation, South Africa, Spain, Zimbabwe |
| Destination countries | Argentina, France, Columbia, India, Liberia, Netherlands, Nigeria, Pakistan, Switzerland, Tonga, United Kingdom, United States | Australia, Austria, France, Ireland, Malawi, New Zealand, Switzerland, Tanzania, United Kingdom |

The data was analysed inductively following the framework approach to data management as described by Ritchie and Spencer (2004). The framework approach is a matrix-based method that uses a thematic framework to classify and organize data according to key themes, concepts and emergent categories. Both field notes and transcripts from audio records were used to analyse the raw data. The online survey, as well as the focus groups and the interviews, was conducted in German and the translation was carried out by the researchers.

### 9.3.1 Limitations of the study

The study is not representative and does not claim to give a comprehensive picture of the migration motivations of health professionals moving to and from Germany. It is a small-scale exploratory study with a limited sample size and restricted resources to recruit participants and conduct focus groups. Even though the researchers tried to recruit participants representing different migrant types and migration motivations, certain groups, which according to anecdotal evidence appear to be gaining in importance, could not be recruited for the study. For example, the researchers faced problems recruiting foreign nurses, especially Eastern European nurses practising in Germany as carers for the elderly and disabled. These nurses were probably not reached by the online questionnaire as it was sent mainly in an electronic format and advertised through professional bodies, hospitals and elderly homes. None of the recruitment agencies specializing in the recruitment of Eastern European nurses for elderly care was willing to provide the contact details of foreign-trained nurses. Using a snowballing sampling method, a few nurses of Eastern European background were contacted directly via the phone or e-mail, but the vast majority were reluctant to share their migration experience. With regard to medical doctors, the researchers could not recruit medical doctors leaving Germany temporarily, for a few months, weeks or weekend shifts.

## 9.4 Results

### 9.4.1 Emigration from Germany

#### German nurses leaving Germany

Most of the German nurses stated they moved out of Germany because they received more attractive job offers abroad, mainly in Switzerland but also in the Scandinavian countries, Australia and New Zealand. Demand for nursing personnel at the destination, and better working conditions in combination with higher remuneration were mentioned among the participants of the study as pull factors for emigration. Those who worked or planned to work in Switzerland particularly explained that higher payment together with a more relaxed working environment was the most decisive factor in their decision to migrate. They claimed that the quality of nursing care in Switzerland is higher than in Germany and that the pace of work is more relaxed, because the patient–staff ratio is lower and health professionals take more time for each patient. Language links and geographical proximity played an important facilitating role in the decision to migrate, especially for nurses living close to the Swiss border.

Active recruitment and the prospect of better employment opportunities were mentioned as major migration motivations by a nurse who was contemplating moving to Norway. She was offered an intensive three-month course in

Germany, targeting primarily nurses and organized by the commune of the potential employer, providing language skills and knowledge about the health system and the work requirements in Norway.

Whereas some destination countries offered attractive employment opportunities, German nurses complained of a perceived effort–reward imbalance in Germany, which involves dissatisfaction with working conditions, remuneration and professional recognition. German nurses deemed these important push factors to leave the country. Participants in the study complained about the long, often unpaid, hours, the many weekend duties and the physical and psychological burden they bear. A nurse working in elderly care complained:

> The working conditions for nurses in elderly care are getting so bad, this can really wear you down, such an ungrateful work, for so little money.

Another nurse explained that an increasing number of nurses, even young people in their late twenties, suffer from burn-out. A third nurse confirmed that absence from illness had increased in her department over the last three to four years, presumably because of an increased level of stress work. Furthermore, participants in the study stated that the time pressure, the lack of personnel, the long hours and the hectic pace of work pose a risk to the patients. A nurse who had left the nursing profession after 20 years of work experience in both Germany and Switzerland stated:

> In my opinion, nursing care in many German hospitals is dangerous; you don't have time to perform your tasks properly. The lack of personnel and the long working hours are real dangers for the patients, especially in the intensive care units.

In the perceived effort–reward imbalance, remuneration plays an important role. A nurse who left to work in Switzerland complained that she was not able to earn more than €1 500 per month in Germany. Another nurse suggested that the relatively low remuneration has an adverse effect on the nurses' work motivation:

> Nurses do not feel responsible for many things. They say, "I am not paid for this, so I am not doing this task, it is the doctors' responsibility". Many say they would work harder if they were paid better and received higher recognition for their work.

Nurses explained that they would like to work abroad also because of the higher recognition of the nursing profession in society and a work organization that promoted less hierarchical structures. A nurse who left to work in Australia claimed that the nursing profession in Australia has a different occupational image; a nurse receives much greater recognition and has a higher social status than in Germany. Another nurse who worked in Switzerland reported that patients in Switzerland appreciated her work more than in Germany. Her impression was that patients in Switzerland valued nurses even more than doctors. In addition, communication between medical doctors and nurses was perceived as more respectful and team oriented than in Germany. In contrast, nurses admitted that communication with medical doctors in Germany often caused frustration:

> In Germany I worked within a very hierarchical structure. In Switzerland we were a team. We all talked to each other on a first-name basis. There was very humane cooperation and open communication.

A few participants explained that the limited scope of responsibility was another motivational factor for them to leave Germany. A nurse working in Germany complained that she did not learn anything new and that her work consisted of routine tasks. In contrast to this, a nurse who worked in Switzerland for many years reported:

> In Switzerland nurses have much greater responsibilities, a broader spectrum of tasks and are more independent in their work. They do counselling and give instructions, which are important for the treatment after the patient's hospital stay. Doctors ask for their opinion, for their judgement.

One nurse explained that the limited competence of German nurses was an obstacle for them to practise in a country like Switzerland where the nurses' scope of responsibility is bigger. She stated that some of the German nurses could not meet the requirements in Switzerland, even though at the beginning they were very confident because in Germany they had to take care of more patients. Her impression was that many German nurses were overwhelmed because they were required to think independently and to bear higher responsibilities. Some of the German nurses were required to take additional training in order to be able to perform their professional duties.

Training and continuing education were deemed by the participants to be a crucial precondition for higher responsibilities. Some participants claimed that nurses in Germany have restricted career options compared with other countries that strongly encouraged "advanced nursing practice" and concepts such as nurse practitioner and nurse clinics. A nurse who worked in New Zealand stated that in New Zealand nurses are better qualified as the emphasis on continuing education is much greater. Nurses needed to apply for the nursing certificate each year and to demonstrate 20 hours of continuing education and 500 clinical hours of relevant professional experience. In her opinion this is an important quality assurance mechanism to keep nurses' knowledge and qualifications up to date.

A young participant stated that she is leaving Germany because she wants to take on bigger responsibilities in her work:

> I am going back to Tanzania, because I will have a much bigger scope of duties and action. I can make diagnoses, work in the laboratory and prescribe medication for tropical diseases such as malaria and tuberculosis. This was a challenge for me; all of a sudden I had to be a midwife. If there is a need, a medical doctor might come, but generally I am much more self-dependent than in Germany.

Some participants said they had left or were planning to leave Germany because of their interest in a foreign country, its language and culture, and the learning experience abroad. One nurse explained she left Germany to work in Ireland because she wanted to improve her English and because she had the wish to change the familiar working environment. She perceived the working conditions in Ireland as worse than in Germany, but that did not discourage her from staying in Ireland.

One nurse who left Germany to work in Malawi and Tanzania explained that she grew up in the German Democratic Republic and, apart from Eastern Europe, foreign countries were hardly accessible for her. She was therefore interested in getting to know countries beyond those of the Soviet Bloc. Another nurse stated that she was eager to experience how the work in Mongolia is organized, what standards are there and generally how the health care system is functioning there.

A few nurses said they had left Germany or plan to leave it (again) because of opportunities for aid work. A nurse who left Germany to work in Tanzania stated that she had always wanted to go to Africa to experience a developing country and help the suffering population there. She applied for a vacancy in a nursing clinic and reported that she sometimes had to bear the responsibility for a whole village, which was a huge challenge for her. Another nurse explained that her religion played an important motivational role in her decision to work abroad. When she learnt about a partnership cooperation between the University of Jena and a hospital in Malawi, she took the opportunity and joined a team of health professionals who went to work in Malawi:

> I am privileged to be born in Germany, one of the richest countries in the world, but I think because of this I have responsibility towards the less privileged. For me it was important to help with what I have – education, money, time. My religion, I am a Christian, was a major motivation.

### German medical doctors leaving Germany

Medical doctors, mainly residents, planning to leave Germany complained about the workload in German hospitals and the work–life imbalance. A medical doctor explained that he was planning to leave Germany because of the high workload and the bad working conditions in his hospital. Because of a shortage of medical personnel he had to work overtime and could often not take proper lunch breaks. One female medical doctor confirmed that the working schedule in German hospitals was incompatible with family and that working time arrangements should be more flexible. Medical doctors, furthermore, complained about the increasing administrative burden they face in their clinical daily routine:

> We don't have time for the patients, because we are occupied with bureaucracy. Everything needs to be documented.

A major factor causing dissatisfaction among young residents in Germany is the hierarchical structure in German hospitals and the leadership style of chief physicians. One participant shared his impression that asking a question during a visit with the head physician was not well received because the chief physician perceived this as a question on his competence. Another medical doctor said he left Germany because of the lack of collegiality and the occurrence of harassment at work. A third participant argued that the higher physician density in Germany sustains outdated hierarchical structures and is a reason for slow career progress. He explained that in the United Kingdom the hierarchy is flatter and junior doctors are allowed to take more responsibilities because there are not as many doctors as in Germany.

The organization and content of specialist training in Germany were criticized by some participants. One medical doctor specializing in neurology and planning to move to the United States complained about the lack of structure in postgraduate training:

> The German specialist training is not well structured, it depends on your own engagement and that of the head of department, but not on the structures within the system. Basically, as a medical doctor you are not entitled to a structured specialist training. The head of department might write that you have done sonography a certain number of times, so that you can get the specialty title, but the truth is that you have done it much fewer times, because you had to manage the daily routine at the ward. In countries such as the US and the Netherlands, the emphasis on training is much bigger.

The lack of structure in the specialist training was perceived as a reason for slow career progress:

> The specialist training here is supposed to last between five and six years including all rotations. However, there is a line of medical doctors who wait to gain experience with functional diagnostics, so I will not be able to obtain

> a specialist title in less than 12 years, even if I work full-time and don't get children during that time.

Another medical doctor explained that he left Germany because he wanted to learn to think in a structured and interdisciplinary way and to gain medical skills that are not limited to one's specialty.

> At the time I left Germany, there were not many vacancies. I was looking for a solid, rudimentary and wide (generalist) education. I wanted to go to a developing country and be able to treat the population there, but I didn't have the feeling the clinical practice in Germany was very pragmatic. In the United Kingdom, the shortage of doctors was so perceptible that medical doctors needed to be trained to treat a wide range of conditions. The structure was based on rotation. We started in the general surgery, then in the vascular surgery, urology, internal medicine, cardiology, gastroenterology, emergency medicine, geriatrics, obstetrics, paediatrics, neurology, psychiatry. The kind of rotation that makes you a family doctor.

The incompatibility of clinical practice and research was a further point of criticism. Research opportunities in other countries, particularly in the United States, seem to attract young and ambitious medical doctors to leave the country.

> In my most productive years between 25 and 45, when I could best work intellectually and carry out research, I will be busy with managing the ward and do things that have little to do with what I studied and what I actually want to do. I want to use my intellectual capacities and contribute to research projects, but I don't have time for this, because in our department we have 130 patients and the length of hospital stay is decreasing. All these patients need to be managed and I am there to steer them through the diagnostic system and release them in the shortest possible time … What I liked about the US is the possibility to start a research project relatively low-threshold, the creative scientific atmosphere and the feeling to be on the playing field of science. This is missing in Germany.

A few participants stated that they left Germany anticipating that they would earn more abroad. However, surprisingly, and contrary to popular expectations and the finding of other research (Ramboll Management, 2004), the majority of participants said that remuneration was not the main reason for emigration. Medical doctors explained that it was rather the combination of better working conditions, fewer patients and less bureaucracy that acted as a decisive pull factor in their decision to migrate. In addition, geographical proximity and language similarities facilitated the migration process to Switzerland. One medical doctor stated that he is planning to leave Germany because of the hierarchical structures in German hospitals, even though he will earn less abroad.

### 9.4.2 Return migration to Germany

#### German nurses returning to Germany

Some of the nurses participating in the study returned to Germany after practising in Austria, France, New Zealand, Malawi, Switzerland, Tanzania, and the United Kingdom. Some had planned to leave Germany for a limited period of time, so returning home was an expected move. Other nurses said they returned to Germany mainly for family reasons. One nurse, who obtained her nursing training in New Zealand and worked there for a few years, stated she returned to Germany in order to nurse her grandmother, who had become sick. She admitted that reintegration in Germany was difficult for her because she was used to greater autonomy, a better occupational image, higher payment and teamwork. Shortly after she returned to Germany, she left the nursing profession. Thanks to her master studies and the higher qualifications she obtained abroad, she was able to find a job as a researcher and studies coordinator in one of the biggest and most renowned hospitals in Germany.

Another nurse who returned to Germany for private reasons after practising in France said she was disappointed to see that not much had changed in Germany. According to her, the nursing profession still has the old occupational image, nurses still perform routine jobs and case management is not applied systematically.

Cultural differences and hierarchical structures in hospitals were mentioned by some participants as an instigating factor in the decision to return to Germany. A German nurse who worked in Vienna for three years stated:

> In Austria, the hierarchical structures are even more pronounced than in Germany. Nursing assistants are below the nurses, i.e. there is another distinct hierarchical level. Native health professionals made it clear that there is a huge difference between the professional groups, reflected in their status and recognition. The doctors behaved as if they were your boss, as if they can dismiss you or at least put that pressure on you. The nursing profession was not appreciated.

Some nurses returned to Germany because of a lack of employment opportunities at the destination. A nurse from Baden-Württemberg, who worked in Switzerland, explained that because of reorganization her position in Switzerland was removed and that this was the reason for her to return to

Germany. She stated that she would not hesitate to move to Switzerland again if she received another opportunity to work there.

A few nurses who returned to Germany were motivated by the wish to complete a Masters' degree, for example in nursing management or medical education. The nurses stated that they planned to stay in Germany only for a limited period of time and to return to Switzerland in the long run, together with their families.

### German medical doctors returning to Germany

Homesickness was mentioned as a major reason for German medical doctors to return to their country of origin. One participant left the United Kingdom and returned to Germany because he felt that Germany was his home country. Financial considerations did not play a role in his decision to return. Despite the fact that he worked in the United Kingdom for more than 10 years, he admitted that he did not feel fully integrated in society there and felt like a "second class doctor". Another interviewee who left the United Kingdom after working there for 14 years said he wanted his children to grow up in Germany. He also admitted that he did not feel fully integrated in British society. In his point of view, German society is more open to foreigners and offers more possibilities for integration than the British. Then he added:

> Although, I have to admit, I would have stayed there if I had my own practice.
> I would have been my own boss, a completely different situation.

Improved employment opportunities in Germany seem to play an important role in the decision of medical doctors to return to Germany. Both medical doctors stated that they left Germany at a time when there was a lack of vacancies for medical doctors in Germany. Between 1982 and 2002, the number of medical graduates exceeded the number of vacancies for medical doctors. Since 2002, however, the trend reversed and a lack of medical doctors became perceptible. Hence, an important factor in the decision of the two interviewees to return to Germany was the increased demand for medical doctors in the country. Both medical doctors felt that their work experience abroad was appreciated in Germany and that it has helped them in their career progress.

One interviewee who was working abroad as a medical doctor specializing in tropical and travel medicine returned to Germany after working in different countries for more than 20 years; his reasons were that working conditions in the operational area worsened and he was approaching retirement age. Another medical doctor returned from France for private reasons and in order to accomplish his specialist training. However, he admitted that he is planning to leave Germany again and would not return unless the hierarchical structures in German hospitals improve.

### 9.4.3 Immigration to Germany

*Foreign nurses moving to Germany*

Higher remuneration and the possibility to save money and send home remittances are important motivations for foreign-trained nurses to come to Germany. A Bulgarian nurse, working in a hospital in southern Germany, reported:

> I had a job as a nurse in Bulgaria, but it was so badly paid. I could not earn more than €250 per month. Here in Germany I earn €1 500. I live in the hospital dormitory; my rent is low. I try to save money which I send home.

She added that she is planning to return to Bulgaria within a year to live with her parents and her son. According to interviews with recruitment agencies and media reports, higher remuneration is the major motivational factor for many Eastern European nurses who provide home-help services in Germany. The vast majority stay in Germany only for a limited period of time and return to their countries once they have saved enough to support their families.

A number of participants came to Germany because of the political and economic conditions in their countries. A male nurse from Iraq, for example, came to Germany even though his professional qualifications were not recognized in Germany. He worked in the construction sector for several years before he completed the nursing training in Germany and was able to work as a nurse. Two participants from Zimbabwe came to Germany as asylum seekers. They obtained their nursing training in Germany. A number of foreign nurses moved to Germany in search of better living conditions. One nurse from Poland stated she moved together with her family because she was dissatisfied with the living conditions in Poland at that time:

> The times in Poland were difficult. Because of the high inflation, we were afraid of losing our savings. Furthermore, we lived close to a chemical plant and I was concerned about the health of my children, but we had no chance to change our apartment. In addition, social services in Poland were bad. Waiting lists for cardiac surgeries were long. Very sick people had to wait, but those who had money or a higher position in the society were taken first. I simply did not want my children to grow up and live in this country.

Family reasons were the major motivational factor in the decision to move to Germany for a few foreign nurses. Nurses from Australia, the Russian Federation, South Africa and Spain admitted they had come to Germany because of their German husbands or wives. One nurse from South Africa observed:

> Because of my husband, I am tied to Germany. Apart from this, I am no longer young enough to be able to work everywhere.

Family appears to be a strong migration motivation, outweighing other factors such as working conditions, remuneration and professional recognition. Hence some nurses accepted worse working conditions, lower remuneration and lower social status. A nurse from Australia, who gained work experience in New Zealand and moved to Germany, stated:

> Remuneration is lower in Germany than in New Zealand. At the ward there is almost always a shortage of personnel, which means stress, and less time for the patients. Nurses in New Zealand and Australia receive higher recognition for their work. My impression is that Germany is 20 years behind other countries in terms of professional image and recognition, social status, training and continuing education, but I work in Germany because my husband and my family is here.

A male nurse from Spain, who moved to Germany for family reasons, stated that he left his job as a nurse in Germany after six months because he was dissatisfied with and could not adapt to the working conditions in Germany.

Once in Germany, foreign nurses face a number of challenges. The most important one was insufficient knowledge of the language. This, nurses admitted, leads to dissatisfaction for themselves, their colleagues and the patients. An African nurse complained that the lack of language skills caused prejudices and unfriendly behaviour among her colleagues. Language and integration courses for foreign-trained nurses are not systematically offered in Germany. Some hospitals offer clinical induction courses. A few study participants reported that some employers offer help with finding accommodation, or provide rooms for their foreign-trained employees.

Most nurses stated that the content of training, the nursing tasks and the responsibilities differed from country to country. On the one hand, some foreign-trained nurses reported that the competences and responsibilities of nurses in their country of training were generally higher than in Germany. On the other hand, foreign nurses complained of not possessing certain clinical, technical and computer skills.

Many of the nurses reported personal contacts and networks as a major factor facilitating migration and successful integration in Germany. A nurse from Kenya confirmed that a network of African friends and acquaintances who were already living in Germany helped her to find her way through the requirements of the German authorities. Eventually, she stayed in Germany because she married a German citizen.

Expert interviews suggested that private recruitment agencies and a bilateral agreement between Germany and Croatia also play a facilitating role in the migration process of foreign nurses. In May 2011, the transitional arrangements on the free movement of labour from the new EU Member States expired (the transitional arrangements for Bulgaria and Romania expired in December 2013 and those for Croatia will expire in July 2020 at the latest), which means that private persons in Germany can directly employ a nurse or a carer from the new EU Member States without using the services of recruitment agencies. However, expert interviews with representatives of recruitment agencies suggest that many families continue paying for the services of private sector intermediaries. In that case, carers are registered as self-employed in their home country and can offer their services if they prove that they have more than one client or they are "delegated" by a company that works with partner agencies in Germany (Ognyanova & Busse, 2011). The carers pay social insurance contributions and taxes in their country of origin and working hours are regulated through the law in their home country. However, it is difficult to monitor if they are kept.

Since the early 1970s, foreign nurses were recruited via so-called bilateral agreements between the German Federal Employment Agency and a number of mainly Eastern European countries. Germany has a bilateral agreement of this type with Croatia, which provides the highest number of foreign nurses and midwives subject to social insurance contributions (Federal Employment Agency's International Placement Services, 2011). In 2013, the Agency also had bilateral agreements with Bosnia and Herzegovina, Serbia, the Philippines, Vietnam and Tunisia (German Federal Employment Agency, unpublished data) (see also Chapter 12).

### Foreign medical doctors moving to Germany

Dissatisfaction with remuneration and the working conditions in the health sector of the home country, on the one hand, and the prospect of higher wages and better working environment in Germany, on the other, were reported as decisive factors in the decision of foreign medical doctors to leave their countries of origin. The majority of foreign medical doctors who participated in the study (from Bulgaria, India, Lithuania, Mongolia, Romania, the Russian Federation, Syria, Ukraine) mentioned higher remuneration as a central factor, or at least a relevant incentive, in the decision to migrate to Germany. One interviewee mentioned that he would have rather moved to the United Kingdom because of higher wages, but that access to the United Kingdom appeared in his case to be more difficult than to Germany.

Many participants complained that the health sector in their countries was underfunded and poorly organized. A medical doctor from Bulgaria observed:

> The wages are low certainly, but also the working conditions are poor, the whole health system. Our psychiatric care is simply very bad, not because medical doctors are not competent enough, but because the system is underfunded.

> I cannot imagine working in Bulgaria as a psychiatrist under such working conditions.

The majority of participants complained that hospitals in their countries of origin are poorly equipped. They reported that the outdated equipment and infrastructure and the lack of modern technologies hindered their career progress.

Specialist training and professional development played an important role in the decision of foreign medical doctors to migrate to Germany. Many medical doctors complained about limited access to specialist training in their home countries (Austria, Syria, India, Iraq, Mongolia, Bulgaria, Latvia) and stated that they migrated to Germany in pursuit of better opportunities for specialist training. One medical doctor from Austria explained:

> Remuneration in Austria is higher than in Germany, you have 14 monthly salaries and there is dismissal pay, but there are fewer vacancies for specialist training than in Germany... Patient access to specialists in Austria is more restricted than in Germany. The fewer specialists you have, the cheaper the health care system.

Specialist training in Germany is attractive for foreign medical doctors because it offers the opportunity to use technologies and equipment that are not available in the country of origin. Generally, foreign medical doctors perceived the quality and management of health care in Germany to be much higher than in their home countries. One participant from Syria stated:

> In Syria the access to modern technology such as PET scans is very limited. Only a few private practices have such technology. Here in Germany I can acquire skills working with new technologies.

The economic and political situation in the home country was an important push factor for migration for a number of medical doctors. One medical doctor from the Russian Federation stated:

> The 1990s in Russia was a difficult time, we had hyperinflation and the system was anything but stable. Furthermore, I wanted my children to grow up in a free and democratic country.

A medical doctor from Ukraine explained:

> I moved because I wanted to treat every person, not only those who could afford to meet a doctor. I never again wanted to have to reject a person because he or she cannot pay the consultation fee.

Some of the participants complained about the high level of corruption in the health system of their home country.

A few of the participants stated that they could easily move to Germany because they were actively recruited or had professional contacts in the country and were offered an employment contract:

> I met a German professor in Bulgaria who was working at the university in Magdeburg and he invited me to come to Germany. He said that I didn't have to take a decision right away, that I should come for three weeks to Germany, familiarize myself with the hospital and the medical staff working there and then take a decision. He would cover all costs, including travel and accommodation.

Only a few of the participants said that they spoke good German before they came to Germany.

Participants from the new EU Member States stated that the free movement of labour and the mutual recognition of professional qualifications in the EU have tremendously facilitated their emigration to Germany. A few medical doctors from the Russian Federation and Ukraine stated that they were able to emigrate to Germany because of the special immigration regulations for Jewish immigrants and ethnic German immigrants.

The majority of non-EU participants perceived the legal framework regulating the immigration of health professionals and the recognition of qualifications as a barrier for migration. They explained that the process of meeting the occupational requirements places a huge burden on non-EU citizens. A medical doctor from India stated that he faced great difficulties in having his medical degree recognized because he had managed to complete his studies in five and a half years, while the German provisions require a study duration of at least six years:

> All the requirements and the bureaucracy of the German authorities prevented me from practising my profession for a long time. The process of obtaining a temporary professional authorization (Berufserlaubnis) should be more transparent. Each state has its own legal provisions. Sometimes qualifications are recognized, sometimes not.

Study participants perceived language barriers as a huge problem. The need for language courses, mentoring and coaching programmes, but also intercultural training, was considered urgent by the participants. A Vietnamese medical doctor admitted:

> Even after a longer period of stay in Germany, I face serious language problems, which hinder communication with my colleagues and with the patients. In addition, my colleagues often use technical terms in Latin which I don't understand. A language course on the technical terminology would have been very helpful.

Another medical doctor confirmed:

> I have difficulties in integrating into the team because I cannot communicate
> very well with my colleagues. Another problem are the documentation
> requirements. German forms are very complicated and extensive.

A number of participants, who were informed about the PROMeTHEUS study
by the VIA Institute for Education and Profession, stated that the integration
course they took at the VIA Institute enabled them to work successfully and
competently in their profession. The course is mainly offered to medical
doctors from non-EU countries and imparts language and medical knowledge.
It facilitates the application and job-seeking process and places medical
doctors in internships. The cost of the course, about €4 500, is covered by
the Federal Employment Agency, but some participants explained that many
job centres are not aware of this possibility. A few participants admitted that
they worked in low-paid jobs before they could practise their profession and
that the integration course helped them to practise their profession again. One
participant reflected:

> This was a very extensive course, not only a language course. It gives you the
> possibility to familiarize yourself with how medicine is practised in Germany.
> You learn what is required to work in a German hospital and how to obtain
> specialist and continuing training. After the course I feel much more confident
> to work as a medical doctor in Germany.

One participant from Kazakhstan took a course with the Otto Benecke
Foundation, commissioned and financed by the state of Brandenburg, which
contains a language course, four months of practical training in a hospital
and a theory part aimed at retraining Jewish immigrants and ethnic German
repatriates and preparing them for the verification of equivalency test.

## 9.5 Discussion and conclusions

At present, the mobility of health professionals to and from Germany is
not a huge and uncontrollable phenomenon for Germany, but the trend is
increasing. The percentage of foreign-national medical doctors registered in
Germany in 2012 was about 7.1% (32 548), a 14.8% increase compared with
the previous year. The percentage of active foreign-national medical doctors
among all active medical doctors in Germany was 8.1% (28 310; a 15.1%
increase compared with the previous year). The total number of foreign medical
doctors in Germany is increasing continuously. In particular, the number
of medical doctors from the new EU Member States (excluding Malta and
Cyprus) is rising rapidly, from 2 548 in 2003 to 9 160 in 2012, an increase of
almost 260%. The number of medical doctors from Romania increased even
further, by 358%, from 635 in 2003 to 2 910 in 2012 (Fig. 9.1). Furthermore,

**Fig. 9.1** *Medical doctors from selected countries registered in Germany, 1995–2012*

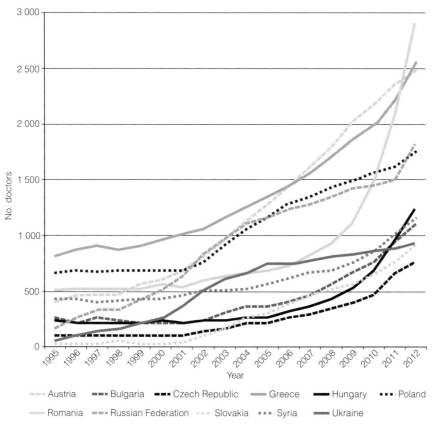

*Source*: German Federal Chamber of Physicians, unpublished data, 2013.

the stock of medical doctors from countries in Asia (Syria) and Africa (Libya, Egypt), but also from European countries such as Greece and Ukraine, has rapidly increased over recent years. Of all foreign medical doctors in Germany in 2012, 73.3% came from Europe, 18.1% from Asia, 4.9% from Africa and 2.9% from the United States.

The annual outflow of medical doctors in 2012 decreased to 2 241 (less than 0.5% of the total number of medical doctors), Germans making up 66.8% of this outflow. In 2011, the annual outflow of medical doctors was higher: 3 410, 68.6% being German. The most attractive destination countries were Switzerland, Austria, the United States and the United Kingdom.

In 2011, about 3 800 vacancies for medical doctors in German hospitals were unfilled, whereas in 2009 and 2010 the numbers were 5 000 and 4 900, respectively (Blum et al., 2011). Despite the slight decrease in the number of vacancies, the shortage of medical doctors in certain, mainly rural and sparsely populated, regions of the country seems to be a persistent problem. At the same time, oversupply of medical doctors can be observed in and around big cities such as Berlin, Munich and Hamburg. Foreign medical doctors play an important role in mitigating the regional shortages of medical doctors in Germany (Ognyanova & Busse, 2011). German hospitals and states affected by the lack of medical personnel are actively recruiting medical doctors abroad. This is often done via the services of private recruitment agencies (Blum & Löffert, 2010).

Because of population ageing, the demand for health professionals is expected to dramatically increase in the future. A study by Ostwald et al. (2010) projects for Germany a shortage of 56 000 medical doctors and 140 000 nurses and other health workers by 2020. By the year 2030, the total shortage of health professionals is expected to almost reach 1 million, including 165 000 medical doctors, 466 000 nurses and auxiliary nurses and 334 000 other health workers. Major determinants for this shortage are the demographic developments in the country, which will increase demand for health and long-term care, and the imminent retirement of health professionals. A study by the German Hospital Institute projects a shortage of 37 400 medical doctors in hospitals by the year 2019 (Blum & Löffert, 2010).

A more recent study suggests a shortage of 570 000 (106 000 medical doctors and 464 000 nurses) by the year 2030. In the worst-case scenario, more than 630 000 full-time health professionals could be missing (every fourth position would be then vacant), because of rising demand, falling number of graduates from 2020 on and the increased retirement of health professionals (PricewaterhouseCoopers, 2012). The European Commission projects a shortage of about 1 million health professionals in the EU in 2020 (590 000 nurses, 230 000 medical doctors and 150 000 dentists, pharmacists and physiotherapists) if no measures are undertaken to counterbalance this trend (European Commission, 2012). Hence, international recruitment in Germany and the wider EU might intensify as a short-term solution to the looming shortages, and migration might increase as a result.

Table 9.3 summarizes the pull and push factors found in this study for the mobility of medical doctors as well as the hurdles and the facilitating factors.

The findings of the study demonstrate that foreign medical doctors face a number of difficulties, including language and cultural barriers, bureaucracy and increased documentation requirements. Simplified and eased labour market and occupational requirements are expected to facilitate the recruitment of foreign non-EU medical doctors. In March 2013, the German Ministry of Health submitted a draft regulation aiming to harmonize nationwide the occupational provisions on the access to the medical profession for foreign-

**Table 9.3** Migration motivations of medical doctors moving to, leaving or returning to Germany

| Migration factors | Migrant type | | |
| --- | --- | --- | --- |
| | Immigrant | Emigrant | Returner |
| Pull | Higher remuneration<br><br>Specialist training and professional development<br><br>Use of modern technology | Attractive employment opportunities (work–life balance)<br><br>Research opportunities | Homesickness<br><br>Employment and career opportunities<br><br>Specialist training |
| Push | Remuneration<br><br>Working conditions<br><br>Economic and political situation | Workload<br><br>Hierarchical structures<br><br>Administrative burden<br><br>Specialist training | Lacking integration in the society<br><br>Working conditions |
| Hurdles | Language barriers<br><br>Occupational requirements for non-EU citizens | Cultural differences | Reintegration |
| Facilitating | Active recruitment and professional contacts<br><br>Free movement of labour and recognition of qualifications in the EU<br><br>Immigration provisions (Jewish immigrants and ethnic German immigrants)<br><br>Integration courses | Language links<br><br>Geographical proximity | Appreciation of work experience abroad |

trained medical doctors, including medical knowledge and language tests. In addition, integration courses providing language skills, as well as cultural, organizational and medical knowledge, play a crucial role in the successful integration of foreign health professionals. The growing number of foreign medical doctors in Germany increases the need to systematically offer such integration courses as a means to enhance quality assurance in the health system.

Successful retention strategies targeting German medical doctors can include administrative work relief and flexible working hours, enabling a better work–life balance; flatter hierarchies and faster career progress; better organized specialist training with opportunities for research; and effective incentives for medical doctors to work in rural and sparsely populated areas. The finding in this study that remuneration is not the main motivation for medical doctors to leave Germany is confirmed by studies demonstrating that remuneration of German doctors is competitive in an international perspective, even though neighbouring countries such as Switzerland and the Netherlands, but also the United Kingdom, pay higher salaries to specialists (Deutsche Krankenhaus Gesellschaft, 2011).

Finally, policy-makers can encourage return migration, which can be beneficial to the German health care system as returners often enrich the system with new experiences, competences and suggestions for improvement, and they can instigate policy learning and transfer. While return migration of medical doctors is not recorded in Germany, and there is a lack of such data, the findings of the study described here indicate that medical doctors are inclined to return to Germany not only because they feel connected to the country but also because their career progression opportunities, as well as remuneration, improve in the later stages of career development.

With regard to nurses, mobility seems to be lower than for medical doctors according to the available official data. The share of foreign nurses and midwives among all nurses and midwives subject to social insurance contributions decreased from 4.8% in 1995 to 3.4% in 2008. This is partly the result of decreased demand for nurses in the country. Between 1996 and 2008, 50 000 full-time positions were abolished in German hospitals under cost-saving measures, especially following the introduction of the German diagnosis-related group system (Isfort et al., 2010). However, the trend reversed in 2009 and the percentage of foreign nurses and midwives among all nurses and midwives has been increasing since then, reaching 3.6% in 2011 and 3.7% in 2012 (Fig. 9.2).

The number of nurses and midwives from the new EU Member States subject to social insurance contributions increased between 1997 and 2011, with Croatia and Poland being major EU source countries in 2012 (Fig. 9.3). However, anecdotal evidence suggests that the number of nurses from Eastern Europe,

**Fig. 9.2** *Percentage of foreign nurses and midwives among all nurses and midwives in Germany, 1995–2011*

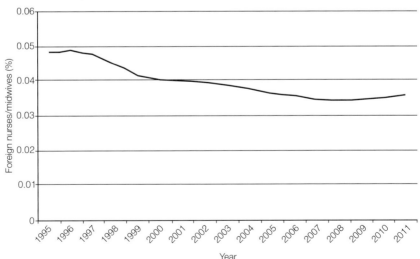

*Source*: Federal Employment Agency, unpublished data, 2013.

*Note*: The classification of professions in Germany was reorganized in 2010, which affects the comparability of data.

**Fig. 9.3** *Nurses from selected major source countries working in Germany, 1997–2012*

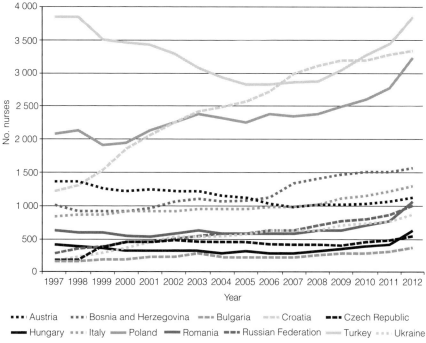

Austria ···· Bosnia and Herzegovina ···· Bulgaria ···· Croatia ···· Czech Republic
Hungary ···· Italy — Poland — Romania ···· Russian Federation — Turkey ···· Ukraine

*Source*: Federal Employment Agency, unpublished data, 2013.

in particular those working in private households as carers for the elderly, has increased much more than the official data suggest (Ognyanova & Busse, 2011). The German Nursing Association estimates that the outflow of nurses from Germany does not exceed 1 000 per year, but official data are not available.

Migration flows of nurses are very likely to increase in the future. Demographic ageing in the country and the fact that Germany lacks a comprehensive system of workforce planning might create perceptible shortages of health professionals in future, nurses for the elderly in particular. Until recently, the current and expected shortage of nurses has not been broached by the media in the way that the shortage of physicians has been debated, which is partly because of the lower organizational capacity of the nursing profession with regard to collective bargaining and its weaker lobbying power. A number of studies exploring the specificities of the nursing profession suggest increasing dissatisfaction with working conditions among nurses (Hasselhorn, Müller & Tackenberg, 2005; Joost, 2007; Dieckmann et al., 2010; Isfort et al., 2010; Zander, Dobler & Busse, 2011). Such developments might lead to increased attrition and outmigration of German nurses and fuel international recruitment at the same time.

The findings of this qualitative study (summarized in Table 9.4) suggest that in order to enhance the attractiveness of the nursing profession policy responses

**Table 9.4** Migration motivations of nurses moving to, leaving or returning to Germany

| Migration factors | Migrant type | | |
| --- | --- | --- | --- |
| | Immigrant | Emigrant | Returner |
| Pull | Higher pay and the possibility to send remittances home | Attractive employment opportunities | Family |
| | Family | Higher recognition and responsibilities | Further qualifications |
| | | Interest in foreign countries | |
| | | Opportunities for aid work | |
| Push | Political, economic and living conditions | Effort–reward imbalance | Cultural differences |
| | | | Hierarchical structures |
| | | | Lack of employment opportunities |
| Hurdles | Language barriers | Differences in content of training and responsibilities | Reintegration |
| | Differences in content of training and responsibilities | | |
| Facilitating | Personal contacts and networks | Language links | Recognition of qualifications and work experience abroad |
| | Private recruitment agencies | Geographical proximity | |
| | Bilateral agreements | Active recruitment | |
| | Support with accommodation | | |

should focus on improving working conditions, increasing remuneration and enhancing competencies, responsibilities and career opportunities for nurses. Advanced competencies and greater responsibilities for nurses should be ensured by appropriate academic and continuing education. Nurses who participated in the study showed a positive attitude towards enhanced responsibilities and a reallocation of tasks from medical doctors to nurses. Many of them lamented the low competence and the low esteem of German nurses and appreciated the wider field of responsibility, scope for decision-making and freedom of action they had abroad. Studies have demonstrated that nurses' participation in decision-making processes has a positive impact on job satisfaction and employee retention (Hasselhorn, Müller & Tackenberg, 2005). The introduction of a chamber of nurses (analogous to the Federal Chamber of Physicians) with mandatory registration would strengthen the position of the relatively weak and poorly organized nursing staff. A few states in Germany have already taken the first steps towards the introduction of a mandatory nurse chamber.

The German Advisory Council on the Assessment of Developments in the Health Care System (2007) recommended a reorganization of the health professions so that certain tasks that were normally performed by physicians could be carried out by non-physicians. As a result, non-physician professions are expected to become more attractive as they will be allowed to take more independent decisions in their professional life, their social status will increase and they will be offered continuing academic education. Furthermore, total health workforce costs are expected to decrease as most non-physician health professionals have shorter training times than physicians and their income is lower. In October 2011, the Federal Joint Committee adopted a Directive according to which, as part of a treatment plan, certain medical tasks can be carried out by nurses who have undergone special training. It is still controversially debated whether the new Directive refers to delegation or substitution of tasks, the latter implying transfer of responsibility, prescribing and billing rights.

The active recruitment of foreign nurses is still not pronounced in Germany, but health professionals from the crisis-hit Southern and Eastern European countries increasingly seek employment in Germany, reflecting a general migration trend towards Germany. In 2012, the annual influx of immigrants amounted to 1 081 000, 13% more than 2011 and the highest number since 1995. Although considerable, the increase in the number of immigrants from Southern Europe remains fairly small in absolute terms compared with the increase in immigration from Eastern Europe (Statistisches Bundesamt, 2013).

A study by Neuhaus, Isfort and Weidner (2009) has suggested that private households already strongly rely on foreign, often irregularly employed, personnel. In view of the demographic changes affecting a number of industrial countries, the international competition for nurses is expected to intensify. This qualitative study demonstrated that language and induction courses play a crucial role in the recruitment and successful integration of foreign-trained personnel and that Germany is lagging behind in this respect.

## References

Advisory Council on the Assessment of Developments in the Health Care System (2007). *Kooperation und Verantwortung. Voraussetzung einer zielorientierten Gesundheitsversorgung. [Cooperation and responsibility prerequisites for target-oriented health care. Report 2007]*. Bonn, Sachverständigenrat zur Begutachtung der Entwicklung im Gesundheitswesen (http://www.svr-gesundheit.de/fileadmin/user_upload/Gutachten/2007/Kurzfassung_2007.pdf, accessed 3 January 2014).

Bijak (2006). *Forecasting international migration: selected theories, models, and methods*. Warsaw, Central European Forum for Migration Research (CEFMR Working Paper 4/2006) (http://www.cefmr.pan.pl/docs/cefmr_wp_2006-04.pdf, accessed 3 January 2014).

Blum K, Löffert S (2010). *Ärztemangel im Krankenhaus – Ausmaß, Ursachen, Gegenmaßnahmen – Forschungsgutachten im Auftrag der Deutschen Krankenhausgesellschaft.* Düsseldorf, Deutsches Krankenhaus Institut (http://www.dki.de/PDF/Zusammenfassung%20Aerztemangel.pdf, accessed 3 January 2014).

Blum et al. (2011). *Krankenhausbarometer 2011.* Düsseldorf, Deutsches Krankenhaus Institut (http://www.dkgev.de/media/file/10655.Krankenhaus_Barometer_2011.pdf, accessed 28 December 2013).

Buchan J (2007). *Health worker migration in Europe: policy issues and options.* London, HLSP Institute (Technical Approach Paper) (http://www.hlsp.org/LinkClick.aspx?fileticket=SM55vQDY0bA%3D&tabid=1702&mid=3361, accessed 2 January 2014).

Deutsche Krankenhaus Gesellschaft (2011). *Gehaltssituation deutscher und europäischer Krankenhausärzte im Vergleich. Ergebnisse der Gutachten von KPMG und DKI zum kaufkraftbereinigten Nettoeinkommen.* Berlin, Deutsche Krankenhaus Gesellschaft (http://www.dkgev.de/media/file/9958.2011-08-18_Grafiken_Arztverguetungen-international.pdf, accessed 2 January 2014).

Dieckmann S et al. (2010). *Balance halten im Pflegealltag.* Berlin, Deutscher Berufsverband für Pflegeberufe (http://www.dbfk.de/verband/bags/BAG-Pflege-im-Krankenhaus/Balance-halten-im-Pflegealltag_final2010-09-02.pdf, accessed 2 January 2014).

di Mattia A, Cassan G (2009). Migration "push" factors in non-OECD countries over the long term. In OECD, ed. *The future of international migration to OECD countries.* Paris, Organisation for Economic Co-operation and Development:139–142 (http://www.iadb.org/intal/intalcdi/PE/2009/03706.pdf, accessed 2 January 2014).

European Commission (2012). *Staff working document on an action plan for the EU health workforce. Towards a job-rich recovery.* Strasbourg, European Commission (http://ec.europa.eu/dgs/health_consumer/docs/swd_ap_eu_healthcare_workforce_en.pdf, accessed 2 January 2014).

Federal Employment Agency's International Placement Services (2011). *Merkblatt zur Vermittlung von Pflegepersonal aus Kroatien nach Deutschland 2011.* Bonn, Bundesagentur für Arbeit Zentrale Auslands- und Fachvermittlung (http://www.arbeitsagentur.de/zentraler-Content/Veroeffentlichungen/Merkblatt-Sammlung/Merkblatt-Vermittlung-Pflegepersonal-Kroatien.pdf, accessed 15 December 2013).

Fellmer S (2008). Germany restricted the freedom of movement for Polish citizens – but does it matter? *EUMAP* (special issue: Across fading borders:

the challenges of east–west migration in the EU) [online] (http://pdc.ceu.hu/archive/00003936/01/fellmer.pdf, accessed 3 January 2014).

Haour-Knipe M, Davies A (2008). *Return migration of nurses.* Geneva, International Centre on Nurse Migration (http://intlnursemigration.org/assets/pdfs/ReturnmigrationA4.pdf, accessed 3 January 2014).

Hasselhorn HM, Müller HM, Tackenberg P, eds. (2005). *Nurses Early Exit Study: NEXT scientific report.* Wuppertal, University of Wuppertal (http://www.econbiz.de/archiv1/2008/53602_nurses_work_europe.pdf, accessed 3 January 2014).

Isfort M et al. (2010). *Pflege-Thermometer 2009: Eine bundesweite Befragung von Pflegekräften zur Situation der Pflege und Patientenversorgung im Krankenhaus.* Cologne, Deutsches Institut für angewandte Pflegeforschung (http://www.dip.de/fileadmin/data/pdf/material/dip_Pflege-Thermometer_2009.pdf, accessed 3 January 2014).

Janus K et al. (2007). German physicians "on strike": shedding light on the roots of physician dissatisfaction. *Health Policy*, 82(3):357–365.

Joost A (2007). *Berufsverbleib und Fluktuation von Altenpflegerinnen und Altenpflegern.* Frankfurt, Wissenschaftliches Zentrum an der Goethe-Universität Frankfurt am Main (http://www.iwak-frankfurt.de/documents/Berufsverbleib.pdf, accessed 3 January 2014).

Kingma M (2006). *Nurses on the move: migration and the global health care economy.* Ithaca, NY, Cornell University Press.

Lowell L (2009). Immigration "pull" factors in OECD countries over the long term. In OECD, ed. *The future of international migration to OECD countries.* Paris, Organisation for Economic Co-operation and Development:51–137 (http://www.iadb.org/intal/intalcdi/PE/2009/03706.pdf, accessed 2 January 2014).

Massey D et al. (1993). Theories of international migration: a review and appraisal. *Population and Development Review*, 19(3):431–466.

Neuhaus A, Isfort M, Weidner F (2009). *Situation und Bedarfe von Familien mit mittel- und osteuropäischen Haushaltshilfen.* Cologne, Deutsches Institut für angewandte Pflegeforschung (http://www.pflege-shv.de/uploads/pflege-shv/Buch-Artikelempflehlungen/dip-Studie-Haushaltshilfen_Bericht0409.pdf, accessed 3 January 2014).

Ognyanova D, Busse R (2011). A destination and a source: Germany manages regional health workforce disparities with foreign medical doctors. In Wismar M et al., eds. *Health professional mobility and health systems. Evidence from 17*

*European countries.* Copenhagen, WHO Regional Office for Europe on behalf of the European Observatory on Health Systems and Policies:211–242.

Ognyanova D et al. (2012). Mobility of health professionals pre and post 2004 and 2007 EU enlargements: evidence from the EU project PROMeTHEUS. *Health Policy*, 108:122–132.

Ostwald D et al. (2010). *Fachkräftemangel. Stationärer und ambulanter Bereich bis zum Jahr 2030.* Frankfurt, WifOR and PricewaterhouseCoopers Wirtschaftsprüfungsgesellschaft (http://www.vpkbb.org/uploads/media/Studie_Fachkraeftemangel_Gesundheit.pdf, accessed 3 January 2014).

PricewaterhouseCoopers (2012). *112 und niemand hilft – Fachkräftemangel: Warum dem Gesundheitssystem ab 2030 die Luft ausgeht.* Frankfurt, PricewaterhouseCoopers.

Ramboll Management (2004). *Gutachten zum "Ausstieg aus der kurativen ärztlichen Berufstätigkeit in Deutschland".* Hamburg, Erstellt im Auftrage des BMGS (https://www.bundesgesundheitsministerium.de/fileadmin/dateien/Publikationen/Gesundheit/Sonstiges/Abschlussbericht_Gutachten_zum_Ausstieg_aus_der_kurativen_aerztlichen_Berufstaetigkeit_in_Deutschland.pdf, accessed 3 January 2014).

Ritchie J, Spencer L (2004). Qualitative data analysis: the call for transparency. *Building Research Capacity*, 7: 2–4 (http://www.tlrp.org/rcbn/capacity/Journal/issue7.pdf, accessed 2 January 2014).

Statistischcs Bundesamt (2013). *Weiter hohe Zuwanderung nach Deutschland im Jahr 2012* [Continuing high level of immigration to Germany in 2012]. Bonn, Statistisches Bundesamt (Press Release 156, 7 June) (https://www.destatis.de/DE/PresseService/Presse/Pressemitteilungen/2013/05/PD13_156_12711.html, accessed 3 January 2014).

Wismar M et al., eds. (2011). *Health professional mobility and health systems. Evidence from 17 European countries.* Copenhagen, WHO Regional Office for Europe on behalf of the European Observatory on Health Systems and Policies.

Zander B, Dobler L, Busse R (2011). Studie spürt Gründen für Burnout nach. Psychische Erkrankungen kommen in der Pflegebranche überproportional häufig vor. *Pflegezeitschrift*, 64(2):98.

16% and consultants by 45% (Department of Health, 2011a). The expansion of the private health sector generated further demand for health workers.

Ireland's economic downturn had an immediate effect on the numbers of non-EU migrant nurses entering Ireland, with the numbers joining the Nursing Register slowing to a trickle from 2008 onwards, following the cessation of active international recruitment campaigns and the implementation of a public sector recruitment embargo (Humphries, Brugha & McGee, 2012). However, the number of non-EU migrant doctors joining the Register of Medical Practitioners (the Register) continued to increase despite the economic downturn. The number of foreign-trained doctors on the Register increased by 15% between 2007 and 2010 (Medical Council of Ireland, 2013). In 2011, Ireland launched international recruitment campaigns in India and Pakistan to recruit doctors into the public health system. It was noted by Ireland's Health Service Executive that the recruitment campaigns, while costly, would provide an opportunity to reduce overtime and agency costs (HSE, 2011). A total of 285 doctors were actively recruited into the Irish health system as a result of the campaigns (Cullen, 2012). By way of comparison, in 2003, there was an intake to Irish medical schools of 315 Irish/EU students (Medical Council of Ireland, 2003).

The active international recruitment of medical doctors was instigated in response to vacant NCHD posts throughout the public hospital system from 2010 onwards (Healy, 2012). The underlying reason for these vacancies is contested. The Health Service Executive attributes the vacancies to the worldwide shortage of doctors, while the Irish Medical Organisation (the national representative organization for doctors in Ireland) "has repeatedly highlighted that it is a retention rather than a recruitment issue" (Irish Medical Organisation, 2011b). The Irish Medical Organisation cites unattractive working conditions, long working hours, inability to access training and the lack of a structured career path for NCHDs as factors that have led to the attrition of doctors from the Irish health system (Irish Medical Organisation, 2011a).

Health information systems in Ireland do not record where non-EU migrant doctors work within the Irish health system. Recent figures from a variety of sources provide some indication of the workplaces of non-EU migrant doctors: of the 4 639 public sector NCHDs in Ireland in 2008, 55% were non-EU (Postgraduate Medical and Dental Board, 2008); 6% of Ireland's 2 245 consultants were non-Irish (EU and non-EU) as were 5% of Ireland's 2 500 GPs (FAS Training and Employment Authority, 2009). These figures suggest that the majority of Ireland's non-EU migrant doctors work in hospitals as NCHDs.

# Chapter 10

# "I am kind of in stalemate". The experiences of non-EU migrant doctors in Ireland

*Niamh Humphries, Posy Bidwell, Ella Tyrrell, Ruairi Brugha, Steve Thomas and Charles Normand*

## 10.1 Introduction

Although historically a source country for health workers, Ireland began actively recruiting health workers internationally in the early 2000s and is becoming the OECD country with the second highest dependency on foreign-trained doctors (OECD, 2010) and the highest dependency on foreign-trained nurses (OECD, 2010). Between 2000 and 2009, 40% of all newly registered nurses in Ireland were from outside the EU (Humphries, Brugha & McGee, 2009). The number of foreign-trained doctors registered on the Irish Medical Register[1] increased by 259% between 2000 and 2010 (Bidwell et al., 2013).

Ireland's increasing dependency on a migrant health workforce drawn largely from outside the EU can be understood in the context of Ireland's economic boom (circa 1995–2007), which enabled increased spending in the Irish health system and necessitated increased staffing levels. Despite recent health cutbacks, the overall numbers employed in the Irish public health system increased between 2002 and 2011 (Department of Health, 2011c): nurses by 8% (Department of Health, 2011b), non-consultant hospital doctors (NCHD)[2] by

---

1 The Register of Medical Practitioners collects data on country of training rather than on nationality.

2 Non-consultant hospital doctors is the term used in Ireland for junior hospital doctors. They may complete initial and higher specialist training to become specialist hospital doctors or GPs or they may work in service or stand-alone posts under the supervision of hospital specialists.

It is clear from the above figures that Ireland has increased its supply of medical doctors via the inward migration of non-EU doctors. Although international recruitment campaigns have played a part in recent years, most of this doctor migration has been initiated by the migrant doctors themselves. In recent years, Ireland has also sought to increase its supply of medical doctors by expanding medical training via the introduction of graduate entry medical programmes and also by increasing the number of medical places at undergraduate and postgraduate level available to EEA students (HSE MET, 2012): of the 831 medical students in the 2003 intake to Irish medical schools, 516 were non-EU students (Medical Council of Ireland, 2003). By 2011, the proportion of medical graduates from Irish medical schools from non-EU countries had fallen to 40% (Higher Education Authority, 2012). Although on paper it would appear that Ireland trains sufficient doctors to meet demand, many emigrate on graduation, particularly those medical students who originate from outside the EU. That non-EU students tend to leave Ireland after graduation is evident in the profile of the 2010 intern cohort, where 76% (411) of interns were EEA nationals and 24% (131) were non-EEA nationals (HSE MET, 2012). That non-EU students tend to leave Ireland after graduation is evident in the profile of the 2010 intern cohort where 76% (411) of interns were EEA nationals and 24% (131) were non-EEA nationals (HSE MET 2012). There were 350 non-EU medical graduates from Irish medical schools in 2010 (Higher Education Authority 2012). Substantial emigration post-graduation is apparent when the number of medical graduates from Irish medical schools in 2010 – 770 - (Higher Education Authority 2012) is compared with the 542 medical graduates who began their internship in 2010 (HSE MET 2012). In 2011, there were 738 medical graduates from Irish medical schools (Higher Education Authority, 2012) while 542 began their internships in the Irish health system in that year (HSE MET 2012).

While the large discrepancy between the number of graduates and number of internship places can be attributed to the departure of non-EU students who had graduated from Irish medical schools, further large-scale emigration of newly qualified doctors was reported in a recent career-tracking exercise which found "clear evidence that around half of the doctors who completed internship in Ireland in mid-2011, have left the country" (HSE MET, 2012). These data suggest large-scale emigration by Irish-trained doctors (including Irish, EU and non-EU nationals) within one to two years of graduation. Ireland is an illustration of an unusual pattern of health professional migration in that, although Ireland trains large numbers of non-EU medical students, the non-EU migrant doctors working in the Irish health system are, for the most part, *not* Irish trained. A 2007 audit of NCHD posts in Ireland revealed that 48%

(1 134) of respondent registrars and senior house officers had graduated from medical schools outside the EU (Royal College of Physicians, 2007).

To place the experiences of non-EU migrant doctors working in Ireland in context, some understanding of the training and medical career pathways in Ireland is necessary. The Republic of Ireland has six medical schools that provide a five or six year undergraduate training programme; five schools also offer a four year graduate entry programme (Thakore, 2009). Graduates of medical schools in Ireland must complete an internship of one year in order to practise medicine in Ireland (HSE MET, 2011). Successful completion of the internship will result in the award of a certificate of experience, which entitles the holder to apply to the Medical Council for registration (HSE MET, 2011). It also entitles the doctor to apply for initial specialist training, of two to four years in duration. While engaged in this training, doctors are ordinarily employed within the public health service at senior house officer level (HSE MET, 2011). Those who successfully complete their initial specialist training and are awarded a certificate of satisfactory completion of basic specialist training, can become a registrar and compete for a place on a higher specialist training programme, which may take a further two to four years to achieve (Irish Medical Organisation, 2011b). Doctors on the higher specialist training programmes are called specialist or senior registrars and remain at this level while completing their training, which can take up to seven years depending on the specialty (Irish Medical Organisation, 2011b). Doctors wishing to become GPs must complete the higher specialist training in general practice, which involves two years of hospital-based training followed by two years of training under the supervision of a GP trainer.

Following completion of higher specialist training and the awarding of a certificate of satisfactory completion of specialist training, doctors are eligible to apply to be formally registered on the relevant specialist division with the Medical Council. Such specialist registration is a requirement to hold a consultant post within the Irish public health service (HSE MET, 2011). However, completion of higher specialist training and the acquisition of specialist registration does not guarantee doctors a consultant post and it has been noted that "there is no further career progression available within the HSE [Health Service Executive] until such time as they are successful in securing a Consultant post via open competition" (Irish Medical Organisation, 2011b). GPs have an equally complex pathway to achieving a GP principal/partner post following completion of their training.

As of 2011, there were 4 751 NCHD posts within the public health system (Department of Health, 2011c), of which 1 278 were not required for participants in initial or higher specialist training (HSE MET, 2011). Recent figures from the Health Service Executive note that 910 NCHDs hold service posts (HSE, 2011). Doctors occupying these posts are not part of the career pathway from internship through initial specialist training, higher specialist training to consultant level. They occupy hospital posts at senior house officer or registrar level, sometimes known as stand-alone posts, as the doctors occupying them work as hospital doctors but do so outside the structured training programme. No career progression is possible outside these structured training programmes. NCHDs in stand-alone posts, which are typically in smaller non-specialist hospitals, undertake many of the basic hospital clinical activities that are also done by those in training programmes. However, staffing, supervision and facilities in these hospitals usually fall well short of what would be required in a structured training programme. Recommendations for the phasing out of NCHD posts with limited training potential (Buttimer, 2006) and for all NCHDs to work in recognized, structured training posts (Royal College of Physicians, 2007) have yet to be implemented, despite recognition that having doctors occupy non-training posts has "serious implications for the provision of quality patient care and clinical decision making" (Hanly, 2003).

The latest available data (from 2007) suggest that non-Irish doctors are more likely to occupy stand-alone posts: a national audit found that 58% of doctors on basic specialist training programmes were Irish, whereas only 25% of doctors occupying stand-alone senior house officer posts were Irish (Royal College of Physicians, 2007). It has been clearly recognized for many years that holding a succession of stand-alone posts has negative career implications for doctors. Media reports on the experiences of non-EU doctors in Ireland suggests that they disproportionately occupy such "hard to fill" (OECD, 2008) or stand-alone posts that are unrecognized for training purposes. This has resulted in a sense of despair among non-EU doctors who feel that they "are being treated like disposable paper cups" (McDonald & Butler, 2006).

All NCHDs are temporary employees holding short-term contracts (Irish Medical Organisation, 2011b). For the most part, hospital doctors do not achieve permanent contracts until they achieve consultant grade. On completion of their training, GPs face similar uncertainty en route to achieving a GP principal/partner post. The career of an NCHD assumes constant rotation on a basis of three, six or twelve months through hospitals across the country (Irish Medical Organisation, 2011b). As a result, many NCHDs move regularly between hospitals and/or geographic locations, particularly in January and July when the new rounds of NCHD contracts are issued. This biannual national movement of doctors has been likened to wildebeest migrations, with the exception that "the great NCHD migration occurs in every direction" (Culliton, 2009). The rotation system continues until NCHDs achieve a permanent post, usually at consultant level and not all doctors achieve this grade. The length of time spent as an NCHD can vary considerably depending on the individual doctor, the speciality chosen, access to training programmes and personal/family circumstances. A 2007 audit found that the average age of a senior house officer was 30 and the average age of a registrar was 38 (Royal College of Physicians, 2007). So, although the NCHD rotation system was designed for doctors in their early postgraduate years, it would appear that some doctors, particularly non-EU migrant doctors, spend long periods of time at NCHD level. An example recently cited was of a doctor who came to Ireland after completing his internship in Pakistan and became a consultant 22 years later (Doctor X, 2007).

Despite recent increases in the number of consultant posts, workforce planning has failed to align training places with the staffing needs of the Irish health system. The result is a career structure that has far more doctors in training than it has specialists (Tussing & Wren, 2006). When compared with the structure in England (Fig. 10.1), it would appear that the Irish system relies more heavily on trainee doctors than does the English system, where the ratio of consultant to junior doctors is greater and where a much higher proportion of junior doctor posts are in training posts. These weaknesses in the Irish health system are widely recognized: "too many trainees, too few trained staff – limited availability of senior clinical decision-making, shortages in particular specialities, bulges and bottlenecks in the career structure" (Forum on Medical Manpower, 2001). They have been clearly identified in policy documents from as early as 2001.

**Fig. 10.1** *Medical posts in England and Ireland 2011*

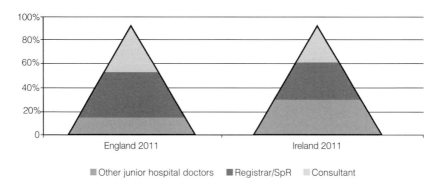

Sources: Department of Health, 2011c; Irish Medical Organisation, 2011b; UK Health and Social Care Information Centre, 2012.

Note: SpR, Specialist registrar.

## 10.2 Methods

### 10.2.1 Study objectives

Despite the major contribution of non-EU migrant doctors to the overall medical workforce in Ireland, little is known about them, their experiences of living and working in Ireland and their plans for the future. Minimal data are available to inform health workforce planners as to the specific roles of these professionals within the health system – such as where in the system they work, at what grades and in what specialist areas. Given the extent to which Ireland relies upon non-EU migrant doctors, their experiences and future migration intentions could have serious repercussions for health workforce planning in Ireland if the migration of non-EU doctors to Ireland was to cease and/or if large numbers of those non-EU doctors currently working in Ireland were to migrate onwards. The need to understand the motivations and future intentions of the non-EU migrant health workforce was highlighted by recent research on non-EU migrant nurses in Ireland, which revealed that many non-EU migrant nurses intended to migrate from Ireland, largely because of poor residency and citizenship entitlements (Humphries, Brugha & McGee, 2009, 2012). This chapter draws on qualitative interviews with non-EU migrant doctors in Ireland and seeks to shed light on the factors influencing their migration decisions: their motivations for coming to Ireland, their reasons for staying in Ireland and the factors that might influence their decisions to leave Ireland, either to return home or to migrate onwards.

### 10.2.2 Study design

Ethics approval for the qualitative research was received from Trinity College Dublin in 2011. In-depth qualitative interviews were conducted with 35 non-EU migrant doctors between November 2011 and March 2012. Interviews were conducted by the research team (PB and NH) and lasted for an average of 35 minutes. Thirty-three interviews were conducted in person and two were conducted over the telephone. Interviews covered a range of topics including respondents' careers and qualifications prior to migration, the decision to migrate, reasons for migrating to Ireland, experiences of working and living in Ireland, ethical issues around health worker migration and the factors influencing their decision to stay and/or their decision to leave Ireland. All interviews were audio-recorded and transcribed in full. Data management and analysis were facilitated by the use of MaxQDA (software for the analysis of qualitative data).

A variety of methods were used to recruit non-EU migrant doctors in Ireland to the study in order to ensure the inclusion of a heterogeneous mix of grades, nationalities, countries of training and arrival years. The recruitment process involved using the Irish Medical Directory (2010) to access non-EU migrant consultants and invite them to participate in the research. An advertisement was placed in the *Irish Medical Times* seeking respondents and an NGO working with immigrants in Ireland also advertised the research on behalf of the research team. Respondents who had taken part in a previous academic study on non-EU migrant doctors in Ireland were invited to take part. Snowball sampling was used throughout the recruitment process. This is a process of chain referral whereby respondents and gatekeepers are used to refer the researcher to other potential respondents (Atkinson & Flint, 2001; Humphries, Brugha & McGee, 2009).

The complexity of doctor migration to Ireland is reflected in the sample. Although all respondents could be categorized as non-EU migrant doctors, not all had trained in non-EU countries: some had trained in Ireland or elsewhere in the EU. Some respondents had come to Ireland upon graduation; others had come to Ireland as specialists. Not all held non-EU citizenship at the time of the interview; some were naturalized Irish citizens while others held dual nationalities. Unpacking the complexity within the non-EU migrant doctor workforce is an important task for health workforce planners in seeking to quantify the non-EU migrant doctor workforce accurately and assess its contribution to the Irish health system. Some non-EU migrant doctors may be rendered "invisible" within the available data sets because they were Irish trained or because they have acquired Irish or EU citizenship.

## 10.3 Results

Of the 35 non-EU migrant doctors interviewed, 31 were currently working as hospital doctors in Ireland; two had registered with the Medical Council of Ireland and were soon to begin working; one was in the process of registering, and one had recently worked as a hospital doctor in Ireland but had since migrated from Ireland. There were 12 women and 23 men. The largest numbers of participants were from Pakistan (10) and Sudan (9), with participants also from India, Nigeria and Iraq and the remainder from eight different non-EU countries. In terms of grades, most respondents were working as NCHDs, with 25 respondents working at senior house officer, registrar or specialist registrar grades; seven worked as hospital consultants. Most respondents (29/35) had come to Ireland since 2000 while the remainder had arrived during the 1980s and 1990s.

### 10.3.1 Motivations for coming to Ireland

The primary reason cited by doctor respondents for migrating to Ireland was in order to obtain postgraduate training and to progress their careers (21/35).

> I came here for two things: experience and qualification. (Doctor 13)

> the fundamental objective to leave [country] and go abroad wasn't looking for easy life or making money, it was for to excel further in our chosen fields (Doctor 2).

Some reported having been dissatisfied with their access to training in their home countries or in other countries to which they had migrated previously. Only seven respondents mentioned either salary levels or a desire for a better life as motivations for their migration to Ireland. These findings immediately challenge the stereotype of a non-EU doctor migrating to Ireland primarily for financial gain. The findings already illustrate two very different perspectives on doctor migration: most respondent doctors came to Ireland to access training and progress their careers, whereas the Irish health system recruits non-EU migrant doctors to fill service posts within the health system (RTE News, 2011). The Health Service Executive (HSE, 2011) explained that active recruitment campaigns were initiated in a 2011 response to difficulties faced by the Health Service Executive in "seeking to attract the quantum and quality of doctors to service related posts to run safe services".

Ireland was frequently selected as a migration destination because of its proximity and perceived similarity to the United Kingdom. Half of all respondents (18/35) had been actively considering migration to the United Kingdom when they decided to come to Ireland instead, sometimes simply because they perceived the registration process to be more straightforward.

> Medical Council registration system was a bit quicker than GMC [UK General Medical Council] registration at that time. (Doctor 33).

Other respondents made a "last minute" switch to Ireland in response to changes in United Kingdom regulations regarding access to training for non-EU migrant doctors.

> I was thinking about go to the UK, but the UK then changed the policy for the non-EU doctors, that …non-EU doctors might not get the training posts … I thought there would be no career progression. So then I decided … to come to Ireland. (Doctor 7).

The proximity of Ireland to the United Kingdom motivated some respondents to migrate to Ireland, particularly those with family/friends in the United Kingdom, while others noted the similarity of the United Kingdom and Irish medical systems. Other respondents came to Ireland to reunite with spouses, colleagues or friends who had previously migrated to Ireland. Three participants noted that their migration to Ireland had been prompted by political upheaval in their countries of origin.

### 10.3.2 Factors influencing the decision to stay

Only nine respondents planned to stay in Ireland and of those, five were working at consultant grade. Several respondents noted that they felt settled in Ireland and this prompted their decision to remain in Ireland, particularly for those who had children.

> I'm very well settled. I think our life is very comfortable. And, well I'm enjoying our presence in this part of the world. Our children are having a good education. We are doing satisfactory job, we are earning reasonable money. (Doctor 15).

> I feel very happy here I had a good working conditions. I was fortunate you know, most of the time, I had a good experience I love to work in here. (Doctor 7).

For some, the decision to remain was something that they had not intended; they had planned to remain for five or ten years and return home, but then remained for family reasons.

> Going back was looking difficult then I decided to stay when the children go the secondary school, it is very difficult to move then. (Doctor 19).

Other more recent migrants were determined to remain in Ireland until they had achieved the training or career progression they had migrated to Ireland to achieve:

> going back home without this exam … it will not help me at all. So I have to pass the exam and then go there. (Doctor 29).

However, for the majority of respondents, the decision to remain permanently in Ireland had not been made. Most were uncertain of their future, waiting to hear the outcome of a recent interview or training application before deciding whether or not they would remain. Although interested in remaining in Ireland, these respondents felt that their onward migration was almost inevitable.

> if something changes I wouldn't … look for another country. I would stay in Ireland. (Doctor 33).

> I'm not really positive that I will get the post. But I'm prepared at this stage to move on. When I finish my fellowship exams I can go … you cannot get older in a registrar post. So I need consultant post. (Doctor 14).

Even those respondents interested in remaining in Ireland appeared resigned to the fact that they would have to leave. Factors such as career progression and the availability of training opportunities featured strongly in those decisions.

### 10.3.3 Factors influencing the decision to leave

Respondents' motivations for leaving Ireland hinged largely on career progression and the perceived lack of opportunities for non-EU migrant doctors to access training or progress their careers in Ireland. They spoke of not progressing (Doctor 33), of being stuck (Doctor 17) and of wasting time (Doctor 21) in Ireland. Each of these issues related to the specificities of medical training in Ireland whereby NCHDs, although officially considered doctors in training, can find themselves in posts that are not recognized for training purposes. Respondents occupying these stand-alone posts were frustrated and sought to emigrate onwards to avail of improved training and career opportunities:

> I don't want to end my career at this level. (Doctor 16)

> it's really tough working … in a job where you … want to succeed and progress and you just keep doing the same job over and over and over and over … it is difficult to stay as an SHO [senior house officer] for 10/20 years but many people are doing that. (Doctor 20).

Those seriously considering onward migration spoke mostly of the United Kingdom as a preferred destination, with a few respondents mentioning Canada, the Gulf States or their home countries as migration options. The overall aim of their migration was to avail of improved training and promotional opportunities.

> I need to get training soon. You need to be on a kind of definite pathway. (Doctor 10).

> I don't think I have any career prospects – that is why we are planning to move. (Doctor 33).

Respondents recognized the career implications of remaining in medical posts unrecognized for training purposes and felt that they were becoming de-skilled as a result. This was something that they felt would have repercussions for their career progression regardless of what country they were in:

> if you are losing your skills you can't work even at home … And you can't work anywhere else. (Doctor 3).

As well as being frustrated about the lack of opportunities for training and career progression, respondents sought to emigrate from Ireland to achieve better working conditions. One doctor spoke of an average working week (including on-calls) of 88 hours and noted that

> we are just working here, we are not living. (Doctor 33).

Others spoke of the difficulties of the six-monthly rotation system, particularly in relation to family commitments. Respondents sought more stability, either in terms of geography and work location or in terms of permanency and job security:

> now my children are here so they are going to school … I don't want to move around much now. (Doctor 3).

> I think I need to find a place to settle down, I think changing the hospital every 6 months I find very hard to adapt and adjust. (Doctor 28).

As was the case with the non-EU migrant nurses (Humphries, Brugha & McGee, 2009), respondent doctors were keenly aware of the opportunities available to them in other countries and comparisons were frequently made, particularly between the United Kingdom and Ireland. The United Kingdom was considered a destination country that was more open to permanent migration.

> I've got a strong feeling that a foreign doctor coming in here and applying for a post and staying forever is not favoured, not in Ireland. The UK it is different. (Doctor 14).

The United Kingdom was also considered to have better career progression and career pathways in comparison with Ireland, as this respondent explained in relation to career progression:

> same thing you can do in UK in 5 years you do 10 years in Ireland. (Doctor 19).

For the most part, respondents were remarkably philosophical about the perceived differences between the opportunities available to them as non-EU migrant doctors and those available to their Irish colleagues. They appeared resigned to the inevitability of it and planned to work around the system by emigrating from Ireland in order to progress their careers.

> they blocked my way at certain point … they blocked my way but that is how system works. It works everywhere like that. (Doctor 4).

> They would like to train their people first then us. (Doctor 14).

Several respondents were at pains to explain that they understood that prioritizing home-trained doctors for training and/or promotions was something that happens everywhere and that similar processes would be in place in their home countries. They were resigned to the fact that they would have to emigrate to progress their careers, but they were disappointed at having to leave Ireland. Other respondents were angrier about the situation, comparing the position of non-EU migrant doctors in Ireland to "being a labourer" (Doctor 16) and "slave labour" (Doctor 32). These doctors had decided to emigrate from Ireland because working conditions were

> very very difficult, prospects were very, very low and supervision was non-existent. (Doctor 32).

## 10.4 Policy implications

The majority of respondents (26/35) were planning to migrate from Ireland. Motivations for moving on related closely to respondents' initial reasons for coming to Ireland, namely to get access to structured training and progress their careers. The findings demonstrate the importance of aligning the needs of the destination country with those of the individual migrant doctor. The mismatch between respondents' desire for training and career progression and the Irish health system's need for doctors to fill stand-alone or service posts meant that dissatisfaction and frustration for respondent non-EU migrant doctors was almost inevitable. Senior figures in the medical establishment have noted that the Irish health system should be obliged to provide postgraduate training opportunities to those recruited from overseas (RTE News, 2011). Respondents echoed similar comments, adding that where recruitment is into service roles, transparency during the recruitment process is essential. The *WHO Global Code of Practice on the International Recruitment of Health Personnel* recommends transparency and fairness in the recruitment process (WHO, 2010).

Respondents' dissatisfaction with the working conditions in the Irish health system, specifically those attached to the NCHD role, was immediately apparent (Table 10.1) and strongly correlated with the reasons cited by the Irish Medical Organisation (2011b) for the emigration of doctors from the Irish health system more generally. In effect, respondents highlight systems' failures that have not been resolved by the inward migration of non-EU doctors. Although willing to come to Ireland to occupy vacancies in the Irish health system, non-EU migrant doctor respondents appear to have encountered similar barriers to their career progression and drawn similar conclusions to those reported by their Irish colleagues – that emigration from Ireland is necessary for career progression (Irish Medical Organisation, 2011a, b). This is borne out by a recent benchmark survey by the Irish Medical Organisation which found that 80% of NCHDs believed that overseas experience would be essential for them to progress their careers in Ireland (Irish Medical Organisation, 2011a). Kingma's statement

**Table 10.1** Factors influencing non-EU migrant doctor decisions to stay or leave Ireland

|  | Endogenous (within the health system) | Exogenous (outside the health system) |
|---|---|---|
| Reasons to leave Ireland | No access to structured training | Instability of frequent moves, particularly for those with families |
|  | Poor quality supervision |  |
|  | Service posts with poor career advancement opportunities | No work–life balance |
|  | Irish favoured for training/promotions | Challenge of being foreign in Ireland |
|  | Long working hours |  |
|  | 6 monthly rotations and relocation for NCHDs |  |
|  | De-skilling (brain waste) |  |
|  | No permanency |  |
| Reasons to emigrate to another country (United Kingdom or elsewhere) | Perception of better training options in the United Kingdom | Perception of better work–life balance in the United Kingdom |
|  | Perception of better career progression opportunities in the United Kingdom | Perception of more equal opportunities for migrants in the United Kingdom than in Ireland |
|  | Perception of shorter working hours in the United Kingdom | Desire to return home |
|  | Career grade option in the United Kingdom |  |
| Reasons to remain in Ireland | May stay if training/promotional opportunities become available | Naturalization process ongoing |
|  | Stay until training completed | Settled in Ireland/children settled |
|  |  | Cannot return home because of instability there |

*Source*: Adapted from Padarath et al., 2004.

that "*injecting migrant nurses into dysfunctional health systems – ones that are not capable of attracting and retaining domestic-educated staff – is not likely to meet the growing health needs of national populations*" (Kingma, 2007) is exemplified well in the Irish experience of doctor migration. Non-EU migrant doctors, like their Irish counterparts, want training opportunities, career progression and a clear career pathway. Most non-EU migrant doctors appear to have migrated to Ireland to achieve these goals and will migrate onwards from Ireland if opportunities are not provided within the Irish health system. Non-EU doctors who find themselves working as NCHDs with limited access to training as well as inadequate supervision and poor working conditions, or who emigrate from Ireland because of lack of opportunities, could be considered casualties of the Irish health system, as could Irish and Irish-trained doctors who do not remain working in the health system within which they trained.

## 10.5 Conclusions

The findings of the study described here illustrate some of the motivations underpinning the migration of non-EU migrant doctors to Ireland and the reasons why they are considering onward migration. If career-tracking data and quantitative data on doctor immigration and emigration can be generated, then combining these with the qualitative results described here has potential to greatly improve our understanding of medical migration and would contribute to better and more efficient health workforce planning and retention in Ireland in the future.

Although this chapter has focused on non-EU migrant doctors, many of the issues they confront are not specific to migrants but rather relate to the structure of the NCHD role and the fact that "many NCHD posts provide no real training" (Tussing & Wren, 2006). Dissatisfaction with the postgraduate training environment for NCHDs has long been recognized as a factor in the "brain drain" from Irish medicine (Buttimer, 2006). Irish doctors emigrate from Ireland because of heavy workloads, pay and working conditions, and because they can achieve a better work–life balance and better training and mentorship in countries such as Australia and New Zealand (Shannon, 2010). Our research has demonstrated that issues of career progression and training structure apply as much to non-EU migrant doctors working in Ireland as they do to Irish-trained doctors.

The need for system-wide reform is self-evident and generally accepted. In the meantime, Ireland has a poorly functioning health workforce system that continues to operate unchanged. Without radical reform, it is likely that Ireland will continue to have both a high dependency on non-EU migrant doctors and to experience the continued high turnover of Irish-trained doctors (non-EU, EU and Irish).

## Acknowledgements

The authors thank the migrant doctors who participated in this research for sharing their stories, and all of those who facilitated the contact between the research team and the migrant doctor respondents. The authors also wish to thank the Irish Health Research Board for funding the Doctor Migration Project under its Health Research Award Scheme (HRA_HSR/2010/10), the Medical Council of Ireland for supplying data and the Higher Education Authority for supplying data on the number of medical graduates from Irish medical schools 2009–2011. The data interpretation and views reported here are solely those of the authors.

## References

Atkinson R, Flint J (2001). Accessing hidden and hard-to-reach populations: snowball research strategies. *Social Research Update*, Issue 3.

Bidwell P et al., (2013). The national and international complications of a decade of doctor migration in the Irish context. *Health Policy*, 110(1): 29–39.

Buttimer J (2006). *The Buttimer report: preparing Ireland's doctors to meet the health needs of the 21st century*. Dublin, Department of Health and Children (Report of the Postgraduate Medical Education and Training Group).

Cullen P (2012). Nearly €2m spent on recruiting doctors in India and Pakistan. *Irish Times*, 16 February.

Culliton G (2009). New procedures mean NCHD problems. *Irish Medical Times*, December.

Department of Health (2011a). Consultant and non-consultant hospital doctors employed within the public health services, 2002 to 2011. Dublin, Department of Health (http://www.dohc.ie/publications/pdf/KeyTrends_2012.pdf?direct=1 [Table 5.2], accessed 3 January 2014).

Department of Health (2011b). *Employment in the public health service by category, 2002 to 2011*. Dublin, Department of Health (http://www.dohc.ie/publications/pdf/KeyTrends_2012.pdf?direct=1 [Table 5.1], accessed 2 January 2014).

Department of Health (2011c). *Health service employment statistics*. Dublin, Department of Health (http://www.dohc.ie/statistics/pdf/stats11_health_service_stats.pdf?direct=1, accessed 3 January 2014).

Doctor X (2007). *The bitter pill: an insider's shocking expose of the Irish Health system*. Dublin, Hachette Books.

FAS Training and Employment Authority (2009). *A quantitative tool for workforce planning in healthcare: example simulations*. Dublin, Training and Employment Authority for the Expert Group on Future Skills Needs.

Forum on Medical Manpower (2001). *Report of the forum on medical manpower*. Dublin, Department of Health and Children.

Hanly D (2003). *Hanly report: report of the national task force on medical staffing*. Dublin, Department of Health and Children.

Healy A (2012). System of recruiting foreign doctors defended. *Irish Times*, 11 January.

Higher Education Authority (2012). *Unpublished statistics.* Higher Education Authority, Dublin.

HSE (2011). *Health Service Executive Briefing for Joint Committee on Health and Children (6th October 2011).* Dublin, Health Service Executive (http://www.oireachtas.ie/parliament/oireachtasbusiness/committees_list/health-and-children/submissionsandpresentations/, accessed 4 December 2013).

HSE MET (2011). *Annual assessment of NCHD posts July 2011 to June 2012.* Dublin, Health Services Executive Medical and Training Unit.

HSE MET (2012). *Implementation of the reform of the intern year. Second interim report.* Dublin, Health Services Executive Medical and Training Unit (http://www.imo.ie/specialty/student/intern-placement-2013/Second-Interim-Implementation-Report-April-2012.pdf, accessed 4 December 2013).

Humphries N, Brugha R, McGee H (2009). "I won't be staying here for long". A qualitative study on the retention of migrant nurses in Ireland. *Human Resources for Health,* 7:68.

Humphries N, Brugha R, McGee H (2012). Nurse migration and health workforce planning: Ireland as illustrative of international challenges. *Health Policy,* 107: 44–53.

Irish Medical Directory (2010). *Irish medical directory. The directory of Irish healthcare.* Dublin, Irish Medical Directory (http://www.imd.ie/index.html, accessed 15 December 2013).

Irish Medical Organisation (2011a). *Benchmark NCHD survey 2011.* Dublin, Irish Medical Organisation.

Irish Medical Organisation (2011b). *Submission to Oireachtas Joint Committee on Health and Children: non-consultant hospital doctors.* Dublin, Irish Medical Organisation.

Kingma M (2007). Nurses on the move: a global overview. *Health Services Research,* 42(3 Part II):1281–1298.

McDonald D, Butler K (2006). Race "block" on Ireland's hospital jobs. *The Sunday Times*, 23 April.

Medical Council of Ireland (2003). *Review of medical schools in Ireland 2003.* Dublin, Irish Medical Council.

Medical Council of Ireland (2013). *Medical workforce intelligence report. A Report on the annual registration retention survey 2012.* Dublin, Medical Council of Ireland.

OECD (2008). *The looming crisis in the health workforce. How can OECD countries respond?* Paris, Organisation for Economic Co-operation and Development (OECD Health Policy Studies) (http://www.who.int/hrh/migration/looming_crisis_health_workforce.pdf, accessed 15 December 2013).

OECD (2010). *International migration of health workers. Improving international co-operation to address the global health workforce crisis.* Paris, Organisation for Economic Co-operation and Development.

Padarath A et al. (2004). *Health personnel in southern Africa: confronting maldistribution and brain drain.* Cape Town, Regional Network for Equity in Health in Southern Africa (EQUINET), Health Systems Trust (South Africa) and MEDACT (UK) (Equinet Discussion Paper Number 3).

Postgraduate Medical and Dental Board (2008). *Survey of NCHD staffing at 1st October 2008.* Dublin, Postgraduate Medical and Dental Board.

Royal College of Physicians (2007). *National audit of SHO and registrar posts. Report of the Audit Steering Group.* Dublin, Royal College of Physicians.

RTE News (2011). Obligation to teach foreign doctors – RCSI. *RTE News* (http://www.rte.ie/news/2011/1013/doctors.html, accessed 3 January 2014).

Shannon J (2010). Ending the NCHD deficit. *Medical Independent,* 25 November.

Thakore H (2009). Medical Education in Ireland. *Medical Teacher,* 31:696–700.

Tussing AD, Wren M-A (2006). *How Ireland cares. The case for health care reform.* Gateshead, UK, New Island.

UK Health and Social Care Information Centre (2012). *NHS workforce: summary of staff in the NHS: results from September 2011 Census.* Leeds, Health and Social Care Information Centre.

WHO (2010). *WHO global code of practice on the international recruitment of health personnel.* Geneva, World Health Organization (Sixty-third World Health Assembly, WHA63.16) (http://www.who.int/hrh/migration/code/WHO_global_code_of_practice_EN.pdf, accessed 1 October 2013).

# Chapter 11

# A multi-country perspective on nurses' tasks below their skill level: reports from domestically trained nurses and foreign-trained nurses from developing countries

*Luk Bruyneel, Baoyue Li, Linda Aiken, Emmanuel Lesaffre, Koen Van den Heede and Walter Sermeus*

## 11.1 Introduction

The 12-country Registered Nurse Forecasting (RN4CAST) study measured and linked organizational features of nurses' workplaces to nurse well-being and patient outcomes in order to challenge assumptions underpinning previous nurse workforce planning efforts (Sermeus et al., 2011). Using a cross-sectional observational design, the study found that deficits in quality of hospital care were common in all countries. Nurse and patient surveys revealed that in hospitals with a good organization of care (improved nurse staffing, better work environments), however, nurse well-being improved and patients were more likely to rate their hospital higher and recommend the hospital to friends and family. Nurses and patients agreed on which hospitals provided good care and should be recommended (Aiken et al., 2012).

From the nurse survey, many demographic characteristics became available, including age, gender, work experience, employment, education and mobility statistics. The last proved interesting to connect with the European Commission's PROMeTHEUS project, which addresses the gaps in knowledge of the numbers and trends for increasing health professional mobility in Europe, and the impact of policy responses to this. This dynamic phenomenon impacts on the composition of the health workforce, which in turn impacts on health system performance (Wismar et al., 2011). The RN4CAST project allows for a specific understanding of this phenomenon among migrated nurse professionals populating about 500 hospitals in 12 European countries. The aim of this chapter is to determine whether there is a difference between domestically trained and foreign-trained nurses from developing countries in nurses' reports on tasks below their skill level performed during their last shift.

Optimizing the full scope of professional nursing practice in institutions that employ nurses educated in other countries is particularly important since the employment of internationally trained nurses may suggest a shortage of nurses at the institutional or national level. Studies, however, have shown that migrant nurses sometimes experience discrimination by means of lower wages and less upward mobility, and may be employed as nursing aides rather than as nurses, which negatively impacts their well-being (Kline, 2003; Centre for Health Workforce Studies, 2008; International Organization for Migration, 2010). Other research suggests that nurses trained abroad aspire to the same professional nursing practice standards common to their country of current employment (Flynn & Aiken, 2002). In light of the increasing international mobility of nurses, Humphries, Brugha and McGee (2009) considered that the evaluation of how migrant nurses' skills are utilized is a prerequisite to incorporating nurse migration into workforce planning. In line with this, Wismar et al. (2011) concluded that health professional mobility can undermine attempts to forecast workforce needs if inflows and outflows are not well understood and factored into planning. According to these authors, inadequate monitoring or a poor understanding of the inflows and outflows of skills of health professionals will reduce the effectiveness of strategies to change skill-mix and task distribution.

Previous studies have shown that nurses' time and energy are often not optimized. When asked about their last shift, nurses across three countries (United States, Canada, Germany) consistently reported high percentages of non-nursing tasks performed, including transporting patients, delivering or retrieving food trays and performing housekeeping activities. At the same time, they reported many nursing tasks that were necessary but left undone because they lacked the time to complete them (Aiken et al., 2001). A time-and-motion study in 36 hospitals found that activities considered by nurses to be wasted time (waiting, looking, retrieving and delivering) consumed 6.6% of reported time in every shift of 10 hours (Hendrich et al., 2008). Another time-and-motion study showed that nurses spent 9.0% of their time during their previous shift on non-nursing tasks, including replenishing charts and forms, tidying rooms, making beds, answering telephones, searching for people, gathering linen and answering call bells (Desjardins et al., 2008).

## 11.2 Methods

### 11.2.1 Study design

The RN4CAST study (Sermeus et al., 2011) favoured a rigorous quantitative multi-country cross-sectional design on the basis of research methods used in a five-nation study of critical issues in nurse staffing and the impact on patient care (Aiken et al., 2001). Data were gathered from four sources (nurse, patient and hospital profile surveys and routinely collected hospital discharge data). The design of the RN4CAST study is described in detail by Sermeus et al. (2011). This analysis used nurse-reported information on migratory status and tasks below skill level that were performed during their last shift.

Depending on national legislation, the study protocol was approved by either central ethical committees (e.g. nation or university) or local ethical committees (e.g. hospitals).

### 11.2.2 Study sample

A minimum of 30 general acute hospitals per country, for a total of 486 hospitals, were sampled as primary sampling units in 12 European countries (Belgium, England, Finland, Germany, Greece, Ireland, the Netherlands, Norway, Poland, Spain, Sweden and Switzerland). In each of the selected hospitals, at least two general medical and surgical nursing units were randomly selected. All staff nurses involved in direct patient care activities served as informants on organization of nursing care, nurse well-being, patient safety and quality of care. The sample consists of 33 731 nurses (62% response rate) from Belgium (3 186), England (2 990), Finland (1 131), Germany (1 508), Greece (367), Ireland (1 406), the Netherlands (2 217), Norway (3 752), Poland (2 605), Spain (2 804), Sweden (10 133) and Switzerland (1 632). Response rates varied from 39% in England to 97% in Poland.

### 11.2.3 Study measures

Nurses were asked to indicate whether they had received their training in the country they were currently working in and, if not, in which country they did receive their training. Based on the World Economic Outlook classification of countries (International Monetary Fund, 2010), nurses were categorized as domestically trained, foreign-trained in a country with an emerging or developing economy (further referred to as foreign-trained in a developing country) or foreign-trained in a country with an advanced economy (further referred to as foreign-trained in a developed country). The International Monetary Fund list of emerging and developing economies (150 out of 184 countries) includes countries from all over the world. Some recent entrants to the EU, for example, have remained classified as emerging economies (e.g. Latvia, Poland).

Within a series of questions about their last shift, nurses were asked to report on a list of tasks below their skill level: whether they had performed these tasks never, sometimes or often during their last shift. The following nine tasks were presented to nurses: routine phlebotomy/blood draw for tests, transporting of patients within hospitals, performing non-nursing care, performing non-nursing services not available on off-hours, delivering and retrieving food trays, answering telephones/clerical duties, arranging discharge referrals and transportation, obtaining supplies or equipment, and cleaning patient rooms and equipment.

Three types of variable were used to control for confounders: the type of last shift worked (morning, evening, night), the number of years worked as a nurse and level of education (bachelor degree or not).

### 11.2.4 Statistical analysis

For each country, the share of foreign-trained nurses and the share of nurses from developing and developed countries was collated plus detailed data on country of origin. The study assessed first whether there were statistically significant differences between domestically trained nurses and foreign-trained nurses from developing countries in reporting type of last shift worked, number of years worked and level of education. Second, nurses' reports on the list of nine tasks performed during their last shift were collated. Third, reports on tasks performed by domestically trained nurses and foreign-trained nurses from developing countries were compared. For analytic purposes, nurses' responses as "never performed" and "sometimes/often performed" were dichotomized. A heat map (Sneath, 1957) was used to graphically compare the reports, with a system of colour coding where a dark grey square indicated that a higher proportion of foreign-trained nurses from developing countries reported this task compared with domestically trained nurses (and a light grey square vice versa). A composite measure of tasks performed during nurses' last shift (minimum 0, maximum 9) was calculated for each individual nurse by taking the sum of the nine dichotomized nursing tasks. This composite measure had a binomial distribution. The overall effect (i.e. over all countries) of nurses' migratory status on this composite measure was estimated using a two-level logistic random effects regression. The country effect was modelled as a fixed effect and the hospitals as a random effect. The intraclass correlation coefficient at the hospital level was calculated as an indication of the degree of homogeneity. The analysis was adjusted for nurses' type of last shift worked, number of years worked as a nurse and level of education. The consistency of the overall effect was analysed by specifying interaction effects between the countries under study and migratory status. A series of similar two-level random effects regression models were constructed to analyse the overall effect of migratory status on each task separately. Despite all efforts to get random effects models with interaction effects to converge, this proved to be hard for four out of the nine tasks for computational issues. Descriptive findings for these tasks showed repetitive high proportions of both domestically trained nurses and foreign-trained nurses from developing countries indicating they had performed these tasks during their last shift. The analysis was repeated comparing nurses' reports on tasks never/sometimes performed and often performed and gave similar findings. The analysis also compared the difference in tasks reported between domestically trained nurses and foreign-trained nurses from a developed country and showed no statistically significant differences. The data analysis used SAS System for Windows version 9.3 (SAS Institute, 2011).

## 11.3 Results

### 11.3.1 Foreign-trained nurses

There were 2 107 nurses (6.2% of the total sample) who indicated that they were trained in a different country from the one where they were currently employed, of which 832 were trained in a developing country (2.5% of total sample). There was large variation in the share of foreign-trained nurses between countries: Ireland (38.6%), Switzerland (22.1%), England (16.7%), Norway (5.5%), Germany (5.1%), Greece (5.1%), Belgium (3.1%), the Netherlands (2.4%), Sweden (2.3%), Spain (1.3%) and Finland (0.9%). In Poland, all nurses that participated in the study were domestically trained nurses and in Greece there were no foreign-trained nurses from developing countries. The share of foreign-trained nurses varied considerably between hospitals in the top three countries with foreign-trained nurses, ranging from 16 to 56% (Ireland), 4 to 50% (Switzerland) and 1 to 52% (England). Countries with low numbers of foreign-trained nurses from developing countries (Finland, Greece, Poland) or high missing values on country of training (Belgium) were dropped from further analysis, which resulted in a total of 813 foreign-trained nurses from developing countries remaining for further analysis. Fig. 11.1 presents the large variation in the share of nurses from developing countries employed in the sample of eight remaining European countries. The percentage of foreign-trained nurses trained in developing countries varied from 11% in Switzerland to as high as 80% in England.

In many countries, a large part of the share of foreign-trained nurses could be explained by mobility between neighbouring countries or countries in the region: 112 of 354 foreign-trained nurses in Switzerland (31.6%) were trained in Germany, 107 (30.2%) in France and 41 (11.6%) in Italy. Nurses trained in developing countries now working in Switzerland included nurses from India (7; 2.0%), the Philippines (4; 1.1%) and Bosnia and Herzegovina (3; 0.85%), among others. In Sweden, 62 of the 231 foreign-trained nurses (26.8%) had obtained their training in Finland and 27 (11.7%) in Germany.

The share of foreign-trained nurses from developing countries was ethnically very diverse, with most nurses trained in Bosnia and Herzegovina (15; 6.5%). In Spain, a different image emerged, with a large share of nurses trained in South American countries, mainly in Peru (8; 21.6%). Norway's largest group of foreign-trained nurses came from Sweden (53 of 231; 26.1%) with 31 (15.3%) from Australia and 31 (15.3%) from Denmark. Nurses from developing countries (200 in total) came from the Philippines (5; 2.5%),

**Fig. 11.1** *Share of foreign-trained nurses from developing and from developed countries*

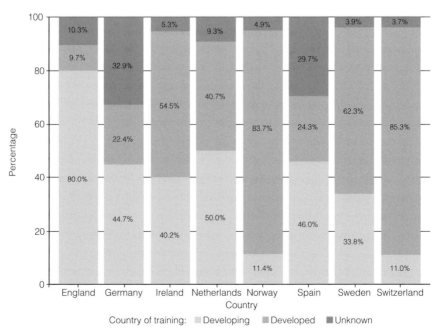

Lithuania (4; 2.0%) and Bosnia and Herzegovina (3; 1.5%), among others. In the Netherlands, after Belgium (7 of 54; 13.0%) and Germany (5; 9.3%), there was a substantial number of nurses from the former Dutch colonies of Suriname (12; 22.2%) and Indonesia (8; 14.8%). Of the 76 foreign-trained nurses in Germany, 13 (17.1%) came from Poland and 4 (5.3%) from Kazakhstan. In England, the main source countries were the Philippines (153 of 494; 31.0%) and India (117; 23.7%) but also nurses from sub-Saharan Africa (Ghana, Kenya, Nigeria, South Africa, Uganda, Zambia and Zimbabwe) accounted for a large proportion (78; 15.8%). As in England, the use of overseas recruiters is widespread in Ireland. Contrary to England, however, Ireland's share of nurses from developing countries was almost completely accounted for by nurses from India (111 of 531; 20.9%) and the Philippines (92; 17.3%) only. The share of European foreign-trained nurses in Ireland (53.2% of total) was almost exclusively made up of nurses who had received their training in the United Kingdom (51.5% of total).

In all eight countries, foreign-trained nurses from developing countries had more years of experience in working as a nurse than domestically trained nurses. These differences were statistically significant across all countries. Statistically significant differences were found for the level of education in England and Ireland, where the share of foreign-trained nurses from developing countries reporting that they had obtained a bachelor level degree in their home country was higher than the share for domestically trained nurses.

### 11.3.2 Nurses' reports on tasks performed during their last shift

Across countries, a high proportion of nurses reported having sometimes or often performed tasks below their skill level during their last shift. Most reported tasks (country-weighted average) were answering telephones/clerical duties (97.4%), performing non-nursing care (90.1%) and obtaining supplies or equipment (71.2%). There was large variability between countries in nurses' reports. For example in Spain, only 16.8% reported having cleaned patient rooms and equipment while in England this was 90% (Table 11.1).

### 11.3.3 Comparison of reports from domestically trained nurses and nurses trained in developing countries

The heat map (Fig. 11.2) shows that in 62 out of 72 cases, higher percentages of nurses from developing countries reported they performed the nine tasks compared with domestically trained nurses (Table 11.1 for detailed findings). Findings were consistent between hospitals and for nurses from the same developing country working in the different countries under study here. For

**Table 11.1** Nurses' reports of tasks below their skill level performed during their last shift for all nurses and by migratory status (trained in a developing country versus domestically trained)[a]

| | Delivering and retrieving food trays (%) | Performing non-nursing care (%) | Arranging discharge referrals (%) | Routine phlebotomy/blood draw for tests (%) | Transport of patients within the hospital (%) | Cleaning patient rooms and equipment (%) | Filling in for non-nursing services not available on off-hours (%) | Obtaining supplies or equipment (%) | Answering phones, clerical duties (%) |
|---|---|---|---|---|---|---|---|---|---|
| *Belgium* | | | | | | | | | |
| Overall (n = 3 038) | 83.8 | 96.8 | 76.9 | 85.8 | 69.9 | 82.6 | 47.6 | 71.6 | 97.9 |
| Domestic (n = 3 021) | 83.7 | 96.9 | 76.9 | 85.8 | 69.9 | 82.7 | 47.5 | 71.5 | 97.9 |
| Developing (n = 17) | 100.0 | 94.1 | 76.5 | 88.2 | 64.7 | 70.6 | 58.8 | 88.2 | 100.0 |
| *Switzerland* | | | | | | | | | |
| Overall (n = 1 274) | 76.7 | 97.2 | 59.8 | 74.3 | 59.3 | 57.0 | 58.6 | 65.8 | 96.9 |
| Domestic (n = 1 246) | 76.6 | 97.3 | 59.7 | 74.1 | 58.9 | 57.2 | 58.6 | 65.5 | 96.9 |
| Developing (n = 28) | 78.6 | 92.9 | 64.3 | 85.2 | 77.8 | 46.4 | 59.3 | 80.0 | 96.3 |
| *Germany* | | | | | | | | | |
| Overall (n = 1 448) | 82.4 | 98.0 | 74.1 | 41.7 | 70.9 | 63.9 | 65.8 | 85.4 | 98.7 |
| Domestic (n = 1 414) | 82.3 | 97.9 | 74.0 | 41.5 | 71.2 | 63.8 | 65.7 | 85.1 | 98.6 |
| Developing (n = 34) | 85.3 | 100.0 | 76.5 | 50.0 | 55.9 | 67.6 | 70.6 | 97.1 | 100.0 |
| *Spain* | | | | | | | | | |
| Overall (n = 2 746) | 44.1 | 91.0 | 57.7 | 86.2 | 45.2 | 16.8 | 22.5 | 72.8 | 98.5 |
| Domestic (n = 2 729) | 44.0 | 91.0 | 57.5 | 86.1 | 45.2 | 16.7 | 22.5 | 72.7 | 98.4 |
| Developing (n = 17) | 68.8 | 88.2 | 76.5 | 94.1 | 52.9 | 37.5 | 23.5 | 87.5 | 100.0 |
| *Finland* | | | | | | | | | |
| Overall (n = 1 070) | 63.3 | 87.2 | 41.6 | 12.8 | 31.7 | 56.4 | 72.1 | 38.6 | 97.8 |
| Domestic (n = 1 068) | 63.3 | 87.2 | 41.6 | 12.8 | 31.5 | 56.5 | 72.1 | 38.6 | 97.8 |
| Developing (n = 2) | 50.0 | 100.0 | 0.0 | 0.0 | 100.0 | 0.0 | 50.0 | 50.0 | 100.0 |

| | | | | | | | | | |
|---|---|---|---|---|---|---|---|---|---|
| *Greece* | | | | | | | | | |
| Overall (n = 335, all domestic trained) | 37.7 | 77.2 | 79.4 | 93.8 | 63.6 | 64.9 | 65.5 | 86.2 | 94.8 |
| *Ireland* | | | | | | | | | |
| Overall (n = 1 061) | 64.2 | 95.2 | 80.7 | 28.5 | 67.5 | 81.6 | 69.2 | 84.3 | 99.1 |
| Domestic (n = 847) | 58.7 | 94.9 | 79.0 | 26.3 | 64.1 | 78.9 | 70.0 | 85.1 | 99.1 |
| Developing (n = 214) | 86.3 | 96.7 | 87.5 | 37.1 | 81.0 | 92.8 | 65.9 | 81.1 | 99.5 |
| *Netherlands* | | | | | | | | | |
| Overall (n = 2 180) | 57.4 | 93.2 | 76.2 | 29.8 | 68.5 | 63.2 | 40.7 | 49.8 | 98.7 |
| Domestic (n = 2 153) | 57.1 | 93.1 | 76.0 | 29.7 | 68.3 | 63.0 | 40.5 | 49.3 | 98.7 |
| Developing (n = 27) | 85.2 | 96.3 | 85.2 | 42.3 | 81.5 | 77.8 | 59.3 | 84.6 | 96.3 |
| *Norway* | | | | | | | | | |
| Overall (n = 3 516) | 78.8 | 71.5 | 64.3 | 39.9 | 42.6 | 68.1 | 59.1 | 63.9 | 97.4 |
| Domestic (n = 3 493) | 78.8 | 71.5 | 64.2 | 39.7 | 42.6 | 68.1 | 59.0 | 63.7 | 97.4 |
| Developing (n = 23) | 82.6 | 78.3 | 69.6 | 69.6 | 34.8 | 73.9 | 65.2 | 87.0 | 100.0 |
| *Poland* | | | | | | | | | |
| Overall (n = 2 593, all domestic trained) | 75.0 | 94.1 | 59.0 | 97.7 | 90.4 | 85.7 | 62.6 | 70.0 | 97.9 |
| *Sweden* | | | | | | | | | |
| Overall (n = 9 913) | 64.5 | 84.2 | 58.1 | 79.5 | 53.4 | 69.5 | 37.7 | 81.3 | 94.6 |
| Domestic (n = 9 837) | 64.4 | 84.1 | 58.0 | 79.4 | 53.3 | 69.4 | 37.6 | 81.2 | 94.6 |
| Developing (n = 76) | 75.7 | 98.6 | 63.0 | 91.9 | 63.0 | 82.4 | 49.3 | 89.2 | 94.7 |
| *England* | | | | | | | | | |
| Overall (n = 2 866) | 66.7 | 96.0 | 83.1 | 54.4 | 60.7 | 90.0 | 63.2 | 85.5 | 99.7 |
| Domestic (n = 2 472) | 63.6 | 96.0 | 82.1 | 51.8 | 57.9 | 89.0 | 62.1 | 85.2 | 99.7 |
| Developing (n = 394) | 86.5 | 95.6 | 89.1 | 71.0 | 78.3 | 96.4 | 70.3 | 87.8 | 99.7 |

[a] Responses were dichotomized as "never performed" and "sometimes/often performed"; migratory status was based on the World Economic Outlook classification of countries (International Monetary Fund, 2010).

**Fig. 11.2** *Heat map comparing reports from domestically trained nurses and nurses trained in a developing country for tasks below their skill level performed during their last shift*

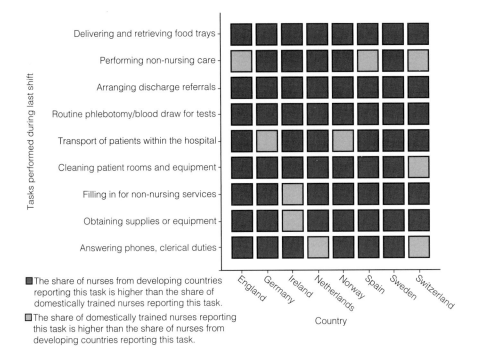

example, 25 English trusts had a total of 153 Philippines employed. In 24 out of 25 trusts, Philippine-trained nurses more often reported that they had delivered and retrieved food trays during their last shift compared with domestically trained nurses. This was also the case in 19 out of 20 Irish hospitals where Philippine-trained nurses were working.

The intraclass correlation coefficient for the nine items varied from 0.08 to 0.35, and was 0.21 for the composite measure, justifying the need for specifying a multilevel model. Table 11.2 shows that, after adjusting for last shift worked, years of experience and level of education, there remained a pronounced overall effect of being a foreign-trained nurse from a developing country and having an increase in reports of tasks performed during the last shift. This overall effect was found for the model testing the association between nurses' migratory status and the composite measure of tasks performed during the last shift. The interaction effect for this analysis was not significant. The series of models to analyse the overall effect of migratory status on each task separately showed that for eight out of nine tasks there was an overall effect of being a foreign-trained nurse from a developing country and an increase in reporting those tasks. Being a foreign-trained nurse from a developing country was a significant predictor of all five tasks for which an interaction effect was specified. The interaction

**Table 11.2** Logistic random effects model estimating the overall effect of nurses' migratory status (trained in a developing country versus domestically trained) across eight countries on task below skill level performed during nurses' last shift[a]

| Tasks performed last shift | Estimate | Odds ratio (95% CI) | p value |
|---|---|---|---|
| Composite measure of nine nursing tasks | 0.74 | 2.10 (1.68–2.61) | <0.0001 |
| Delivering and retrieving food trays[b] | 1.65 | 5.21 (4.04–6.72) | <0.0001 |
| Performing non-nursing care[c] | 0.53 | 1.70 (1.13–2.56) | 0.014 |
| Arranging discharge referrals[b] | 0.89 | 2.44 (1.92–3.08) | <0.0001 |
| Routine phlebotomy/blood draw for tests[b] | 0.90 | 2.46 (1.91–3.17) | <0.0001 |
| Transport of patients within the hospital[c] | 0.73 | 2.08 (1.71–2.52) | <0.0001 |
| Cleaning patient rooms and equipment[b] | 0.64 | 1.90 (1.44–2.50) | <0.0001 |
| Filling in for non-nursing services not available off-hours[c] | 0.19 | 1.21 (0.99–1.47) | 0.048 |
| Obtaining supplies or equipment[b] | 0.30 | 1.35 (1.03–1.78) | 0.033 |
| Answering phones, clerical duties[c] | 0.53 | 1.70 (0.70–4.10) | 0.235 |

[a]Model adjusted for reported last shift worked (morning, evening, night); number of years worked as a nurse and degree obtained (bachelor degree or not); trained in a developing country versus domestically trained based on the World Economic Outlook classification of countries (International Monetary Fund, 2010); eight countries covered were England, Germany, Ireland, the Netherlands, Norway, Spain, Sweden, Switzerland; [b]Interaction effect specified; [c]No interaction effect specified because of computational problems.

effect was non-significant for three tasks (arranging discharge referrals, routine phlebotomy/blood draw for tests, cleaning patient rooms and equipment). For "delivering and retrieving food trays" and "obtaining supplies or equipment", the interaction effect was significant. For three out of four tasks for which no interaction effect could be specified, being a foreign-trained nurse from a developing country was a significant predictor (performing non-nursing care, transport of patients within the hospital, filling in for non-nursing services not available at off-hours). Migratory status failed to predict the task of "answering telephones, clerical duties", for which in each country at least 90% of both domestically trained nurses and foreign-trained nurses reported they had performed this task during their last shift.

## 11.4 Conclusions

This study documented high proportions of nurses across 12 countries indicating that they had performed tasks below their skill level during their last shift. These findings support the previous studies of Aiken et al. (2001), Desjardins et al. (2008) and Hendrich et al. (2008) in which nurses reported much time spent on non-nursing tasks or much time wasted during their last shift.

Findings also revealed that, while a high share of all nurses reported having performed tasks below their skill level during their last shift, being a foreign-trained nurse from a developing country was a significant predictor of performing tasks below skill level. The consistency in results across countries and hospitals makes these findings compelling.

In 2010, the World Health Assembly adopted the *WHO Global Code of Practice on the International Recruitment of Health Personnel* (WHO, 2010). The ambition of this first Code, global in scope, is for WHO Member States to refrain from the active recruitment of health personnel from developing countries facing critical shortages of health workers. The Code also emphasizes the importance of equal treatment for migrant health workers and the domestically trained health workforce.

The RN4CAST data provided an opportunity to contribute to our understanding of this limited area of research (Sermeus et al., 2011). The mix of countries participating in this study reflects the diversity of health systems in Europe, ensuring a rich perspective of nursing workforce issues from all angles. Robust statistical techniques were used to analyse the differences among domestically trained nurses and foreign-trained nurses from developing countries. Several limitations, however, warrant consideration. First, the measure of migratory status used may not have captured adequately the nationality of the nurses since only the country of training was known. Second, although these tasks were defined as non-nursing tasks in previous research (Aiken et al., 2001; Desjardins et al., 2008; Hendrich et al., 2008), it is conceivable that some tasks in certain situations of care were indeed nursing tasks. Third, not all tasks below nurses' skill level may have been captured adequately, since the response was limited to a list of nine tasks. Fourth, in this multi-country European context, the context in which nurses performed these tasks can be very diverse. The influence of professional practice standards, skill levels of foreign-trained nurses from developing countries and values attached to these tasks resulting from previous work experiences in their home countries was unknown. It was not known, for example, whether foreign-trained nurses from developing countries were more likely than domestically trained nurses to be assigned to perform tasks below their skill level or whether foreign-trained nurses were more task oriented and brought the customs and roles of nursing from their developing country backgrounds into developed countries, and thus were more prone to voluntarily take on tasks below their skill level. The differences found between reports from domestically trained nurses and foreign-trained nurses were, however, not attributable to a lower level of education or fewer years of experience. To the contrary, in each country the foreign-trained nurses from developing countries had significantly more experience in working as a nurse than the domestically trained nurses. However, it was not known how long they had been working as a nurse in their destination country.

Stepping back from the limitations, the findings from this study provide evidence that there remains much room for improvement to optimize the use of nurses' time and energy. Hospital human resource management should give more attention to professional socialization and lifelong learning for nurses to improve their priority setting and time management as well as ensuring that non-nursing resources are used for tasks that do not require the unique training of professional nurses. The findings suggest that nurses from developing countries, particularly, tend to accept less skilled work, making their roles in the hospital complementary (nursing aides rather than nurses) to those of the skilled native workers. The complements and substitutes analysis from the economic theory of labour markets shows that it is entirely possible that everyone gains from such matching (Baldwin & Wyplosz, 2009). Such reasoning would imply that native nurses are generally better educated. Although our comparison of the proportion of nurses with a bachelor's degree who are native or foreign-trained suggests otherwise, it could indeed be questioned whether nurses' training and competences are equivalent across the countries presented in this study. Nurses from developing countries outside the EU, particularly, may be in need of continuing education on professional nurse roles and responsibilities in complex health care settings. As discussed above, countries such as Latvia and Poland have remained classified as developing countries despite having joined the EU in the 2004 enlargement. Labour market integration associated with this enlargement calls for harmonization of education. Since the free movement of workers is the cornerstone of EU integration, Directive 2005/36/EC on the recognition of professional qualifications lays down the right for workers to pursue a profession in a Member State other than the one in which they have obtained their professional qualifications (European Commission, 2005). The intention is to allow workers to find the jobs that best suit their skills and expertise while simultaneously allowing firms to hire the most appropriate workers (Baldwin & Wyplosz, 2009). The analysis here indicates that being a foreign-trained nurse was a significant predictor of performing tasks below skill level also for nurses from the new EU Member States that are classified as developing countries. An example of this is a Polish midwife who returned to Poland after working in France, stating that the work she was doing "did not match her professional competence" (Kautsch & Czabanowska, 2011). If nurses from developing countries were to have the same nursing skills and expertise as their native-trained colleagues, however, there are still other factors that may have caused them to perform tasks below their skill level, pulling them away from direct patient care. For example, Ognyanova and Busse (2011) concluded from previous research that inadequate language skills of foreign health professionals are problematic for both patients and colleagues in Germany. Another area of interest is different cultural perceptions of professional roles (e.g. scope of practice, levels of autonomy, holistic versus task-oriented care). For the United Kingdom as a major destination country, Young (2011) concluded that one challenge associated with mobility is the potential impact on practice of these cultural perceptions. Further research should, therefore, aim for a better understanding of the conditions under which foreign-trained nurses from developing countries performed the tasks associated with a professional role in their destination country. This knowledge will support workforce strategies to optimize migrated nurses' skills and to achieve effective employment of foreign health professionals already in the country (Wismar et al., 2011).

## Acknowledgements

The research leading to these results has received funding from the EU Seventh Framework Programme (FP7/2007–2013) under grant agreement 223468. More information on the RN4CAST project is given at http://www.rn4cast.eu.

## References

Aiken LH et al. (2001). Nurses' reports on hospital care in five countries. *Health Affairs*, 20(3):43–53.

Aiken LH et al. (2012). Patient safety, satisfaction, and quality of hospital care: cross-sectional surveys of nurses and patients in 12 countries in Europe and the United States. *British Medical Journal*, 344:e1717.

Baldwin R, Wyplosz C (2009). *The economics of European integration*, 3rd edn. London, McGraw-Hill Higher Education.

Center for Health Workforce Studies (2008). *The hospital nursing workforce in New York: findings from a survey of hospital registered nurses*. Rensselaer, NY, Center for Health Workforce Studies at the University of Albany (http://www.albany.edu/news/pdf_files/0805_Hospital_Workforce_Survey.pdf, accessed 3 January 2014).

Desjardins F et al. (2008). Reorganizing nursing work on surgical units: a time-and-motion study. *Nursing Leadership,* 21(3):26–38.

European Commission (2005). *Directive 2005/36/EC on the recognition of professional qualifications*. Brussels, European Commission (http://ec.europa.eu/internal_market/qualifications/policy_developments/legislation/index_en.htm, accessed 5 August 2013).

Flynn L, Aiken LH (2002). Does international nurse recruitment influence practice values in U.S. hospitals? *Journal of Nursing Scholarship*, 34(1):65–71.

Hendrich A et al. (2008). A 36-hospital time and motion study: how do medical-surgical nurses spend their time? *The Permanente Journal*, 12(3):25–34.

Humphries N, Brugha R, McGee H (2009). *Career progression of migrant nurses in Ireland*. Dublin, Royal College of Surgeons in Ireland (Nurse Migration Project Policy Brief 5).

International Monetary Fund (2010). *World economic outlook April 2010. Rebalancing growth*. Washington, DC, International Monetary Fund (http://www.imf.org/external/pubs/ft/weo/2010/01/pdf/text.pdf, accessed 3 January 2014).

International Organization for Migration (2010). *The role of migrant care workers in ageing societies; report on research findings in the United Kingdom, Ireland, Canada and the United States*. Geneva, International Organization for Migration (IOM Migration Research Series No. 41) (http://publications.iom.int/bookstore/free/MRS41.pdf, accessed 3 January 2014).

Kautsch M, Czabanowska K (2011). When the grass gets greener at home: Poland's changing incentives for health professional mobility. In Wismar M et al., eds. *Health professional mobility and health systems. Evidence from 17 European countries*. Copenhagen, WHO Regional Office for Europe on behalf of the European Observatory on Health Systems and Policies:419–448.

Kline DS (2003). Push and pull factors in international nurse migration. *Journal of Nursing Scholarship*, 35(2):107–111.

Ognyanova D, Busse R (2011). A destination and a source: Germany manages regional health workforce disparities with foreign medical doctors. In Wismar M et al., eds. *Health professional mobility and health systems. Evidence from 17 European countries*. Copenhagen, WHO Regional Office for Europe on behalf of the European Observatory on Health Systems and Policies:211–242.

SAS Institute (2011). *SAS system for windows, SAS/STAT software*, version 9.3. Cary, NC, SAS Institute.

Sermeus W et al. (2011). Nurse forecasting in Europe (RN4CAST): rationale, design and methodology. *BMC Nursing*, 10(6):1–9.

Sneath PH (1957). The application of computers to taxonomy. *Journal of General Microbiology*, 17(1):201–226.

WHO (2010). *WHO global code of practice on the international recruitment of health personnel*. Geneva, World Health Organization (Sixty-third World Health Assembly, WHA63.16). (http://www.who.int/hrh/migration/code/WHO_global_code_of_practice_EN.pdf, accessed 1 October 2013).

Wismar M et al. (2011). Health professional mobility and health systems in Europe: an introduction. In Wismar M et al., eds. *Health professional mobility and health systems. Evidence from 17 European countries.* Copenhagen, WHO Regional Office for Europe on behalf of the European Observatory on Health Systems and Policies:3–22.

Young R (2011). A major destination country: the United Kingdom and its changing recruitment policies. In Wismar M et al., eds. *Health professional mobility and health systems. Evidence from 17 European countries.* Copenhagen, WHO Regional Office for Europe on behalf of the European Observatory on Health Systems and Policies:295–335.

# Part IV
# Policy responses in a changing Europe

# Chapter 12

# The unfinished workforce agenda: Europe as a test-bed for policy effectiveness

*Diana Ognyanova, Evgeniya Plotnikova and Reinhard Busse*

## 12.1 Introduction

Strengthening the health workforce in Europe is an unfinished agenda. This is one of the messages emanating from the chapters of this book and the first PROMeTHEUS volume (Wismar et al., 2011). In order to address mobility, attrition, maldistribution and many other pressing workforce issues, a lot remains to be done. This chapter demonstrates that Europe is a test-bed for developing policies and practices addressing key health workforce challenges, many of which go beyond mobility. There are plenty of relevant policies, strategies and interventions implemented at different levels in European countries aiming at strengthening the health workforce. Countries can learn from each other's experience and build on these achievements.

To harness these experiences and to mobilize the tacit knowledge in countries, the European Commission together with the Member States under the leadership of the Belgian Government launched a Joint Action on Health Workforce Planning and Forecasting (2013), facilitating the exchange of best practices and consolidating the achievements by developing European guidance on the topic. In addition, new policy-oriented research was commissioned in 2013 by the European Commission to map and analyse effective policies, strategies and interventions on health workforce recruitment and retention in countries.

The purpose of this chapter is to provide an insight into the achievements and diversity in Europe when dealing with mobility of health professionals.

It should encourage further exchanges of experiences in Europe on the international, national, regional and organizational level. Health professional mobility is a fast-moving topic and so are the developments in health workforce policies and interventions in different countries. In this regard, the chapter is neither comprehensive nor totally systematic as it is based on the experiences in just 17 European countries as published in 2011 (Wismar et al., 2011). It therefore represents a certain "point in time". While there are certainly new developments covered in some of the thematic chapters of this volume, this panorama provides added value and encouragement for exchange, research and action.

Governments, states, regions and health care providers have all attempted to "manage" or steer the mobility of health professionals in order to address such health workforce challenges. The chapter presents a broad overview of such interventions, drawing from evidence accumulated in the first volume (Wismar et al., 2011). It looks first at general health workforce policies that indirectly affect mobility of health professionals (i.e. self-sufficiency, retention and health workforce planning) and then at health workforce mobility policies (e.g. international (ethical) recruitment) before examining bilateral agreements classified by their primary aim: ethical recruitment, international development, common labour markets and optimization of health care in border regions. The role of recruitment agencies in health workforce mobility is discussed before concluding with key observations and a summary of findings.

## 12.2 Workforce policies affecting mobility of health professionals

This section reviews policies implemented at national, regional and health provider level, reported in 17 European countries, that have influenced the mobility of health professionals. While policies explicitly targeting mobility of health professionals exist in only a few countries, general health workforce policies that do not focus on mobility of health professionals primarily can have a substantial effect on mobility. Such policies include health workforce sustainability/self-sufficiency policies and retention policies, but also workforce planning.

For the purposes of analysis and reporting, the chapter classifies the 17 countries into those that are either mainly source countries (Estonia, Hungary, Lithuania, Poland, Serbia, Romania, Slovakia, Turkey) or mainly destination countries (Austria, Belgium, Finland, France, Germany, Italy, Spain, Slovenia, United Kingdom), based on the mobility profiles described in the country case studies, while recognizing that all countries have a mixed mobility profile.

Self-sufficiency policies are discussed primarily in the context of destination countries, while retention policies are considered mainly in the context of source countries but also, to a lesser degree, in destination countries characterized by regional maldistribution of health professionals. Table 12.1 gives an overview of the various policies and practices that influence mobility of health professionals.

**Table 12.1** Policies and practices that influence the mobility of health professionals, by level of decision-making

| Level of decision-making | Policy type | | |
| --- | --- | --- | --- |
| | **General health workforce policies in destination countries** | **Mobility policies and instruments/flows** | **General health workforce policies in source countries** |
| National | Self-sufficiency and sustainability policy | International (ethical) recruitment | Retention policy |
| | Retention policy | | |
| | Workforce planning | Bilateral agreements | Workforce planning |
| | | International recruitment | |
| | | International development | |
| | | Common labour market | |
| | | Optimization of health care | |
| Federated state/region/ health provider | Retention policy | (Temporary) placements of staff | Retention policy |
| | | Educational programmes for students | |
| | | Twinning | |
| Private sector | | International recruitment through agencies | |

### 12.2.1 General health workforce policies

#### Sustainability and self-sufficiency policies

Health workforce sustainability and self-sufficiency policies strive to attain a sustainable stock of domestic health professionals to meet service requirements without significant reliance on foreign health professionals (Little & Buchan, 2007). "Self-sufficiency" was an explicit or implicit policy goal in a number of countries as a way of reducing reliance on international recruitment, motivated by a desire either to reduce the potential negative impact of such recruitment on source countries or to reduce the vulnerability of domestic workforce planning to unmanaged international flows. More recently the phrases "health workforce sustainability" and "sustainable workforce" have generally replaced "self-sufficiency", reflecting the use of the former phrases in the *WHO Global Code of Practice on the International Recruitment of Health Personnel* (WHO, 2010b). It should be noted that none of these phrases is clearly or precisely defined. As such, the extent to which countries have actually developed detailed policies in this area is quite limited; more often it is a loosely expressed policy goal.

Fig. 12.1 presents the percentage of foreign (national/trained/born) medical doctors among the total stock of medical doctors in selected EU countries in 2007.[1] This gives an idea of the relative reliance on foreign medical doctors in these countries. However, this indicator falls short of measuring workforce sustainability, as it does not tell anything about the effectiveness of the current staff mix and profile, or the distribution of the health workforce.

**Fig. 12.1** *Percentage of foreign (national/trained/born) medical doctors among all medical doctors in selected EU countries, 2007*

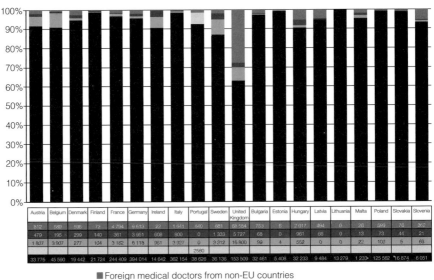

| | Austria | Belgium | Denmark | Finland | France | Germany | Ireland | Italy | Portugal | Sweden | United Kingdom | Bulgaria | Estonia | Hungary | Latvia | Lithuania | Malta | Poland | Slovakia | Slovenia |
|---|---|---|---|---|---|---|---|---|---|---|---|---|---|---|---|---|---|---|---|---|
| | 812 | 589 | 595 | 72 | 4 794 | 9 613 | 22 | 1 641 | 640 | 681 | 68 554 | 753 | 6 | 2 017 | 494 | 0 | 20 | 599 | 78 | 262 |
| | 479 | 195 | 299 | 140 | 361 | 3 951 | 608 | 800 | 0 | 1 333 | 5 727 | 68 | 0 | 961 | 66 | 0 | 13 | 73 | 44 | 21 |
| | 1 837 | 3 907 | 277 | 104 | 3 182 | 6 118 | 961 | 3 027 | 0 | 3 312 | 16 800 | 99 | 4 | 562 | 0 | 0 | 22 | 103 | 5 | 63 |
| | | | | | | | | | 2580 | | | | | | | | | | | |
| | 33 775 | 45 590 | 19 442 | 21 724 | 244 409 | 394 014 | 14 642 | 362 154 | 38 626 | 36 136 | 153 509 | 32 461 | 5 408 | 32 233 | 9 484 | 13 279 | 1 233 | 125 562 | 16 874 | 6 051 |

■ Foreign medical doctors from non-EU countries
■ Foreign medical doctors from new EU Member States (EU12)
■ Foreign medical doctors from old EU Member States (EU15)
▨ Foreign medical doctors from all EU Member States
■ Domestic doctors

*Source*: PROMeTHEUS database.

Fig. 12.1 shows that the United Kingdom has the highest reliance on foreign-trained doctors to meet its requirements. However, it is important to complement this indicator by reliable data on annual flows in order to assess trends: in other words, is the country clearly moving towards or away from self-sufficiency in terms of its relative reliance on health professionals from domestic and international sources.

The United Kingdom example shows a discernible reduction in reliance on international inflows in recent years (Buchan & Seccombe, 2013). However,

1 Data for foreign nationality for Austria, Belgium, France, Germany, Hungary, Italy, Poland and Slovakia; data for country of training for Denmark, Estonia, Finland, Ireland, Latvia, Malta, Portugal, Slovenia, Sweden and United Kingdom; country of birth for Bulgaria. For a methodological discussion on the use of different indicators see Chapter 3.

this is not just the result of a deliberate attempt to become self-sufficient. As noted in Chapter 1, it also reflects tougher immigration laws for non-EU migrants and reduced funding availability, which restricts any additional workforce expansion (see also Young, 2011).

A policy orientation towards self-sufficiency can be observed in Slovenia. Following an unsuccessful attempt to recruit internationally between 2000 and 2004, the country moved towards a policy of self-sufficiency. Attempts to make Slovenia self-sufficient have included expansion of training capacities through the opening of an additional medical faculty and four additional nursing schools (Albreht, 2011).

Austria has a self-sufficiency policy at the national level but planning decisions are taken by the states and, as a result, the country still has a relatively high intake of internationally recruited health professionals. The quota regulation for medical universities represents a self-sufficiency instrument at a national level to ensure that a certain defined percentage of medical training places are reserved for Austrian citizens in order to meet domestic workforce requirements (Offermanns, Malle & Jusic, 2011).

### Retention policies

Retention of employees is the systematic effort to create and foster an environment that encourages employees to remain employed by having policies and practices in place that address their needs (WHO Regional Office for Europe, 2011). While not necessarily implemented with the primary goal of managing health professional mobility, retention policies can have a distinct effect on migration flows. Retention policies in source countries can play an essential role in mitigating the losses caused by outmigration, which typically are greatest in rural and remote areas. As almost all countries suffer from maldistribution characterized by urban concentration and rural deficits, effective retention of health professionals in remote and rural areas in destination countries can also impact on mobility by reducing the demand for international recruitment (WHO, 2006, 2010a). Evidence in countries suggests that foreign health professionals tend to fill vacancies in rural and remote areas (Ognyanova & Busse, 2011).

Retention policies have been developed and implemented in source countries within the EU, such as Estonia, Lithuania, Poland, Slovakia and (locally) Hungary. While these interventions were not always a direct response to health professional mobility, they may have subsequently had an impact on the migration decisions of individual health professionals and therefore reduced international outflow. Each of these cases will be looked at below, starting with national level followed by the regional and organizational level.

*Retention policies at the national level*

In Estonia, salary increases for health professionals have been the main instrument used to reduce emigration in recent years. On 1 January 2005, a minimum salary level agreement came into force between health professionals (medical doctors and nurses), trade unions, health care provider associations and the state. It is assumed that this has had a retention effect on health professionals. A further agreement was signed in January 2006 to provide additional annual increases of minimum income in 2006, 2007 and 2008.

The salaries of health professionals showed higher increases than the national gross average income in Estonia. This was the outcome of a policy aimed at prioritizing health professionals and was further supported by additional revenues generated in the health insurance system during the period of economic growth. However, the economic crisis then led to reductions in salaries. Overall, however, the health sector has seen smaller salary decreases and lower levels of unemployment than other economic sectors (Saar & Habicht, 2011).

In Lithuania, a health care reform implemented in two stages (2003–2005, 2006–2008) contributed to significant changes in working conditions as well as better distribution of the services and duties of health professionals. While not an explicit response to outmigration, representatives of the health professions (mainly associations of medical doctors and nurses) had been pressing the Ministry of Health not only to restructure health care institutions and improve infrastructure but also to increase salaries. In 2005, the Ministry of Health and the associations signed a memorandum on salary increases (20% annually for medical doctors and nurses in 2005–2008). This is likely to have had a positive influence on reducing the high rates of dropout from medical studies, attrition to other better paid professions and emigration rates. Incentive schemes have been used to address regional maldistribution and promote deployment in remote areas. Medical doctors who practise in rural areas receive financial bonuses (Padaiga, Pukas & Starkienė, 2011).

Financial support from EU structural funds has been used to modernize and develop the public health care infrastructure and in particular the cardiology infrastructure in the south-eastern region of Lithuania. This enabled renovation of most hospitals and supply of new medical equipment, and supported improvement to GP and primary health care facilities. Further measures to ensure available and high-quality essential health care services had been envisaged by the government, but the global economic crisis has raised some barriers against reaching the anticipated goals of the reform (Padaiga, Pukas & Starkienė, 2011).

In Poland, different and unrelated initiatives have been implemented in order to enhance retention of health workers. In 2001, the government raised the salaries of all fully contracted health professionals in public health care institutions by 203 zloty (about €56) per month – whatever their positions, years of work experience, qualifications or the implications for their health care institutions. However, it was not specified how the pay rise was to be financed and the initiative left numerous health care institutions in debt. Other interventions before EU accession aimed to reduce the number of health professionals in order to improve the income and employment opportunities for the remaining health workforce and for newcomers. The main policy tool was state reimbursement of the redundancy payments made by public health care institutions (Kautsch & Czabanowska, 2011).

Another initiative was offering preferred "start up" loans to health professionals who decided to leave the public sector and start their own health provision. This might have indirectly contributed to reducing the outmigration of Polish health professionals by creating financial, career-related and entrepreneurial incentives that influenced domestic opportunities for professional development.

National intervention took place also with regard to the training capacities for health and health-related studies in Poland. Based on the assessment of needs for graduates in given studies, the health minister determined the quotas for candidates in public and private higher education. As a result, academic facilities increased the number of enrolled medical students in 2005 but there was only a small increase in the financial subsidy for medical universities. At the postgraduate level, the health minister issued the list of priority specializations. Medical doctors undertaking specialist training in the priority areas were offered higher pay (Kautsch & Czabanowska, 2011).

In Slovakia, retention policies have focused on better remuneration, improved social recognition of health professionals, improved working conditions and education (including continuing medical education), enhanced transparency on the work of ethical committees and the modernization of health care facilities. The gradual increase of health insurance funds has allowed for an increase in the salaries of health professionals. The average monthly salary of medical doctors was 181.6% of the average monthly salary in Slovakia in 2005 but rose to 214.7% by 2009. The average salary for nurses was 84.6% of the average monthly salary in 2005, rising to 98.8% in 2009.

It is probable that improved salaries have contributed to the reduction in the number of applications for equivalence confirmations in Slovakia, which is one indication of the migration intention of health professionals. Further increases in salaries were constrained by the economic crisis and so other retention options, such as non-financial incentives and housing support, have been discussed (Beňušová et al., 2011).

Slovakia has embarked on a programme to make health facilities more attractive for patients and the health workforce by reducing inequalities in the distribution of resources and technical capacities. Funded by the European Social Fund's Operational Programme Education and the European Regional Development Fund's Operational Programme Health, €250 million was invested in the modernization of Slovak health care providers between 2007 and 2013. This is expected to reduce the level of emigration motivated by dissatisfaction with working with outdated or inadequate equipment in health care facilities.

The Operational Programme Education intervention focuses on the retention of specialist medical doctors, aiming to balance the regional differences in available workforce capacities in Slovakia and EU Member States. Specialized training is funded on the condition that the enrolled medical doctors work in Slovakia for a specified period of time after the successful completion of their studies. Those who fail to meet this obligation must repay their EU grant so that funding may be used for another specialist. After successful evaluation of the pilot project for medical doctors in 2008, the Ministry of Health announced that the self-governing regions (excluding Bratislava) could apply for financial support for specialized training for all health professionals. All the eligible self-governing regions have implemented projects based on the second Operational Programme Education (Beňušová et al., 2011).

In Hungary, there has been growing awareness of the problem of outmigration but interventions so far have concentrated on attempts to limit outflows through administrative measures. A new system of postgraduate medical training was introduced in 2009, presumably in response to increasing concern over the outmigration of Hungarian health professionals, mainly medical doctors (Eke, Girasek & Szócska, 2011). The new system authorizes health care institutions to apply to the Ministry of Health for resident places, according to their needs. Related finance is allocated according to the number of resident places.

Residents contract with the institutions at the start of their residencies. On top of their salary, they are eligible to apply for financial support for their specialist training. In return, they agree a specified length of service required following qualification as a specialist. If doctors decide to migrate to another country upon qualifying in their specialization without fulfilling the requirement to work in the domestic system, they are obliged to repay the financial support. In addition, the Ministry of Health steers young medical doctors into identified shortage specialties by increasing the remuneration (Eke, Girasek & Szócska, 2011).

*Retention measures at regional and organizational level*

In some countries, measures to retain health professionals are typically implemented at the local and/or health care provider level, either in the absence of a national policy-led approach or because individual organizations and local government authorities can be responsive to local labour market challenges. In Hungary, for example, local government authorities collaborate with health care providers to offer incentives in rural areas, where an undersupply of health professionals is a long-standing problem. These efforts are mainly local, individual and non-coordinated. In addition, some health care providers in Hungary offer higher salaries and financial compensations to attract and retain specialists in the most critical fields, such as anaesthetics and pathology. Support for accommodation is the most common non-financial incentive (Eke, Girasek & Szócska, 2011). Similarly, in Lithuania, some hospitals in rural areas offer free accommodation and transportation services for medical doctors.

In Poland, in order to meet the increased financial expectations of medical doctors who might otherwise change employer or emigrate, some managers of provider institutions are offering changes in employment status – from full-time employment contract to fee-for-service self-employment agreements (with smaller mandatory insurance contributions) (Kautsch & Czabanowska, 2011).

In Germany, some hospitals in the eastern states are trying to attract and retain young medical doctors with offers of extra bonuses such as cheaper loans, lower rent and mortgages. There are also efforts by rural hospitals to attract and retain staff with improved work–life balance and family-friendly working conditions, such as child care or specific working time arrangements.

### Workforce planning

Appropriate workforce planning (i.e. the process of aligning the numbers, skills and competencies of health professionals with the aims, priorities and needs of the health system) can play a significant role in avoiding health workforce imbalances, such as under- or oversupply of health professionals and skill-mix imbalances. To this end, workforce monitoring, analyses and forecasts are conducted using a variety of methodologies. Workforce planning furthermore aims to guide the development of educational and training contents and capacities. However, in most countries, workforce planning is an underdeveloped issue. In practice, the process is complex and includes many actors with conflicting interests, which is particularly evident in decentralized systems.

There is growing interest in workforce planning and the application of sophisticated forecasting methodologies in a few EU countries, such as Belgium,

Estonia, Finland, Lithuania, Spain and the United Kingdom. Some countries have no nationwide planning but use procedures at the regional level, as in Austria; others disperse planning across different sectors, as in Germany.

Mobility of health professionals is a factor of uncertainty in workforce planning. Even when countries have workforce planning mechanisms, problems arise from the possible lack of data on mobility and the limitations of the standard mobility indicators in measuring labour mobility, which make it difficult to factor in the loss or gain of health professionals. Only a few countries take mobility of health professionals into account in the planning process. This does happen in Estonia, for example, where the continuous planning and monitoring of health professionals takes place at the state level led by the Ministry of Social Affairs in coordination with the Ministry of Education and Research and the training institutions. The planning process includes analysis of the dynamics of the number of professionals who have migrated and the number who are working outside the health sector. Furthermore, the Ministry of Social Affairs has financed several studies to explore the emigration intentions of health professionals and their satisfaction with the working environment in Estonia (Saar & Habicht, 2011). Lithuania has conducted studies on health professional mobility to factor outflows into workforce planning (Padaiga, Pukas & Starkienė, 2011).

Workforce planning may extend beyond the health system, as in Finland, where decision-makers introduced a comprehensive workforce planning system that included other sectors in addition to health care in order to cover competing labour market demands (Kuusio et al., 2011). However, in most countries, workforce planning is an underdeveloped policy tool or there remains a significant disconnect between workforce planning and the development of training capacities, as is the case in Serbia (Jekić, Katrava & Vučković-Krčmar, 2011) and Romania (Galan, Olsavszky & Vladescu, 2011).

### 12.2.2 Health workforce mobility policies

*International recruitment*

International recruitment has been a solution for domestic health workforce imbalances in a number of destination countries. The most prominent country that has pursued a policy of international recruitment for decades is the United Kingdom, where more than a third of medical doctors and every tenth nurse registered are internationally trained (Young, 2011).

International recruitment has also been a means of filling shortages of health professionals in other European countries. Slovenia has been a destination country for health professionals from the countries of former Yugoslavia for several decades. Faced with a shortage of key health professional groups, Slovenia has relied to a considerable extent on foreign doctors from this source. In 2003–2008, every fifth medical doctor practising in Slovenia was foreign-trained, particularly from neighbouring countries. Overall, about 80% of all immigrant doctors and dentists in Slovenia come from three sources: Croatia, Serbia and Bosnia and Herzegovina (Albreht, 2011).

In Finland, active measures for recruiting foreign health professionals have increasingly been employed over the past few years. The Government Migration Policy Programme issued in October 2006 also emphasized active recruitment of a migrant labour force. The National Institute for Health and Welfare and Helsinki University Central Hospital have launched a pilot project to recruit nurses from other EU countries. The project aims to develop ethical recruitment among health care personnel (Kuusio et al., 2011).

### Ethical international recruitment

International recruitment is increasingly being linked to ethical considerations of the impact of health workforce migration on source countries, especially in the developing world. As discussed in Chapter 8, concerns in the United Kingdom about the impact on the health systems of those countries that are the main migration sources led to various codes of practice on international recruitment being developed, but the impact of these policy instruments is difficult to measure (Young et al., 2008; Buchan et al., 2009).

Codes on ethical recruitment also exist in other countries. In Italy, there is a code to reduce immigration from non-EU countries but it is not clear whether this applies only to health professionals. A national code on ethical recruitment exists in Austria, even though planning and recruitment take place at regional and local levels and the effects of this code are not assessed (Wismar et al., 2011).

Efforts to enhance ethical recruitment have also been made at the international level. In 2010, the World Health Assembly adopted the *WHO Global Code of Practice for the International Recruitment of Health Personnel*. The Code discourages recruitment from countries with workforce shortages and provides guidance to strengthen the workforce and health systems across the globe, including an emphasis on improving staff retention, workforce sustainability and effective workforce planning (WHO, 2010b).

### Bilateral agreements on mobility of health professionals

Countries (or actors within different countries) can conclude agreements specifically targeting health professionals. The agreements are negotiated between two or more parties at the national, regional or health care provider level. These arrangements appear in the form of bilateral labour agreements, letters of intent, twinning schemes, memoranda of understanding and informal (non-written) communication between involved stakeholders. In terms of the content, such agreements may perform differing, but not mutually exclusive and often overlapping, functions, including active international recruitment, promotion of ethical principles in the recruitment of foreign health workers, assistance in international development by means of educational support and sharing of expertise, the creation of a common labour market and optimization of health care in border regions. Annex 12.1 illustrates the geographical and functional diversity of bilateral arrangements seen at national, regional and health provider levels. Chapter 14 has a more detailed analysis of bilateral agreements.

Bilateral agreements have in the past typically focused on recruitment of foreign health professionals, but since the early 2000s their recruitment function has reduced in importance while ethical recruitment and assistance in international development have increasingly come to the fore.

*Agreements at national level*

The United Kingdom's experience with bilateral agreements is discussed in detail in Chapter 14. However, as highlighted in Annex 12A.1, other countries also have a long track record in using this type of policy instrument. For example, bilateral agreements for the recruitment of nurses have been in place in Germany since the early 1970s – first to recruit nurses from the Republic of Korea and then with a number of eastern European countries. Since 2005, Germany has had a bilateral agreement of this kind with Croatia, and about 131 nurses were recruited from Croatia within the framework of the bilateral agreement between 2009 and 2011 (Deutscher Bundestag, 2012). In December 2012, Croatia was the second major source country after Turkey for nurses and midwives subject to social insurance contributions, with a total stock of 3 337 nurses and midwives (German Federal Employment Agency, unpublished data). In 2013, the German Federal Employment Agency concluded bilateral agreements on the recruitment of nurses with Serbia, the Philippines and Bosnia and Herzegovina. The recruitment and integration of the foreign health workforce are carried out by the German Society for International Cooperation in the framework of a so-called "Triple Win" project. By September 2013, only 389 nurses had taken part in the project (273 from Bosnia and Herzegovina, 93 from Serbia and 23 from the Philippines), but the goal is to expand and recruit nurses from Vietnam, Indonesia, Tunisia and Albania as well. Another project-related cooperation, between the German Federal Employment Agency and the Chinese employment agency (implemented by the German Association of Employers in Social and Health and Elderly Care and the German Confederation of German Employers), facilitated the recruitment of 150 Chinese nurses in elderly care (Deutscher Bundestag, 2013). As part of a pilot project initiated by the German Ministry of Economics and Technology (2013), 100 Vietnamese nurses have started training as nurses for the elderly in Germany.

An agreement between Spain and France was signed in early 2000, which allowed for Spanish nurses to work in France at a time when French hospitals were facing difficulties recruiting nurses. This led the French Federations of Hospitals to cooperate with the Ministry of Health in order to recruit 770 Spanish nurses. Local hospital managers were required to give written guarantees to smooth the arrival and integration of Spanish nurses and to help them in their work (Delamaire & Schweyer, 2011).

An agreement between Spain and the Philippines, which was signed in June 2006, allows entry of up to 100 000 Filipino health workers into Spain, where they are afforded the same social protections as Spanish workers. Spain signed agreements also with Morocco and with Colombia, which incorporate concepts of migration and human capacity development (Dhillon, Clark & Kapp, 2010).

To facilitate mobility of health professionals and international recruitment, some countries have concluded bilateral agreements on the recognition of qualifications. France has bilateral agreements (*conventions d'établissements*) with Morocco and Tunisia providing for recognition of qualifications. There are furthermore state agreements with several countries in Africa (the Central African Republic, Chad, Democratic Republic of the Congo, Gabon, Mali and Togo). Medical doctors from the countries listed can practise in France if they have a French medical degree or other titles mentioned in the Code de la Santé Publique. In practice, the policy is vague with room for flexibility: the state can issue derogations in some cases. Some foreign health professionals work as medical doctors but are officially classified as students (Delamaire & Schweyer, 2011). A bilateral agreement signed between Belgium and South Africa in 1965 establishes a system of mutual recognition of basic medical diplomas and has been in use for 40 years (Safuta & Baeten, 2011).

*Agreements at regional and institutional level*

In Germany, the states of Thüringen, Mecklenburg-Vorpommern, Brandenburg, Sachsen and Sachsen-Anhalt concluded an informal agreement with the Austrian chamber of physicians in order to tackle a shortage of medical doctors in Eastern Germany. These arrangements enable young Austrian medical doctors to work in German hospitals (Offermanns, Malle & Jusic, 2011).

In Italy, some regions have agreed bilateral educational programmes with foreign nursing institutes in order to recruit qualified foreign health professionals and to secure the language and professional skills required to work in the destination. For example, SkyNurse is an experimental project involving 180 Romanian candidates in a 14-month training programme that includes three months of online distance learning between classrooms in Padua and the partners' institutes in Bucharest and Pitesti. The final one month training is organized in the Veneto Region (Bertinato et al., 2011).

The Province of Parma has a bilateral agreement for cooperation in nurse training with the Province of Cluj-Napoca. The bilateral agreement between the two local authorities and the respective nurse training institutes started in the 2003–2004 academic year. Fully funded by the Province of Parma, the project added modules to the existing Cluj nurse training programme, covering the Italian language and Italian health regulations and professional standards. While the long-term goal is to support the Cluj University in the development of a joint degree in nursing, recognized according to EU standards, the cooperation has already led to recruitment of nurses. In 2005, 26 Romanian nurses moved to Italy and about 40 in 2006 (Chaloff, 2008).

### Bilateral agreements on international development

*Agreements at national level*

Another type of bilateral agreement primarily focuses on international development through educational support and sharing of expertise. Some of the United Kingdom bilateral agreements, discussed in more detail in Chapter 14, have been set within the context of the wider policy on international development (see also Dhillon, Clark & Kapp, 2010; Young, 2011).

France has signed agreements with Benin and Senegal that address migration flows with a particular focus on health professionals and support for human resources for health development. The France–Senegal agreement aims to encourage migration that is favourable for each country's economic, social and cultural development and should not lead to a loss of skilled resources for the country of origin. The aim is to achieve the opposite result: migration should encourage an increase in development in the country of origin not only through the remittances of migrants but also through the training and experience acquired by migrants during their stay in the destination country (Dhillon, Clark & Kapp, 2010).

Concrete mechanisms to achieve this include the creation of a migration observatory and the exchange of information, including details on health sector cooperation such as the creation of a joint French–Senegalese faculty of medicine, support for reintegration of health professionals and other efforts to ensure that migrant health personnel can contribute to broader development in source countries. The last includes a programme with matching funds that the Senegalese diaspora in France make available for development in Senegal. France's agreement with Benin similarly places a very specific focus on addressing the negative effects for Benin of the international migration of its health professionals (Dhillon, Clark & Kapp, 2010).

In Turkey, the employment of foreign health professionals is prohibited by law and therefore there are no bilateral agreements on health professional mobility between Turkey and other countries. However, Turkey started the Great Student Project in 1992–1993 with the aims of enhancing the relationship with the Turkic Republics, Turks and relative communities,[2] helping them to meet their educated workforce needs and promoting the Turkish language and Turkish culture. The Great Student Project is carried out within the framework of cooperation agreements, protocols and relevant legislation. Turkey provides scholarships to students according to these agreements and by 9 September 2009, a total of 5 347 students had studied in Turkey under the Project (Yildirim & Kaya, 2011).

*Agreements at regional or health care provider level*

Support for the development of modern institutions in the beneficiary country is sometimes organized at the subnational level. For example, in the United Kingdom there were Royal College sponsorship schemes for medical doctors as well as exchange agreements and twinning or staff volunteering partnerships between local NHS organizations and overseas providers and regional governments (Sloan, 2005). At the time, this allowed the NHS organizations to employ individuals from outside the United Kingdom and EEA for up to 24 months as part of a government-authorized exchange programme (NHS Employers, 2008).

Initiatives in other countries also focus on educational support and sharing of expertise through staff exchange. There are several examples in Belgium. In 1990, the French-speaking Catholic University of Louvain and the Romanian University of Medicine and Pharmacy "Gr.T. Popa" Iaşi signed an agreement allowing Romanian medical students in their third or fourth years to spend one year (potentially extendable to two years) of their specialization in one of the Belgian hospitals. By 2009, some 450 Romanian interns had taken part in the programme. Before Romania's accession to the EU, participants could undertake part of their specialization in Belgium under the responsibility of a qualified doctor without possessing a certificate of equivalence of their diploma and a licence to practise (Safuta & Baeten, 2011).

---

2 These include Turkic Republics: Azerbaijan, Kazakhstan, Kyrgyzstan, Turkmenistan, Uzbekistan; Balkan and Asian countries: Afghanistan, Bosnia and Herzegovina, Bulgaria, Islamic Republic of Iran, Iraq, Lebanon, Romania, the Syrian Arab Republic, the former Yugoslav Republic of Macedonia; the Russian Federation: over 60 communities.

Some other hospitals signed similar cooperation agreements. For example, a university hospital in Liège signed such an agreement with a Vietnamese hospital. The French-speaking University of Brussels runs the Fonds de Soutien à la Formation Médicale scholarship programme. In 2005, the University Hospital of Antwerp hosted several Polish nursing students as part of an exchange programme and, more recently, nurses from the Philippines (Safuta & Baeten, 2011). In France, there was an agreement between Lille Regional University Hospital and a hospital in Poland that facilitated the temporary placement of 20 Polish nurses in 2004 (Delamaire & Schweyer, 2011).

### Bilateral agreements on common labour market

Another type of agreement aims to create a common labour market between countries.[3] The mobility and mutual recognition of health professionals has been relatively open and well established between the Nordic countries since the 1950s, enabled by a framework of agreements allowing broader mobility across countries. The first agreement on the common Nordic labour market was introduced in 1954 and amended in 1982. The agreement for particular health professionals was specified in 1993 and amended in 1998. These have been negotiated as part of a broader set of agreements and cooperation between the Nordic countries. It is likely that the existence of common labour markets has contributed to the mobility of health professionals, particularly when there have been large salary differences (Kuusio et al., 2011).

The Socialist Federal Republic of Yugoslavia signed bilateral agreements that are still active, even if losing relevance. Together with the adoption of rules regarding the mutual recognition of degrees between the countries of the former Yugoslavia, these agreements ensure automatic recognition of the degrees of all graduates from the former USSR and from the area of the former Yugoslavia for those who graduated before 25 June 1991. The main aim of this bilateral agreement was to enable health professionals to move freely between the countries and facilitate access to the wider labour market (Albreht, 2011).

Some accession countries signed bilateral agreements that allowed temporary opening of certain EU15 labour markets to accession countries until enlargement was finalized and full mobility established. Such agreements were signed between Poland and some EU15 countries. As a result, countries such as Ireland, the Netherlands, Spain and the United Kingdom opened their markets to Polish health professionals. They entered into bilateral agreements with Poland to recruit staff for a fixed period of time and to provide cultural adaptation support (Kautsch & Czabanowska, 2011).

---

3 The EU regulations on the single market, which covers labour mobility, are beyond the scope of this chapter.

## Bilateral agreements on optimization of health care in border regions

### Agreements at national level

Another type of agreement aims to optimize health care in border regions. The Sanicademia and the Healthregio project are examples of bilateral agreements between Austria and its neighbouring regions. The Healthregio project (Regional Network for the Improvement of Healthcare Services) is implemented under INTERREG III A, the external border programme of the EU. It aimed to optimize the structure of health care provision in the border regions of Austria, the Czech Republic, Slovakia and Hungary in order to create a quality location for health care services in central Europe. The project priorities are the mobility of patients and health professionals; education and skills development for health professionals; legislative changes and progress in national health care systems; and comparable statistical data on the region (Healthregio, 2004).

Austria collaborated with Slovenia and Italy in a cross-border cooperation project called INTERREG IV, which ran from 2007 until 2013 and dealt with health professional mobility in the region. The project aimed to enhance and harmonize training and specialization of health professionals in the different countries and regions. Furthermore, it aimed to harmonize quality management systems at hospital level. It offered exchange programmes for health professionals and organized thematic seminars and language courses (Sanicademia, 2011).

France and Germany have signed an agreement on cooperation and provision of health care in border regions that allows a two-way movement of staff, in particular ambulance and emergency staff (Wiskow, 2006).

A *convention médicale transfrontalière* that France has signed with Monaco and with Switzerland enables medical doctors who work next to the French border to practise on the other side of the border under specific conditions included in the contract. In addition, France signed an *accord de réciprocité* with Monaco in 1938 which allows equal numbers of French and Monegasque doctors to work and settle in the host country (Delamaire & Schweyer, 2011).

### Agreements at regional/professional body level

The two medical chambers of South Tyrol in Italy and Tyrol in Austria developed a special model of cross-border collaboration. The Südtirol Enquête was established in 1987 in order to ensure that medical doctors can be trained in South Tyrolean hospitals in accordance with Austrian law and receive the Austrian licence to practise medicine (approbation). In this way, Austrian medical training is secured for South Tyrolean graduates and Austrian medical doctors gain training possibilities in South Tyrol (Offermanns, Malle & Jusic, 2011).

### The role of recruitment agencies

In many countries, active recruitment of health professionals takes place via the services of private recruitment agencies. Health care providers facing shortages of health professionals pay these agencies to recruit foreign health workers. These agencies may have specific detailed knowledge of foreign labour markets and already established recruitment networks. They act as intermediaries in the recruitment process, making the connection between the employer and the potential recruits.

In Belgium, some hospitals recruit nursing staff by using the services of liaison or temporary work agencies that recruit abroad. Several Brussels hospitals have used this method to hire Romanian or Lebanese nurses. Such private companies provide Belgian hospitals not only with nurses but also with specializing foreign medical doctors, who work as assistants in Belgium. Private companies not only recruit in the country of origin but often also arrange travel, accommodation and administrative requirements (such as residence permits, diploma recognition/equivalence) for their recruits. Hospitals that have hired foreign-trained nurses evaluate these experiences overall as positive or mixed, mentioning communication difficulties because of insufficient command of the hospital's working language (Safuta & Baeten, 2011).

In Italy, private hospitals and nursing homes largely recruit health professionals from Albania through private agencies. The nursing sector is one where Albanian agencies have been able to establish a niche. The agency La Speranza, for example, has an office in Tirana and an office in Milan and handles only nursing personnel. It sent about 500 nurses from Albania to northern Italy between 1999 and 2008. The Milan office contacts private hospitals and nursing homes. The Tirana office verifies the qualifications – only the new post-1995 Albanian nursing schools are recognized in Italy – and prepares the documentation for recognition of nursing skills. The agency also provides language lessons and preparation for the nursing examination in Italy.

Nursing is a traditional profession for Albanian women, but about half of the agency's clients are men. According to the agency, these men went to nursing school in order to emigrate. Hence it is most probable that the expansion of the nursing education sector in Albania to a point where new supply exceeds domestic demand is the result of emigration opportunities. La Speranza reports that not one of the nurses sent to Italy has returned to Albania. Some nurses report having to pay high fees to the agencies and complain about finding themselves stuck in unpleasant working conditions in private structures where their contract is not respected (Chaloff, 2008). Recruitment agencies deny this, as the International Labour Organization Private Employment Agency Convention of 1997, which Albania ratified in 1999, prohibits workers from paying fees, requiring the employer to cover the costs.

The public sector in Italy also uses private agencies for recruitment. One example is a protocol signed in 2004 between the Modena USL (Health Service) and a private Romanian recruitment agency, International Staffing. Under the terms of the protocol, the latter provides 80 hours of Italian language training so that the nurses can pass the language examination once in Italy. The private agency also supports all bureaucratic steps in the recruitment, recognition and visa process. The nurses pay only administrative and travel costs, but they sign a contract stating that if they withdraw from the process they must pay a penalty. The Italian region pays the agency €600 for each nurse who actually starts working in public structures in Italy (Chaloff, 2008).

A number of private agencies recruit health professionals in Eastern Europe for eastern German hospitals that are unable to recruit sufficient medical doctors. Furthermore, a growing number of agencies provide home-help services by nurses from Eastern European countries. The recruitment through these agencies takes place in a legal grey area. Very often carers are registered as self-employed in their home country and can offer their services if they prove that they have more than one client or they are "delegated" by a company that works with partner agencies in Germany (Ognyanova & Busse, 2011). The carer pays social insurance contributions and taxes in their country of origin and working hours are regulated through the law in their home country. However, it is not possible to monitor if these requirements are adhered to. Usually the carer lives with the family of the person in need of care, which suggests constant addressability, as well as disguised self-employment, as there is only one employer.

Recruitment agencies play an important role also in other countries such as Austria, where the placement of home-care staff from the Czech Republic and Slovakia is organized largely through such agencies, and in France, where hospitals pay private agencies to attract foreign health workers. Recruitment agencies employ Estonian and Lithuanian nurses to cover workforce shortages in Norwegian facilities. Spain and the United Kingdom gained important inflows of medical doctors from Poland and Romania partly through the active roles of recruitment agencies targeting these countries.

The importance of recruitment agencies in stimulating and enabling the flow of health professionals to the United Kingdom was recognized when the NHS Code on International Recruitment was extended to cover the practices of recruitment agencies acting on behalf of NHS employers (Buchan et al., 2009). A voluntary code of practice for recruitment agencies has also been established in the United States of America (Alliance for Ethical International Recruitment Practices, 2013).

## 12.3 Discussion and conclusions

Overall, there are substantial variations among countries in the levels of activity and interventions influencing mobility of health professionals. This chapter has illustrated the wide variation in policy responses that have been adopted in different countries and at different levels – national, regional and/ or health care provider. While international recruitment remains a political and managerial response to workforce shortages in a number of countries, a policy leaning towards health workforce sustainability/self-sufficiency and ethical recruitment can be observed more recently in some countries. At the same time, retention policies that reduce flows out of the workforce by creating effective incentive systems, such as improving salaries and working conditions of health professionals, have been employed in some countries.

The review of different agreements used to facilitate the mobility of health professionals has shown that, apart from recruitment to fill domestic shortages, bilateral agreements can also pursue differing, but not mutually exclusive and often overlapping, goals such as international development and health human resources development, the creation of a common labour market and optimization of health care in border regions. Alongside bilateral agreements concluded at the national level, there are a number of cross-border arrangements between European countries at the regional and/or health care provider level. Furthermore, the role of private sector recruitment agencies contributes to the mobility of health professionals, and in some countries this has led to attempts to extend coverage of codes of practice to their activities.

As discussed in Chapter 1, the international mobility of health professionals raises difficult questions of ethics and international equity, in particular when there are persistent net flows of staff from poorer to richer countries. Managing mobility of health professionals involves balancing the freedom of individuals to pursue work where they choose with the need to reduce excessive losses from both internal and international mobility. Outmigration of health professionals can exacerbate existing imbalances in health human resources such as shortages and regional maldistribution, creating a need for measures to ensure workforce retention.

At the same time, international migration of health professionals can increase the flexibility of labour markets, especially in the short term, by speeding up the process of reaching equilibrium. Bilateral agreements at the national, regional or institutional level have the potential to improve the management of international mobility of health workers and reduce adverse consequences, especially if they include clauses whereby a recipient country agrees to underwrite the costs of training additional staff; and/or recruit staff for a fixed period only, prior to their returning to the source country; and/or recruit surplus staff in source countries (Buchan, 2008). However, as the detailed assessment of bilateral agreements in the United Kingdom in chapter 14 shows, this has not always been the case in practice.

Appropriate workforce planning that takes into account the migration of health professionals plays a significant role in avoiding health workforce imbalances. Growing interest in workforce planning and the application of sophisticated forecasting methodologies can be observed in a few countries. Sharing information on workforce planning methodologies and projections of workforce supply, demand and needs could help to steer mobility of health professionals in mutually beneficial directions.

## Annex 12.1 Bilateral arrangements

Table 12A.1 shows examples at the levels of national, regional and health provider to illustrate geographical and functional diversity of bilateral arrangements. Where available, data on migratory flows have been added to attempt to trace the effect of the agreements on migration flows. Chapter 14 has a more detailed analysis of bilateral agreements.

**Table 12A.1** Examples of bilateral agreements on mobility of health professionals

| Countries | Date of signature/current status | Type and focus | Migration flows |
|---|---|---|---|
| Germany–Croatia | 2005 | Bilateral agreements between the German Federal Employment Agency and national authorities on the recruitment of nurses | 131 Croatian nurses were recruited within the framework of the agreement between 2009 and 2011 |
| Germany–Bosnia and Herzegovina, Serbia, the Philippines | 2013 | Bilateral agreements between the German Federal Employment Agency and national authorities on the recruitment of nurses | By September 2013, 273 nurses from Bosnia and Herzegovina, 93 from Serbia and 23 from the Philippines had been recruited |
| Germany–Vietnam, China, Tunisia | | Bilateral agreements between the German Federal Employment Agency and national authorities on the recruitment of nurses | |
| Germany–Vietnam | | Pilot project of the German Ministry of Economics and Technology for the recruitment and training of nurses for the elderly from Vietnam | 100 Vietnamese enrolled in training as nurses for the elderly in Germany |
| United Kingdom–Spain | 2000/expired | Agreement on recruitment of Spanish health professionals (primarily nurses) | Estimated number recruited, 1 300 |
| United Kingdom–Indonesia | 2002/expired | Memorandum of understanding on the recruitment and employment of health professionals | Only a pilot cohort of Indonesian nurses recruited |
| United Kingdom–Philippines | 2002/expired | Bilateral agreement on promotion of employment opportunities for Filipino health professionals (primarily nurses) | In 2001–2002, the number of newly registered Filipino nurses reached 7 235 while in the reporting year prior to the agreement (2000–2001) only half of this number was registered, namely 3 396[a] |
| United Kingdom–Philippines | 2003/expired | Memorandum of understanding on bilateral cooperation in health care to slow down the active recruitment of Filipino nurses and to strengthen the ethical principles in recruitment and employment of foreign health workers | Since 2003, the number of Filipino nurses registered with the NMC began to decrease and by 2005 fell by 2 521[a] |

| | | | |
|---|---|---|---|
| United Kingdom–China | 2005/expired | Letter of intent on cooperation in recruiting Chinese health professionals with certain limitations (except from rural areas); agreement aimed to promote ethical principles in recruitment of foreign health workers | No precise data available on number of recruits but, based on anecdotal information, this agreement brought a small number (pilot cohort ) of Chinese nurses |
| United Kingdom–India | 2001/expired | Exchange of letters (no written agreement) on recruitment of Indian nurses (except from the regions Andhra Pradesh, Madhya Pradesh, Orissa, West Bengal) | Number of newly registered nurses from India increased from 96 (in 1999–2000) to 289 (2000–2001) and reached 3 690 in 2004–2005[a] |
| Poland–Netherlands | 2002 | Covenant on migrant health workers on recruitment of Polish nurses | 91 nurses moved to practise in the Netherlands |
| France–Germany | 2005 | Agreement on cooperation and provision of health care in border regions | Ambulances and emergency staff (two-way movement of labour force) |
| France–Spain | 2002 | Bilateral agreement on active recruitment of Spanish nurses and cross-border cooperation | 770 Spanish nurses recruited between 2002 and 2004 |
| France–Morocco | | *Conventions d'établissements* providing for recognition of qualifications | |
| France–Tunisia | | *Conventions d'établissements* providing for recognition of qualifications | |
| France–Central African Republic, Chad, Democratic Republic of Congo, Gabon, Mali, Togo | | State agreements ensuring that medical doctors from the countries listed can practise in France if they have a French medical degree or other titles mentioned in the Code de la santé publique | |
| Spain–Philippines | 2006 | Bilateral agreement on active recruitment of Filipino health workers | Allowed entry of up to 100 000 Filipino health workers into Spain |
| Belgium–South Africa | 1965 | Bilateral agreement on recognition of qualifications to facilitate mobility | |

**Table 12A.1** contd

| Countries | Date of signature/ current status | Type and focus | Migration flows |
|---|---|---|---|
| Former Yugoslavia–the former USSR | | Agreement ensures automatic recognition of the degrees of all graduates who graduated before 25 June 1991 | |
| Spain–Colombia | | Bilateral agreement on migration and human capacity development | |
| Spain–Morocco | | Bilateral agreement on migration and human capacity development | |
| United Kingdom–South Africa | 2003/ prolonged until 2013 | Memorandum of understanding on international development and sharing of expertise; time-limited placements of health professionals | Pilot cohort of 18 South African nurses recruited to work in London in an NHS Trust for two years; all nurses returned to South Africa when their employment contracts expired; 70 British health professionals practised in South Africa in 2003–2004; a further 259 British placements were organized in South Africa in 2004–2005 |
| France–Benin | | Focus on international development and support for human resources for health development | |
| France–Senegal | 2006 | Focus on international development and support for human resources for health development | |
| Austria–the Czech Republic–Slovakia–Hungary | 2004/ expired | Healthregio project; optimization of health care provision in border region, facilitating mobility of health professionals, education and skills development | |
| France–Monaco | 1938 | *Accord de réciprocité* facilitating the establishment of medical doctors on the other side of the border | Currently 14 French and Monegasque doctors take part in the agreement |
| France–Switzerland | | *Convention médicale transfrontalière* facilitating the establishment of medical doctors on the other side of the border | |

| | | |
|---|---|---|
| Austria–Italy | 1987 | Collaboration between the medical chambers of South Tyrol in Italy and Tyrol in Austria |
| Italy–Romania | 2002 | Focus on recruitment and educational support in bilateral programmes between regions and nursing institutes: Padua–Bucharest, Pitesti Cluj–Parma Province, Veneto Region–Timis County | Romania is the most important source country for nurses in Italy (8 497 nurses; 25% of foreign-registered nurses); as part of the Cluj–Parma nurse-training cooperation, 26 nurses moved to Italy in 2005 and about 40 in 2006 |
| Belgium–Romania | 1990 | Agreement between the Catholic University of Louvain in Belgium ((UCL) and the University of Medicine and Pharmacy (UMF) in Romania allowing Romanian medical students in third or fourth years to spend one year (potentially extendable to two years) of their specialization in one of UCL's hospitals | By 2009, some 450 Romanian students had taken part in the programme |
| France–Poland | 2004 | Agreement between Lille Regional University Hospital and a hospital in Poland | Facilitated the temporary recruitment of 20 Polish nurses in 2004 |
| Turkey–Turkic Republics | 1992–1993 | The Great Student Project aimed to enhance the relationship to the Turkic Republics, Turks and relative communities and help them to meet their educated workforce needs by providing scholarships to students from these countries | As of 9 September 2009, the Project had enabled a total of 5347 students to study in Turkey |

Sources: OECD, 2004, 2008; Dumont & Zurn, 2007; Dhillon, Clark & Kapp, 2010; Aspen Institute, 2011; Wismar et al., 2011; International Organization for Migration, 2005.

Notes: NHS, National Health Service; NMC, Nursing and Midwifery Council; ªEstimation based on the UK Nursing and Midwifery Council (NMC) registration records. However, there is no precise information and/or distinction between the recruitment through bilateral agreements and other channels such as private recruitment agencies. The statistics provided in the NMC reports cover the year from March to April next year.

## References

Albreht T (2011). Addressing shortages: Slovenia's reliance on foreign health professionals, current developments and policy responses. In Wismar M et al., eds. *Health professional mobility and health systems. Evidence from 17 European countries.* Copenhagen, WHO Regional Office for Europe on behalf of the European Observatory on Health Systems and Policies:511–537.

Alliance for Ethical International Recruitment Practices (2013). [web site]. Washington, DC, Alliance for Ethical International Recruitment Practices (http://http://www.fairinternationalrecruitment.org/, accessed 10 January 2014).

Aspen Institute (2011). *Databank of bilateral agreements.* (http://www.aspeninstitute.org/policy-work/global-health-development/news/hwmi-databank-bilateral-agreements, accessed 3 January 2014).

Beňušová K et al. (2011). Regaining self-sufficiency: Slovakia and the challenges of health professionals leaving the country. In Wismar M et al., eds. *Health professional mobility and health systems. Evidence from 17 European countries.* Copenhagen, WHO Regional Office for Europe on behalf of the European Observatory on Health Systems and Policies:479–510.

Bertinato L et al. (2011). Oversupplying doctors but seeking carers: Italy's demographic challenges and health professional mobility. In Wismar M et al., eds. *Health professional mobility and health systems. Evidence from 17 European countries.* Copenhagen, WHO Regional Office for Europe on behalf of the European Observatory on Health Systems and Policies:243–262.

Buchan J (2008). *How can the migration of health service professionals be managed so as to reduce any negative effects on supply?* Copenhagen, WHO Regional Office for Europe on behalf of the European Observatory on Health Systems and Policies (HEN–OBS Joint Policy Brief No. 7).

Buchan J, Seccombe I (2013). The end of growth? Analysing NHS nurse staff. *Journal of Advanced Nursing,* 69(9):2123–2130.

Buchan J et al. (2009). Does a code make a difference: assessing the English code of practice on international recruitment. *Human Resources for Health,* 7:33.

Chaloff J (2008). *Mismatches in the formal sector, expansion of the informal sector: immigration of health professionals to Italy.* Paris, Organisation for Economic Co-operation and Development (Health Working Paper No. 34).

Delamaire ML, Schweyer FX (2011). Nationally moderate, locally significant: France and health professional mobility from far and near. In Wismar M et al., eds. *Health professional mobility and health systems. Evidence from 17 European countries.* Copenhagen, WHO Regional Office for Europe on behalf of the European Observatory on Health Systems and Policies:181–210.

Deutscher Bundestag (2012). *Antwort der Bundesregierung auf die Kleine Anfrage der Abgeordneten Dr. Marlies Volkmer, Karin Roth (Esslingen), Mechthild Rawert, weiterer Abgeordneter und der Fraktion der SPD – Drucksache 17/9208 – Umsetzung des globalen Verhaltenskodex der Weltgesundheitsorganisation für die grenzüberschreitende Anwerbung von Gesundheitsfachkräften durch die Bundesregierung [Reply of the Federal Government to the minor members of parliament Dr. Marlies Volkmer, Karin Roth Esslingen), Mechthild Rawert, other MPs and the parliamentary group of the SPD – Printed Matter 17/9208 – Implementation of the global code of the World Health Organization for cross-border recruitment of health professionals by the Federal government].* Berlin, Deutscher Bundestag (http://dipbt.bundestag.de/dip21/btd/17/093/1709314.pdf, accessed 10 January 2014).

Deutscher Bundestag (2013). *Antwort der Bundesregierung auf die Kleine Anfrage der Abgeordneten Niema Movassat, Annette Groth, Heike Hänsel, weiterer Abgeordneter und der Fraktion DIE LINKE – Drucksache 17/14579 – Abwerbung von Fachkräften aus den Ländern des Südens im Pflege- und Gesundheitsbereich [Reply of the Federal Government to the minor deputies Niema Movassat, Annette Groth, Heike Hänsel, other MPs and DIE LINKE – Printed matter 17/14579 – Brain drain from the countries of the South in the care and health sector].* Berlin, Deutscher Bundestag (http://dip21.bundestag.de/dip21/btd/17/147/1714716.pdf, accessed 10 January 2014).

Dhillon IS, Clark ME, Kapp RH (2010). *Innovations in cooperation: a guidebook on bilateral agreements to address health worker migration.* Washington, DC, Aspen Institute. (http://aspeninstitute.org/sites/default/files/content/docs/pubs/Bilateral%20Report_final%20code.pdf, accessed 10 January 2014).

Dumont JC, Zurn P (2007). Immigrant health workers in OECD countries in the broader context of highly skilled migration. In OECD, ed. *International migration outlook,* 2nd edn. Paris, Organisation for Economic Co-operation and Development:161–228.

Eke E, Girasek E, Szócska M (2011). From melting pot to laboratory of change in central Europe: Hungary and health workforce migration. In Wismar M et al., eds. *Health professional mobility and health systems. Evidence from 17 European countries.* Copenhagen, WHO Regional Office for Europe on behalf of the European Observatory on Health Systems and Policies:365–394.

Galan A, Olsavszky V, Vladescu C (2011). Emergent challenge of health professional emigration: Romania's accession to the EU. In Wismar M et al., eds. *Health professional mobility and health systems. Evidence from 17 European countries.* Copenhagen, WHO Regional Office for Europe on behalf of the European Observatory on Health Systems and Policies:449–478.

German Ministry of Economics and Technology (2013). *Pflegekräfte aus Drittstaaten gewinnen [Attract nurses from third countries].* Berlin, Bundesministeriums für Wirtschaft und Technologie (http://www.fachkraefte-offensive.de/DE/Service/Meldungen/2013/bmwi-studie-2013-01-03.html, accessed 10 January 2014).

Healthregio (2004). *Abstract.* Vienna, Healthregio (http://www.healthregio.net/healthregio.htm, accessed 10 January 2014).

International Organization for Migration (2005). *Monitoring of the pilot project Polish nurses in the Netherlands; development of competencies.* The Hague, International Organization for Migration (Final report to the Ministry of Health Care of the Netherlands).

Jekić IM, Katrava A, Vučković-Krčmar M (2011). Geopolitics, economic downturn and oversupply of medical doctors: Serbia's emigrating health professionals. In Wismar M et al., eds. *Health professional mobility and health systems. Evidence from 17 European countries.* Copenhagen, WHO Regional Office for Europe on behalf of the European Observatory on Health Systems and Policies:541–568.

Joint Action Health Workforce Planning and Forecasting (2013). [web site]. Brussels, Joint Action Health Workforce Planning & Forecasting (http://euhwforce.weebly.com/, accessed 10 January 2014).

Kautsch M, Czabanowska K (2011). When the grass gets greener at home: Poland's changing incentives for health professional mobility. In Wismar M et al., eds. *Health professional mobility and health systems. Evidence from 17 European countries.* Copenhagen, WHO Regional Office for Europe on behalf of the European Observatory on Health Systems and Policies:419–448.

Kuusio H et al. (2011). Changing context and priorities in recruitment and employment: Finland balances inflows and outflows of health professionals. In Wismar M et al., eds. *Health professional mobility and health systems. Evidence from 17 European countries.* Copenhagen, WHO Regional Office for Europe on behalf of the European Observatory on Health Systems and Policies:163–180.

Little L, Buchan J (2007). *Nursing self sufficiency/sustainability in the global context.* Geneva, International Centre for Human Resources in Nursing (http://www.icn.ch/images/stories/documents/pillars/sew/ICHRN/Policy_and_Research_Papers/Nursing_Self_Sufficiency.Sustainability_in_the_Global_Context.pdf, accessed 3 January 2014).

NHS Employers (2008). *The points-based system: how the immigration overhaul affects NHS recruitment.* Leeds, NHS Employers (Briefing 55) (http://www.nhsemployers.org/Aboutus/Publications/Documents/The%20points-based%20system.pdf, accessed 10 January 2014).

OECD (2004). *Migration for employment: bilateral agreements at a crossroads.* Paris, Organisation for Economic Co-operation and Development.

OECD (2008). *The looming crisis of the health workforce: how can OECD countries respond?* Paris, Organisation for Economic Co-operation and Development.

Offermanns G, Malle EM, Jusic M (2011). Mobility, language and neighbours: Austria as source and destination country. In Wismar M et al., eds. *Health professional mobility and health systems. Evidence from 17 European countries.* Copenhagen, WHO Regional Office for Europe on behalf of the European Observatory on Health Systems and Policies:89–128.

Ognyanova D, Busse R (2011). A destination and a source: Germany manages regional health workforce disparities with foreign medical doctors. In Wismar M et al., eds. *Health professional mobility and health systems. Evidence from 17 European countries.* Copenhagen, WHO Regional Office for Europe on behalf of the European Observatory on Health Systems and Policies:211–242.

Padaiga Ž, Pukas M, Starkienė L (2011). Awareness, planning and retention: Lithuania's approach to managing health professional mobility. In Wismar M et al., eds. *Health professional mobility and health systems. Evidence from 17 European countries.* Copenhagen, WHO Regional Office for Europe on behalf of the European Observatory on Health Systems and Policies:395–418.

Saar P, Habicht J (2011). Migration and attrition: Estonia's health sector and cross-border mobility to its northern neighbour. In Wismar M et al., eds. *Health professional mobility and health systems. Evidence from 17 European countries.* Copenhagen, WHO Regional Office for Europe on behalf of the European Observatory on Health Systems and Policies:339–364.

Safuta A, Baeten R (2011). Of permeable borders: Belgium as both source and host country. In Wismar M et al., eds. *Health professional mobility and health systems. Evidence from 17 European countries.* Copenhagen, WHO Regional Office for Europe on behalf of the European Observatory on Health Systems and Policies:129–162.

Sanicademia (2011). *Crossborder health education.* Villach, Sanicademia (http://www.sanicademia.at/index.php?view=article&catid=77&id=68&lang=de, accessed 10 January 2014).

Sloan J (2005). *NHS links: a new approach to international health links.* BMJ Careers, 19 February (http://careers.bmj.com/careers/advice/view-article. html?id=680, accessed 10 January 2014).

WHO (2006). *Working together for health: world health report 2006.* Geneva, World Health Organization.

WHO (2010a). *Increasing access to health workers in remote and rural areas through improved retention: global policy recommendations.* Geneva, World Health Organization (http://whqlibdoc.who.int/publications/2010/9789241564014_ eng.pdf, accessed 10 January 2014).

WHO (2010b). *WHO global code of practice on the international recruitment of health personnel.* Geneva, World Health Organization (Sixty-third World Health Assembly, WHA63.16) (http://www.who.int/hrh/migration/code/ WHO_global_code_of_practice_EN.pdf, accessed 1 October 2013).

WHO Regional Office for Europe (2011). *Technical meeting on health workforce retention in countries of the South-eastern Europe Health Network, Bucharest, 28– 29 March.* Copenhagen, WHO Regional Office for Europe (http://www.euro. who.int/__data/assets/pdf_file/0018/152271/e95775.pdf, accessed 10 January 2014).

Wiskow C, ed. (2006). *Health worker migration flows in Europe: overview and case studies in selected CEE countries: Romania, Czech Republic, Serbia and Croatia.* Geneva, International Labour Organization (Working Paper 245) (http://www.ilo.org/wcmsp5/groups/public/---ed_dialogue/---sector/ documents/publication/wcms_161162.pdf, accessed 14 December 2013).

Wismar M et al., eds. (2011). *Health professional mobility and health systems. Evidence from 17 European countries.* Copenhagen, WHO Regional Office for Europe on behalf of the European Observatory on Health Systems and Policies.

Yıldırım HH, Kaya S (2011). At the crossroads: Turkey's domestic workforce and restrictive labour laws in the light of EU candidacy. In Wismar M et al., eds. *Health professional mobility and health systems. Evidence from 17 European countries.* Copenhagen, WHO Regional Office for Europe on behalf of the European Observatory on Health Systems and Policies:569–597.

Young R (2011). A major destination country: the United Kingdom and its changing recruitment policies. In Wismar M et al., eds. *Health professional mobility and health systems. Evidence from 17 European countries.* Copenhagen, WHO Regional Office for Europe on behalf of the European Observatory on Health Systems and Policies:295–335.

Young R et al. (2008). *International recruitment into the NHS: evaluation of initiatives for hospital doctors, general practitioners, nurses, midwives and allied health professionals.* London, Florence Nightingale School of Nursing and Midwifery, King's College London, with Open University Centre for Education in Medicine, Manchester Business School and NPCRDC, University of Manchester (Report submitted to the Department of Health).

# Chapter 13

# Policy responses facilitating mobility or mitigating its negative effects: national, EU and international instruments

*Sherry Merkur*

## 13.1 Introduction

When considering health professional mobility, the international and European landscape must be considered alongside national policies and guidance. Two types of instrument will be identified and discussed in this chapter: (1) tools which aim at mitigating potential negative effects of migration in sending countries, which are non-binding; and (2) instruments which aim at facilitating mobility/migration and are binding. The former includes codes of practice, guidance and policy statements related to the ethical recruitment of health professionals, which started to emerge at the national level around 2000 and have also been produced by professional bodies and other institutions. Since then, some countries have provided guidance to their national health system and health employers. On the supranational level, the European Health Policy Forum (2003) recommendations on the mobility of health professionals, the European Commission's Green Paper on the European Workforce for Health (European Commission, 2008b) and the *WHO Global Code of Practice on the International Recruitment of Health Personnel* (WHO, 2010a) have taken discussions on ethical recruitment to an international audience. The second group, tools that facilitate mobility and migration, includes EU legislation and GATS (WHO, 1995), which allows for a freer flow of service workers (mode 4) and has the potential to be used for health care professionals. Within the European Single Market, health professionals have the freedom to move and to provide services in another Member State. The Directive on the recognition of professional qualifications has been undergoing modernization since 2011 (European Commission, 2011b), and the various stakeholders have different perspectives on the proposed changes.

This chapter is intended to provide a detailed exposition of the evolution of national and international instruments that relate in different ways to the mobility of health professionals. The focus is mainly on EU Member States for the national instruments, but organizations around the world are included under the international instruments presented in Table 13.1.

The material for this chapter was compiled using searches of the literature. Articles needed to have been written in the English language and relate to health professional mobility, international ethical recruitment, and instruments, codes of practice, guidance or policy statements. Preference was given to peer-reviewed articles in well-respected journals, although literature and web sites from relevant professional bodies, associations, organizations and ministries (the "grey literature") were also considered. The main limitation of this chapter could be that sources in languages other than English were not considered.

The first section maps national codes and global instruments that aim at mitigating the potential negative effects of migration in vulnerable countries. Following this, the tools that focus on facilitating the mobility of health professionals are presented: the relevance of GATS to health services and personnel, and the importance of the recognition of professional qualifications in the EU to support mobility.

## 13.2 Ethical international recruitment: mapping national codes and global instruments

Recently, many developed countries, including some in Europe, have been undertaking large-scale, targeted international recruitment efforts to address domestic shortages. Although working abroad can benefit recruited health care professionals in terms of enhancing professional experience and a chance to increase their quality of life, concerns related to the impact upon the health systems of developing countries also need to be addressed. Emigration is thought to be one cause of skills shortages in developing nations, the "brain drain" (Wiskow, 2006; Robinson, 2007). This phenomenon has led to calls to protect developing countries' health systems from losing their skilled health personnel.

**Table 13.1** Selected European and international instruments for ethical recruitment, presented chronologically

| Instrument | Aim | Organization | Date Adopted | Type |
|---|---|---|---|---|
| International Council of Nurses (2007): *Position Statement: Ethical Nurse Recruitment* | Call for a regulated recruitment process based on ethical principles that guide informed decision-making and reinforce sound employment policies on the part of governments, employers and nurses, thus supporting fair and cost-effective recruitment and retention practices | The International Council of Nurses represents more than 130 national nurses associations | 2001, revised and reaffirmed in 2007 | Position statement |
| World Organisation for Family Doctors (2002): *A Code of Practice for the International Recruitment of Health Care Professionals (Melbourne Manifesto)* | To promote the best possible standards of health care around the world; to encourage rational workforce planning by all countries in order to meet their own needs; to discourage activities which could harm any country's health care system | The World Organisation for Family Doctors has 120 member organizations (national colleges, academies or organizations concerned with the academic aspects of general family practice) in 99 countries | May 2002 | Code |
| Commonwealth Secretariat (2003): *Commonwealth Code of Practice for the International Recruitment of Health Workers* | To discourage the targeted recruitment of health workers from countries that are themselves experiencing shortages; to safeguard the rights of recruits and the conditions relating to their profession in the recruiting countries | Adopted by the Commonwealth Health Ministers, representing 54 countries | May 2003 | Code |
| World Medical Association (2003): *Statement on Ethical Guidelines for the International Recruitment of Physicians* | Calls for every country to do its utmost to educate an adequate number of physicians taking into account its needs and resources; a country should not rely on immigration from other countries to meet its need for physicians | World Medical Association represents physicians; members include 95 national medical associations | September 2003 | Position statement |
| European Federation of Nurses Associations (2004): *Practice Guidance for International Nurse Recruitment* | Sets out the key considerations for ensuring both ethical recruitment and employment of internationally recruited nurses in Europe (based on the Royal College of Nurses *Good Practice Guidance*) | The European Federation of Nurses Associations represents more than 1 million European nurses | May 2004 | Guidance |

**Table 13.1** contd

| Instrument | Aim | Organization | Date Adopted | Type |
|---|---|---|---|---|
| World Federation of Public Health Associations (2005): *Ethical Restrictions on International Recruitment of Health Professionals from Low-income Countries* | Recommends health employers voluntarily adopt a code of ethics to judiciously manage the employment of health professionals from abroad, including not recruiting from developing countries (based on the United Kingdom's list of countries) unless a bilateral agreement is in place; governments should take an active lead by clearly requiring all public health services to adopt the code of ethics | The World Federation of Public Health Associations has 70 members including national and regional public health associations and regional associations of schools of public health | May 2005 | Code |
| International Labour Organization (2006): *Action Programme on the International Migration of Health Service Workers: The Supply Side* | Presents the ceding nation's perspective on the management of health services migration that could be shared with other supplying countries | The International Labour Organization (ILO) is a United Nations tripartite agency with government, employer and worker representatives and 185 Member States | 2006 | Action programme |
| World Dental Federation (2006): *Ethical Recruitment of Oral Health Professionals* | Calls on national dental associations to collaborate with governments to ensure that an adequate number of dentists are educated and licensed to practise; promote policies and strategies that enhance effective retention of dentists in their countries; promote strategies with partners to lessen the adverse effects of emigration; and encourage their governments to provide employment rights and protections equivalent to other oral health professionals in their countries | World Dental Federation represents more than 200 member national dental associations and specialist groups, covering more than 1 million dentists worldwide | September 2006 | Policy statement |
| European Commission (2006): *Programme for Action (PfA) to Tackle the Shortage of Health Workers in Developing Countries 2007–2013* | To protect against health personnel shortages in non-EU countries | Economic and political partnership between 27 Member States | December 2006 | Action programme |

| | | | | |
|---|---|---|---|---|
| EPSU–HOSPEEM (2008): Code of Conduct and Follow up on Ethical Cross-border Recruitment and Retention in the Hospital Sector | To establish in the European hospital sector social dialogue a full commitment to promote ethical recruitment practices at European, national, regional and local level; fully implemented in EU Member States by April 2011 | European Federation of Public Service Unions (EPSU) includes 8 million public service workers from over 250 trade unions and the European hospital and health care employers' association (HOSPEEM) | April 2008 | Code |
| WHO (2010a): Global Code of Practice on the International Recruitment of Health Personnel | To establish and promote voluntary principles and practices for the ethical international recruitment of health personnel; to serve as a reference for Member States; to provide guidance for the formulation and implementation of bilateral agreements and legal instruments; to facilitate and promote international discussion and advance cooperation | WHO is the directing and coordinating authority for health within the United Nations and is made up of 194 Member States; its decision-making body is the World Health Assembly | May 2010 | Code |

Since 1999, codes of practice and other instruments for ethical international recruitment have been produced by countries, international organizations and professional associations with the aim to reduce the negative impact of health professional mobility on vulnerable health systems in developing countries. Codes may be directed at a particular health professional (e.g. nurses) or at the spectrum of health personnel and can have multiple aims, such as protecting specific countries from aggressive recruitment of their health personnel, ensuring that professionals are properly prepared for the job (e.g. participate in supervised practice) and protecting professionals from dishonest employers.

This section explores the codes, guidance and policy statements at the national, European and international level.

### 13.2.1 National codes of practice, guidance and policy statements

On the national level, some European countries have introduced codes of practice and other instruments to discourage the active recruitment of health personnel from developing countries and to promote recruitment via bilateral agreements. Examples are in place in England, Scotland and Ireland, while the Netherlands and Norway provide a clear policy stance.

The Department of Health in England was the first organization to produce an international recruitment guidance; this covered the NHS and was based on ethical principles, including being sensitive to local health care needs abroad. It was also the first to develop a robust code of practice for international recruitment (1999).[1] In its 1999 code on nursing recruitment (Department of Health, 1999), NHS employers were instructed to ensure that they did not actively recruit nurses and midwives from developing countries who were experiencing nursing shortages, in particular from South Africa or the West Indies. In 2001, the Department of Health widened the scope to discourage the recruitment of all health personnel from developing countries unless there was a formal agreement between the Department of Health and the country in question.

The Department of Health published the revised *Code of Practice for the International Recruitment of Healthcare Professionals* (Department of Health, 2004) to promote high standards of practice in the ethical international recruitment of health care professionals. It covered a wide range of health personnel including medical staff, nurses, dentists, radiographers, physiotherapists, occupational therapists and all other allied health professionals. The Department of Health also identified a list of developing countries from which health professional recruitment should be restricted (Box 13.1) (NHS

---

1 Earlier guidance was produced on the immigration and employment of overseas medical and dental students, doctors and dentists (Department of Health, 1998), recruiting overseas physiotherapists (Chartered Society of Physiotherapy, 1998) and international nursing recruitment (Department of Health, 1999).

---

**Box 13.1** *Developing countries restricted for recruitment of health professionals*

In 2004, the English Department of Health identified 153 countries for restricted recruitment (Department of Health, 2004). Since then, a few countries have asked to be removed from the list, including all Indian states (except the four that receive aid from the Department for International Development), China (except in small rural areas), Pakistan (for a period of time) and the Philippines (except the United Kingdom can recruit registered nurses and other health care professionals that are regulated by appropriate professional bodies in both countries, e.g. physiotherapists, radiographers, occupational therapists, biomedical scientists).

This list is dynamic such that NHS Employers have been charged with reviewing and updating the list over time (NHS Employers, 2013).

---

Employers, 2013). This edition further applies to recruitment through agencies of temporary/locum health care professionals as well as permanent staff and also applies to all health care organizations, including the independent sector.

Compliance with the Code was required if recruitment agencies were to act on behalf of the NHS, and recruitment agencies were given one year to comply. A review of the new Code was planned for June 2011, but no additional information on this process was available at the time of writing. The NHS Employers web site (2013) provides information on organizations that comply with the Code. Additionally, the Department of Health provides further guidance on its web site and has also adopted a related code of practice for the supply of temporary staff (Department of Health, 2013a, b).

The Scottish Executive introduced a *Code of Practice for the International Recruitment of Healthcare Professionals in Scotland* in March 2006. The Code endeavours to guide Scottish health care organizations and recruitment agencies in ethical international recruitment practices; raise awareness of health worker migration and to mitigate the adverse effects; and set benchmarks to support the international health care professional by recommending robust induction procedures, mentoring support and provision of professional programmes (Scottish Executive, 2006). Furthermore, NHS Employers has a partnership agreement with the Scottish Executive to monitor arrangements for the Code of Practice.

Other countries, as discussed below, implement guidance rather than a formal code. For example, in Ireland, the Department of Health and Children recommended in 2001 that Irish employers only actively recruit (nurses and midwives) in countries where the national government supports the process (Department of Health and Children of Ireland, 2001).

The Netherlands' Ministry of Health, Welfare and Sport produced an action plan in 2007 called *Working on Care*. The plan stated that the recruitment of health workers from outside the EU should be a last resort and only undertaken when all institutions have extensively tried the other solutions nationally, such as retaining and training. The Ministry encourages employers to establish a code of conduct and not proactively recruit health workers from developing countries or from countries with their own health worker shortages.

In 2007, Norway developed a framework on global solidarity, where it pledged to refrain from recruiting health workers from developing countries (Norwegian Directorate of Health, 2007). Actions were proposed for three areas: balancing domestic capacity, targeting development assistance at measures to increase receiving countries' capacity for training and retention, and creating both national and international guidelines with mechanisms for compensation.

### 13.2.2 European and international instruments

Other efforts towards the international ethical recruitment of health professionals include initiatives taken by the EU and WHO. Additional instruments, including codes, guidance, policy statements, position statements and action programmes, by other organizations are listed in Table 13.1. Since 2000, there has been a surge of these instruments, which signals increased awareness about ethical considerations when recruiting health professionals from abroad. Professional bodies, including those representing family doctors, nurses, dentists and health workers, have all produced guidance, which principally cover three areas: (1) to limit the recruitment of health professionals from countries which are at risk of (or are already) experiencing a shortage; (2) to promote good recruitment and retention practices in these countries; and (3) to encourage rational workforce planning. There is great diversity in the signatories, such as trade unions, professional organizations and countries themselves (Table 13.1).

### *EU*

The EU has recognized its responsibility to protect some non-EU countries from worsening health personnel shortages in several initiatives. In December 2005, it adopted the *Strategy for Action on the Crisis in Human Resources for Health in Developing Countries* (European Commission, 2005b), and in 2006, the *Programme for Action to Tackle the Shortage of Health Workers in Developing Countries (2007–2013)* (European Commission, 2006). Furthermore, the European Commission's vision for a common immigration policy presents approaches to avoid undermining development prospects of third countries by instead promoting circular migration (European Commission, 2008a).

Circular migration is defined as when a health worker moves to another country to obtain training or gain experience and then returns to their home country with improved knowledge and skills; however, the benefits of circular migration continue to be debated in the literature (Agunias & Newland, 2007). Following this, the 2008 *Green Paper on the European Workforce for Health* (European Commission, 2008b) trialled the possibility of a more broad-reaching EU-level code, but the European Commission has indicated that it will put this on hold until the *WHO Global Code of Practice* is assessed.

Specifically for the hospital sector, the agreement in 2008 between EPSU and HOSPEEM included a code of conduct and follow-up on ethical cross-border recruitment and retention (EPSU–HOSPEEM, 2008).

### *WHO Global Code of Practice*

A resolution to adopt the voluntary *WHO Global Code of Practice on the International Recruitment of Health Personnel* was unanimously passed in May 2010 at the 63rd World Health Assembly (WHO, 2010b). The *Global Code of Practice* applies to all health personnel and to all WHO Member States.[2] It discourages countries from actively recruiting from poor nations facing critical staff shortages and also calls for countries that recruit staff from poorer countries to provide technical assistance, support and training of health professionals in those countries, although there is no explicit mention of financial compensation.

The Code builds on existing regional and bilateral agreements, memoranda of understanding and national and regional codes of practice, the collaborative work of many stakeholders, a public hearing and input from the WHO Executive Board. Intense negotiations in the Assembly included strong inputs from countries with both positive and negative net migration of health professionals, including Botswana, Brazil, Kenya, Norway, the Philippines, South Africa, the United Kingdom and Zambia as well as the EU (Zarocostas, 2010).

The *Global Code of Practice* is based on 10 articles that outline a range of issues, including guiding principles (article 2), health workforce development and health systems sustainability (article 5) and implementation of the Code (article 8). Emphasis is placed on the need for Member States to build on bilateral agreements and improve their workforce planning and retention of staff, with the aim of achieving a sustainable workforce. The key argument in the *Global Code of Practice* is that there is a need for Member States, where they are able, to take more responsibility for planning and meeting their staffing requirements from their own resources (WHO, 2011).

---

2 In 1981, the World Health Assembly voted to adopt the WHO's only other voluntary code of ethical practice, the Code of Marketing of Breast-milk Substitutes.

Although the Code is voluntary, WHO Member States are asked to periodically report on measures, results, difficulties, lessons and data on the international migration of health workers (see Chapter 5). The first report on the *Global Code of Practice* to the World Health Assembly was planned for 2013, with further reports produced every three years (WHO, 2010a).

## 13.3 Instruments facilitating the international free movement of health professionals

### 13.3.1 GATS

GATS is a treaty of the World Trade Organization that was created to extend the multilateral trading system to the service sectors. The General Agreement on Tariffs and Trade (GATT) provides such a system for merchandise trade. Before the World Trade Organization's Uruguay Round negotiations began in 1986, public services such as health care, postal services and education were not included in international trade agreements. As a result of the Uruguay Round negotiations, GATS entered into force in January 1995.

GATS may relate to health through its four modes of liberalization of trade in services.

1. Cross-border delivery of services: e-health (Oh et al., 2005).

2. Consumption of services abroad: health tourism.

3. Commercial presence: foreign direct investment in hospitals, clinics, insurance or contracts for such facilities, which can be a joint venture between foreign and domestic partners (Smith, 2004).

4. The presence of natural persons, as in the temporary movement of health professionals from one country to another.

GATS mode 4 deals with the movement of natural persons who supply services in the territories of other World Trade Organization members. Proponents of GATS argue that the Agreement has the potential to liberalize the temporary movement of people between countries, enhancing skilled people's knowledge and competence as well as raising their earnings. The GATS process claims to be one of "brain circulation" not "brain drain". However, an opposing view, specifically for public services, considers that professionals will move from vulnerable countries to richer countries, thus increasing the brain drain, even though GATS only applies to those working on a temporary basis. Also, through increased efforts towards privatization, governments could lose their ability to manage some public services. Opponents of GATS argue that it has the potential to push the privatization of services that are currently provided by governments and minimize the ability for state regulation of health services (WHO, 1995).

There is little evidence of the effects of the Agreement on the movement of health workers (WHO, 2006). Smith, Chanda and Tangcharoensathien (2009) have emphasized the need for those engaged in the stewardship of a domestic health system to have an advanced understanding of how trade in health services affects a country's health system and policy, both now and in the future. Although mode 4 can relate to health professional mobility directly, the effects of European legislative frameworks are considered more important in the context of EU Member States.

### 13.3.2 The recognition of professional qualifications in the EU

In the EU, the mutual recognition of diplomas, certificates and other evidence of formal qualifications exists in order to assist the free movement of professionals throughout the EU. This upholds one of the fundamental freedoms of the single market – the right of EU citizens to establish themselves and to provide services anywhere in the EU.

Directive 2005/36/EC on the recognition of professional qualifications (European Commission, 2005a) facilitates the mutual recognition of professional qualifications and enables the free movement of health care professionals across the EEA. The intention is to make it easier for qualified professionals to practise their professions in European countries other than their own with a minimum of bureaucracy but with appropriate safeguards for public health and safety and consumer protection. The Directive was adopted on 7 September 2005 and was meant to be transposed into domestic law by Member States by October 2007; however, it was not until September 2010 that all 27 Member States had complied with the Directive (European Commission, 2010).

According to the Directive, individuals must submit an application along with documents and certificates to the competent authority in the host Member State. The authority then has one month to acknowledge receipt of the application and flag up any missing documents, and it must make a decision within three months after the full application has been received. Individuals are then entitled to use the professional title from the host Member State. However, if a profession is regulated in the host Member State by an association or organization, the individual has to register with or be approved by the professional regulator, council or chamber. For doctors, this means registering with, for example, the General Medical Council in the United Kingdom, Bundesärztekammer (the German Medical Association) in Germany, or Conseil National de l'Ordre des Médecins (the French Order of Doctors) in France.

The Directive provides for the harmonization of minimum training requirements and the automatic recognition of professional qualifications. Specifically for health professionals in the EU, Directive 2005/36/EC considered the so-called "sectoral" directives, which covered doctors, general nurses, midwives, veterinary surgeons, dental surgeons and pharmacists up until transposition.[3] However, the 2005 Directive went further to specify both the minimum number of years and the minimum number of hours for training doctors and general care nurses (the sectoral directives only specified the former).

Regarding transposition for the EU12, differences in training requirements have been largely compensated by recent professional experience – the acquired rights regime. Also, bridging programmes have been in place to upgrade qualifications, specifically for nurses and midwives who qualified in Poland prior to accession.

### *The revision process for Directive 2005/36/EC on professional qualifications*

At the time of writing, Directive 2005/36/EC was under review by the EU legislators with a view to modernization (European Commission, 2011a). In March 2010, the European Commission initiated an evaluation process to review the Directive. Following a first report on national implementation (European Commission, 2010), the Commission launched a consultation process from January to March 2011 to gather suggestions for amendments to the Directive. Some 400 responses from competent authorities, professional associations (for medical doctors, nurses, pharmacists, dentists, etc.), the public and other stakeholder groups were collected. In June 2011, the Commission published its Green Paper on modernizing the Professional Qualifications Directive, followed by a legislative proposal at the end of 2011 (European Commission, 2011b).

From the Commission side, the proposed changes to the Directive as presented in the June 2011 Green Paper included the introduction of a European Professional Card, improved communication between Member States regarding information held on professionals, and modernizing automatic recognition. The underlying principle of all these changes is to make recognition of qualifications easier in order to make working in another Member State simpler and faster (European Commission, 2011b).

During the consultation, even between the different professional groups, similar challenges and potential benefits have emerged in several areas, including outdated standards for training, the lack of exchange of information between Member States on fitness to practise, the recognized potential of the Internal

---

3 Directive 2005/36/EC abrogated previous sectoral directives relating to the recognition of diplomas for the purposes of establishment from 20 October 2007.

Market Information system to facilitate information sharing between Member States; support for the assessment of CPD across the EU; and consideration of the language skills of health professionals crossing borders (Goodard, 2011).

Much of the discussion for doctors has focused on the need to move forward from simply acknowledging the length of professional training and rather to focus on competencies stemming from experience and ongoing professional development. Despite this apparently positive step, challenges remain with the Green Paper's proposals on key issues. First, the expertise of, and reliance on, "National Contact Points" for each Member State (who are meant to serve as a central point of access, and provide advice and individual assistance for professionals) is uncertain given the wide diversity of medical specialties. Next, although the need to demonstrate CPD in the home country is proposed, there remains huge diversity of requirements in different EU Member States (Merkur et al., 2008). Furthermore, some doctors have argued that rather than developing a new European Professional Card or similar system, thus increasing bureaucracy, the Internal Market Information system could be used to improve communication, such as providing alerts regarding individual doctors (Goodard, 2011).

For nurses, who are the single largest professional group affected by Directive 2005/36/EC, some wide-reaching positive effects have been observed since transposition, including extending the years of education for girls and women, with positive societal effects; providing an impetus to establish regulatory functions and authorities where they were previously lacking; and protecting the professional title of nurse. Nevertheless, concerns have been raised about the proposed increased reliance on, and competency of, the variety of regulators for nurses as well as acknowledging the importance of retaining and potentially updating the minimum content of nurse education and training (the Annex) particularly for the newer Member States (Keighley & Williams, 2011). For nurses and midwives, the Commission has proposed an increase to the minimum duration of general education from 10 to 12 school years, and the minimum training required remains set at three years.

From the perspective of the regulators and competent authorities, some specific challenges have been identified concerning the need to strike the necessary balance between protecting the public by ensuring professionals are appropriately fit to practise while being required to accept a professional's qualifications without being able to check their education, training, practical experience or language skills (Dickson, 2011). On the latter point, the General Medical Council in the United Kingdom has expressed concern as under Directive 2005/36/EC it is prevented from testing the language skills of doctors applying for registration from EEA countries even though international medical graduates from elsewhere are required to show that they have the necessary knowledge of the English language to practise (Bruce et al., 2011). On this point, the Green Paper does flag the potential for language testing for doctors who have direct contact with patients.

Some regulators have also showed interest in increased sharing of information through the Internal Market Information system, which they consider a more cost-effective resource than the introduction of professional cards, particularly in relation to suspended doctors through the implementation of proactive sharing of information and obligatory alerts.

The European Council, in its conclusion of 23 October 2011, underlined that all efforts should be made to ensure agreement on the 12 priorities of the Single Market Act (to which a modernization of Directive 2005/36/EC belongs) by the end of 2012 (European Council, 2011). A few weeks later, on 19 December 2011, the European Commission released its legislative proposal (European Commission, 2011b). The Commission suggested simplifying the recognition and registration procedures for doctors from the EEA and increasing the use of e-government tools, such as the European Professional Card and the Points of Single Contact. The Commission identified the Internal Market Information system as having considerable potential to facilitate communication between competent authorities. In an attempt to combat public concerns about patient safety, the Commission proposed provisions on effective and proportionate checks of migrant health professionals' language knowledge and the introduction of an EU-wide proactive alert mechanism for professionals who have been banned from practice (Tiedje & Zsigmond, 2012).

In response to the Commission proposal, the European Parliament published two reports in July 2012 on the recognition of professional qualifications Directive from the Internal Market and Consumer Protection Committee (Vergnaud, 2012) and the Environment, Public Health and Food Safety Committee (Weisgerber, 2012). These reports put forward some amendments to the legislative proposal as follows: stronger recommendations for verifying language competence following recognition, slight increases to the deadlines for recognition under the European Professional Card, and the extension of an alert mechanism to all sectoral professionals. Furthermore, the Internal Market and Consumer Protection report proposed additional proportionate (post-recognition) controls on professionals if they had not worked for the previous four years. The two Committees plan to adopt their final reports in November 2012 and agree the final text by 2013.

It is expected that formal adoption of the modernized Directive will take place in 2013, with national transposition planned for 2015–2016 (Tiedje, 2011).[4]

## 13.4 Discussion

When examining the multitude of instruments to promote the ethical recruitment of health personnel, certain trends can be identified. These include:

- pressure by governments and professional organizations on employers to not recruit from developing countries, particularly those with health worker shortages, unless intergovernment bilateral agreements have been negotiated;

- the promotion of improved employment rights and protections by governments facing health worker emigration in order to retain their health personnel;

- pressure by organizations such as the Commonwealth and WHO on countries to focus on self-sufficiency and sustainability of their health workforce; and

- the need for monitoring uptake and adherence to guidance.

Taking each of the above points in turn: first, since 2000, a surge in the development of instruments can be observed, which signals the increasing importance placed by national bodies, governments and international organizations on the ethical dimensions of international recruitment. At the national level, it seems to be only northern European countries that are developing codes and other tools. Further, these ethical recruitment principles do not apply to mobility between EU Member States, but rather only to migration from outside the EU.

Second, governments can provide incentives for circular migration, such that agreed career pathways are determined so that when a migrant health worker considers returning to their home country there are relevant posts available and a salary level that reflects their experience gained abroad.

With regard to self-sufficiency and sustainability, the onus is placed back on to the countries themselves to work to achieve a sustainable workforce (Little & Buchan, 2007; Buchan, Naccarella & Brooks, 2011). Towards this

---

4 Since the writing of this chapter, Directive 2013/55/EU amending Directive 2005/36/EC on the recognition of professional qualifications and Regulation (EU) No 1024/2012 on administrative cooperation through the Internal Market Information System was published on 20 November 2013. Relevant features include: a pro-active fitness to practise alert mechanism; the ability for competent authorities to assess the language competence of professionals after recognition but before access to the profession; a requirement for member states to encourage CPD; the option of a European Professional Card; and continuing professional education and revised minimum training requirements for some health-care professionals.

aim, countries need to focus on workforce planning and retention of staff, in particular from their own national resources, where possible.

Finally, although many instruments recognize the need for monitoring uptake and adherence, very few can actually take these forward because of the voluntary nature of most codes. Few countries have codes of ethical recruitment in place, and many EU Member States rely on developments of the *WHO Global Code of Practice*. Furthermore, the EPSU–HOSPEEM Code of Conduct (2008) has received little attention on the national level. Only the Departments of Health in England and Scotland actually share prescriptive country lists for non-recruitment. Therefore, there are challenges facing whether these codes and other instruments actually work in practice. Because these instruments are voluntary, feasibility depends largely on the developed country adhering to the Code (Scott et al., 2004) given that incentives or sanctions for adherence or non-adherence remain highly unlikely.

The weakness of codes is also related to difficulties in implementing and monitoring them (Buchan et al., 2009; Connell & Buchan, 2011). To better facilitate implementation, more information needs to be disseminated to the competent authorities on the desired aims of any code of practice. Support systems need to be put in place; specifically, this may entail explaining to health care managers the practical application of the code for their organization. This can be achieved through additional written information or training. Moreover, because the implementation of voluntary codes of practice on a country level requires extensive systems development, countries in the process of major structural reforms are at risk (Martineau & Willetts, 2006). In countries with a federated regulatory structure or multiple independent sector providers, a single country code may not have the required reach. For developing countries, good visibility of codes is necessary for all stakeholders involved: policy-makers, employers and potential recruits (Buchan et al., 2009).

Despite the continued interest in developing these instruments, research is lacking on the effectiveness of implementation. Research in this area is particularly challenging because of the dynamic nature of health workforce recruitment patterns, which vary greatly over time.

Studies on the English codes have flagged up several obstacles in assessing impact, including lack of monitoring, inappropriate data sets and disentangling other reasons for the increase or decline of inflow of health professionals beyond the code (Buchan et al., 2009; Young, Weir & Buchan, 2010). Given these challenges, the potential impact of international codes remains uncertain. However, if a clear link is identified between the explicit objectives and relevant monitoring capacity, then it may be possible to assess the impact of these instruments in the future (Buchan et al., 2009).

It is also important to highlight that there is additional difficulty when considering a multi-country instrument, as in the case of Europe or the *WHO Global Code of Practice*. A single country code only focuses on the approach of employers and one government, and it can be relatively straightforward to develop, adapt (where necessary) and monitor. However, where many countries are concerned, it can be much more difficult to get agreement, which poses a risk that the final code will be diluted to get universal support.

As the WHO tries to establish the *Global Code of Practice*, WHO Member States are invited to periodically report on its implementation. The first round of national self-assessment reports were to be completed by June 2012 (see Chapter 5). If there is a supervisory or monitoring system in place, then monitoring may be possible and it may create an incentive for countries to provide reports to international bodies. The challenges in attributing changes to the impact of a code are inherent in any code and not related to multi-country or global coverage.

## 13.5 Conclusions

Health professional mobility, whatever the net direction, is an important policy consideration in many countries. The need to recruit and maintain a qualified, competent and highly skilled workforce, which is up to date in its medical knowledge and fit to practise, is a relevant consideration in every country. Despite this uniform need, the methods by which health professional recruitment is carried out vary greatly.

Although there is increased acknowledgement in many countries of the need to undertake ethical recruitment when hiring medical staff across a border, there is great divergence in whether such efforts are governed by a direct code or through more subtle guidance. Overall, the instruments of international, national and professional bodies that aim at mitigating the potential negative effects of migration in sending countries are non-binding.

Health professional groups – doctors, nurses, dentists – are becoming increasingly vocal in stating their position on ethical recruitment. What was once a domain of national concern has now reached international attention, specifically with the launch of the *WHO Global Code of Practice*. This is an ambitious instrument that will require careful analysis of its success following its implementation and over time. Only longitudinal analysis, both quantitative (on the actual net change of health professionals departing from vulnerable countries) and qualitative (on any changes in methods used for recruitment) will provide clarity on the effectiveness of such an instrument.

When considering binding tools that aim at facilitating mobility and migration, although GATS provides direct modes of liberalizing trade in services, which clearly relate to the health sector, it does not appear as a prominent mechanism or consideration in European health professional mobility. Rather, in the EU, the Single Market Act, within which the Professional Qualifications Directive sits, provides entitlements for health professionals to take up work in other EU Member States.

At EU level, the legislative process for modernizing Directive 2005/36/EC on the recognition of professional qualifications has been ongoing since December 2011. Clear vested interests became apparent in the position statements of various stakeholders during the consultation process on the Directive. Although there remains some divergence of opinion regarding specific points (e.g. the need for language testing, the need for a professional card), all stakeholders have declared that they are seeking an appropriate balance between protecting the safety of the public (through ensuring the provision of high-quality care by highly qualified health professionals), and further clarifying the requirements for health professionals to practise in a host Member State, and upholding the individual right to move within the EU.

The Internal Market Information system appears to be an underutilized resource for information sharing, but to realize its potential some improvements will be necessary in terms of the type of information and the way this can be shared in order to broaden its use among many national authorities. The use of pilot projects for interested professions has the potential to make some strides in this direction.

A significant divergence between EU Member States, for both doctors and nurses, is their stance on needing to encourage high-quality CPD. Whether such requirements are mandatory, and how often and how much CPD is required, remains a topic that requires additional attention and consideration at the national and then EU level. Next, on the issue of competent authorities, further development is clearly needed particularly in relation to the regulation of the nursing profession, and how the proposed National Contact Points can add additional clarity on the Member State level. As stated by the Commission, the modernization of Directive 2005/36/EC offers the potential for developing new approaches to enhance mobility, but countries and national authorities need to be mindful of how these movements can affect the structure of their domestic health workforce and of the implications of the new EU legislation for health professionals.

# References

Agunias D, Newland K (2007). *Policy Brief: circular migration and development: trends, policy routes, and ways forward*. Washington, DC, Migration Policy Institute (http://www.migrationpolicy.org/pubs/MigDevPB_041807.pdf, accessed 3 January 2014).

Bruce L et al. (2011). *The state of medical education and practice in the UK*. London, General Medical Council (http://www.gmc-uk.org/State_of_medicine_Final_web.pdf_44213427.pdf, accessed 3 January 2014).

Buchan J et al. (2009). Does a code make a difference: assessing the English code of practice on international recruitment. *Human Resources for Health*, 7:33.

Buchan JM, Naccarella L, Brooks PM (2011). Is health workforce sustainability in Australia and New Zealand a realistic policy goal? *Australian Health Review*, 35(2):152–155.

Chartered Society of Physiotherapy (1998). *Recruiting overseas physiotherapists: a guide for therapy services managers*. London, Chartered Society of Physiotherapy.

Commonwealth Secretariat (2003). *Commonwealth code of practice for international recruitment of health workers*. London, Commonwealth Secretariat (http://secretariat.thecommonwealth.org/files/35877/FileName/CommonwealthCodeofPractice.pdf, accessed 3 January 2014).

Connell J, Buchan J (2011). The impossible dream? Codes of practice and the international migration of skilled health workers. *World Medical and Health Policy*, 3(3):1–17.

Department of Health (1998). *Guide to immigration and employment of overseas medical and dental students, doctors and dentists in the UK*. London, HMSO.

Department of Health (1999). *Guidance on international nursing recruitment*. London, HMSO (http://webarchive.nationalarchives.gov.uk/20130107105354/http://www.dh.gov.uk/prod_consum_dh/groups/dh_digitalassets/@dh/@en/documents/digitalasset/dh_4034794.pdf, accessed 3 January 2014).

Department of Health (2001). *Code of Practice for NHS Employers involved in international recruitment of healthcare professionals*. London, The Stationery Office.

Department of Health (2004). *Code of practice for the international recruitment of healthcare professionals*, revised edition. London, The Stationery Office (http://www.idcsig.org/DoH%20International%20Recruitment.pdf, accessed 8 October 2013).

Department of Health (2013a). *Code of practice for the supply of temporary staffing*. London, DH Publications.

Department of Health (2013b). *International recruitment: NHS employers web page*. London, Department of Health (http://www.nhsemployers.org/RecruitmentAndRetention/InternationalRecruitment/Code-of-Practice/Pages/Code-practice-international-recruitment.aspx, accessed 3 January 2014).

Department of Health and Children of Ireland (2001). *Guidance for best practice on the recruitment of overseas nurses and midwives*. Dublin, Department of Health and Children of Ireland (http://www.dohc.ie/publications/pdf/bpronm.pdf?direct=1, accessed 3 January 2014).

Dickson N (2011). The free movement of professionals: a UK regulator's perspective. *Eurohealth*, 17(4):3–5.

EPSU–HOSPEEM (2008). *EPSU–HOSPEEM code of conduct and follow up on ethical cross-border recruitment and retention in the hospital sector*. Brussels, European Federation of Public Service Unions and European Hospital and Healthcare Employers' Association (http://www.epsu.org/a/3715, accessed 2 January 2014).

European Commission (2005a). *Directive 2005/36/EC on the recognition of professional qualifications*. Brussels, European Commission (http://ec.europa.eu/internal_market/qualifications/policy_developments/legislation/index_en.htm, accessed 5 August 2013).

European Commission (2005b). *Strategy for action on the crisis in human resources for health in developing countries*. Brussels, European Commission (COM(2005) 642).

European Commission (2006). *Programme for action (PfA) to tackle the shortage of health workers in developing countries 2007–2013*. Brussels, European Commission (COM(2006) 870).

European Commission (2008a). *A common immigration policy for Europe: principles, actions and tools*. Brussels, European Commission (COM(2008) 359 final).

European Commission (2008b). *Green Paper on the European Workforce for Health*. Brussels, European Commission (COM(2008) 725 final) (http://ec.europa.eu/health/ph_systems/docs/workforce_gp_en.pdf, accessed 2 January 2014).

European Commission (2010). *Commission Staff working document on the transposition and implementation of the professional qualifications directive*. Brussels, European Commission (SEC(2010) 1292 final).

European Commission (2011a). *Green paper on modernising the professional qualifications directive*. Brussels, European Commission (COM(2011) 367 final).

European Commission (2011b). *Proposal for a Directive of the European Parliament and of the Council amending Directive 2005/36/EC on the recognition of professional qualifications and regulation on administrative cooperation through the Internal Market Information System*. Brussels, European Commission (COM(2011) 0883) (http://www.europarl.europa.eu/sides/getDoc.do?type=REPORT&reference=A7-2013-0038&language=EN, accessed 3 January 2014).

European Council (2011). *Conclusions*. Brussels, European Council (EUCO 52/1/11 REV 1).

European Federation of Nurses Associations (2004). *EFN good practice guidance for international nurse recruitment*. Brussels, European Federation of Nurses Associations (http://efnweb.be/wp-content/uploads/2011/11/EFN_Good_Practice_Guidance_Recruitment.doc).

Goodard AF (2011). The Professional Qualifications Directive Green Paper: the UK physician's perspective. *Eurohealth*, 17(4):7–10.

International Council of Nurses (2007). *Position statement: ethical nurse recruitment*. Geneva, International Council of Nurses (http://www.icn.ch/images/stories/documents/publications/position_statements/C03_Ethical_Nurse_Recruitment.pdf, accessed 9 October 2013).

International Labour Organization (2006). *Orientation to social dialogue for countries participating in the Action Programme on International Migration of Health Care Workers: the supply side. 2006*. Geneva, International Labour Office (http://www.ilo.org/sector/activities/action-programmes/health-services/WCMS_161955/lang--en/index.htm, accessed 5 December 2013).

Keighley T, Williams S (2011). Regulating nursing qualifications across Europe: a case of unintended consequences. *Eurohealth*, 17(4):11–14.

Little L, Buchan J (2007). *Nursing self sufficiency/sustainability in the global context*. Geneva, International Centre for Human Resources in Nursing (http://www.icn.ch/images/stories/documents/pillars/sew/ICHRN/Policy_and_Research_Papers/Nursing_Self_Sufficiency.Sustainability_in_the_Global_Context.pdf, accessed 3 January 2014).

Martineau T, Willetts A (2006). The health workforce: managing the crisis ethical international recruitment of health professionals – will codes of practice protect developing country health systems? *Health Policy*, 75(3):358–367.

Merkur S et al. (2008). *Do lifelong learning and revalidation ensure that physicians are fit to practise?* Copenhagen, WHO Regional Office for Europe on behalf of the European Observatory (http://www.euro.who.int/__data/assets/pdf_file/0005/75434/E93412.pdf, accessed 10 December 2013).

Netherland Ministry of Health, Welfare and Sport (2007). *Werken aan de zorg [Working on Care]*. The Hague, Ministry of Health, Welfare and Sport.

NHS Employers (2013). *Code of practice: list of developing countries*. Leeds, NHS Employers (http://www.nhsemployers.org/RecruitmentAndRetention/InternationalRecruitment/Code-of-Practice/Pages/developing-countries.aspx, accessed 8 October 2013).

Norwegian Directorate of Health (2007). *Recruitment of health workers: towards global solidarity*. Oslo, Norwegian Directorate of Health (http://helsedirektoratet.no/english/publications/recruitment-of-health-workers-towards-global-solidarity/Sider/default.aspx, accessed 3 January 2014).

Oh et al. (2005). What is eHealth: a systematic review of published definitions. *Journal of Medical Internet Research*, 7:e1.

Robinson R (2007). *The costs and benefits of health worker migration from East and Southern Africa (ESA): a literature review*. Harare, Equinet (Equinet Discussion Paper 49) (http://www.equinetafrica.org/bibl/docs/DIS49HRrobinson.pdf, accessed 3 January 2014).

Scott ML et al. (2004). Brain drain or ethical recruitment? Solving health workforce shortages with professionals from developing countries. *Medical Journal of Australia*, 80(4):174–176.

Scottish Executive (2006). *Code of practice for the international recruitment of healthcare professionals in Scotland*. Edinburgh, Scottish Executive (http://www.scotland.gov.uk/Resource/0041/00412480.pdf, accessed 1 October 2013).

Smith RD (2004). Foreign direct investment and trade in health services: a review of the literature. *Social Science and Medicine*, 59:2313–2323.

Smith RD, Chanda R, Tangcharoensathien V (2009). Trade in health-related services. *Lancet*, 373(9663):593–601.

Tiedje J (2011). Revision of the professional qualifications directive. London, Royal College of Physicians (Presentation by Jürgen Tiedje, DG Internal Market and Services, 11 July) (http://www.rcplondon.ac.uk/sites/default/files/jurgen_tiedje_presentation_by_european_commission.pdf, accessed 3 January 2014).

Tiedje J, Zsigmond A (2012). How to modernise the professional qualifications directive. *Eurohealth*, 18(2):18–22.

Vergnaud B (2012). *Project report on legislative proposal to Directive 2005/36/EC.* Brussels, Internal Market and Consumer Protection Committee (http://www.europarl.europa.eu/sides/getDoc.do?pubRef=-//EP//NONSGML+COMPARL+PE-494.470+01+DOC+PDF+V0//FR, accessed 3 January 2014).

Weisgerber A (2012). *Project report on legislative proposal to Directive 2005/36/EC.* Brussels, Environment, Public Health and Food Safety Committees (http://www.europarl.europa.eu/sides/getDoc.do?pubRef=-//EP//NONSGML+COMPARL+PE-494.475+01+DOC+PDF+V0//DE, accessed 3 January 2014).

WHO (1995). *General agreement on trade in services (GATS).* Geneva, World Health Organization (http://www.who.int/trade/glossary/story033/en/index.html, accessed 3 January 2014).

WHO (2006). *International migration of health personnel: a challenge for health systems in developing countries.* Geneva, World Health Organization (Fifty-ninth World Health Assembly, A59/18) (http://apps.who.int/gb/archive/pdf_files/WHA59/A59_18-en.pdf, accessed 3 January 2014).

WHO (2010a). *Global code of practice on the international recruitment of health personnel: implementation by the Secretariat.* Geneva, World Health Organization (http://www.who.int/hrh/resources/Code_implementation_strategy.pdf, accessed 3 January 2014).

WHO (2010b). *WHO global code of practice on the international recruitment of health personnel.* Geneva, World Health Organization (Sixty-third World Health Assembly, WHA63.16) (http://www.who.int/hrh/migration/code/WHO_global_code_of_practice_EN.pdf, accessed 1 October 2013).

WHO (2011). *User's guide to the WHO global code of practice on the international recruitment of health personnel.* Geneva, World Health Organization (http://whqlibdoc.who.int/hq/2010/WHO_HSS_HRH_HMR_2010.2_eng.pdf, accessed 4 December 2013).

Wiskow C, ed. (2006). *Health worker migration flows in Europe: overview and case studies in selected CEE countries: Romania, Czech Republic, Serbia and Croatia.* Geneva, International Labour Organization (Working Paper 245) (http://www.ilo.org/wcmsp5/groups/public/---ed_dialogue/---sector/documents/publication/wcms_161162.pdf, accessed 14 December 2013).

World Dental Federation (2006). *Ethical recruitment of oral health professionals.* New Delhi, World Dental Federation (Adopted by the FDI General Assembly, Shenzhen, China, 24 September).

World Federation of Public Health Associations (2005). *Ethical restrictions on international recruitment of health professionals from low-income countries.* Geneva, General Assembly of the World Federation of Public Health Associations.

World Medical Association (2003). *Statement on ethical guidelines for the international recruitment of physicians.* Helsinki, World Medical Association (Adopted at the Fifty-fourth General Assembly, September) (http://www. wma.net/en/30publications/10policies/e14/index.html.pdf?print-media-type&footer-right=[page]/[toPage], accessed 3 January 2014).

World Organisation for Family Doctors (2002). *A code of practice for the international recruitment of health care professionals (Melbourne manifesto).* Singapore, World Organisation for Family Doctors (Adopted at the 5th Wonca World Rural Health Conference, Melbourne, 3 May) (http://www.acrrm.org. au/files/uploads/pdf/advocacy/melbourne-manifesto_wonca.pdf, accessed 9 October 2013).

Young R, Weir H, Buchan J (2010). *Health professional mobility in Europe and the UK: a scoping study of issues and evidence.* Southampton, UK, National Institute for Health Research (Research Report for the Service Delivery and Organisation Programme).

Zarocostas J (2010). WHO agrees new code on ethical recruitment of international health personnel. *British Medical Journal,* 340:c2784.

# Chapter 14

# The role of bilateral agreements in the regulation of health worker migration

*Evgeniya Plotnikova*

## 14.1 Introduction

This chapter reflects on the role of bilateral agreements in the regulation of cross-border mobility of health workers. These bilateral labour agreements are a commonly used tool in the context of cross-border labour migration and are defined as, "… all forms of arrangements between countries, regions and public institutions that provide for the recruitment and employment of foreign workers" (Bobeva & Garson, 2004, p. 11).

The discussion in this chapter is based on an analysis of policy reports produced by international organizations as well as by findings of a qualitative case study on bilateral labour agreements negotiated between the British Government and a number of source countries – the Philippines, India, Spain and South Africa.

The contemporary policy discourse is concerned with effective measures for the regulation of health worker migration (Stilwell et al., 2004; Bomba, 2009; OECD, 2010; Connell & Buchan, 2011). In fact, migration of health workers has become a complex and a very dynamic process that can include many stops in the migratory route, where one country often becomes a stepping stone for a move to another state. This multilevel nature of contemporary migration is only one of the challenges in regulating health worker mobility. Other challenges include an increasing number of health worker migrants, a lack of data documenting migratory paths and a diverse number of stakeholders involved in this process, often with conflicting interests. These stakeholders are international organizations, migrant health workers and patients, government authorities, trade unions, professional organizations and regulatory bodies in both destination and source countries.

The problem of managing cross-border mobility of health workers has posed a number of questions on how to balance economic needs and negative public discourse around migration, and on how to ensure coherence of professional qualifications of foreign health workers with national standards, particularly when automatic recognition of qualifications is promoted at the European level. Finally, since migration of health workers involves and affects many stakeholders, the core of the regulatory problem is how to manage migration with recognition of the individual interests of patients and health workers, the needs of the national health systems in both source and destination countries and the international norms – the right to health care of patients in source and destination countries and the right to freedom of movement and labour rights of migrant health workers.

A number of regulatory measures have been proposed in response to these challenges (see Chapters 12 and 13). As previous chapters have shown, the contemporary regulatory framework in the migration of health workers comprises many layers of regulation, which may be introduced at the national, bilateral, regional or international levels.

A number of instruments at the international level apply to health workforce migration, and organizations such as WHO, the International Council of Nurses and the World Trade Organization have introduced a number of instruments relevant to health workforce migration: the *WHO Global Code of Practice* (WHO, 2010), the International Council of Nurses *Position Statement on Ethical Recruitment* (International Council of Nurses, 2001) and mode 4 on the free flow of service workers in the GATS (WHO, 1995). Regional actors, such as the North American Free Trade Agreement members, the Caribbean Community, Commonwealth countries, the Asia–Pacific Economic Cooperation and the EU, have also become active agents producing mechanisms to facilitate the migration of health workers. With more regulatory tools being introduced at the international level, and international agencies becoming more visible and, some might argue, more influential in facilitation of labour migration, the early signs of an emerging global governance framework can be observed, although it is still lacking coherence. The picture of existing international arrangements in management of health worker mobility outlined above would be incomplete without consideration of the role of bilateral government arrangements in managing cross-border mobility of health workers.

## 14.2 Bilateral agreements in regulation of the cross-border mobility of health workers

The negotiation of bilateral government agreements on workforce mobility is a well-established practice in international relations that dates back to the late 19th century when the earliest versions of labour recruitment programmes were initiated between countries. At that time, the United States signed a number of trade agreements on commerce and navigation that also allowed entry to foreign workers with a limited right of residence in the party countries (International Organization for Migration, 2003). In Europe, the early examples of bilateral labour agreements were concluded to address the demographic challenges after the First World War (Mullan, 1998). However, the active period in negotiation of bilateral labour schemes occurred after the Second World War when many European countries experienced a significant labour shortage as a result of population decline, mass emigration and relocation induced by the war. Among other Western European states, Belgium, France, Germany, the Netherlands and Switzerland became active in the negotiation of labour agreements. These countries operated a number of bilateral schemes with Ireland, countries in southern Europe (Greece, Italy, Portugal and Spain), Turkey, the former Yugoslavia and countries in north Africa (Algeria, Morocco and Tunisia). The purpose of these agreements was to recruit low-skilled labour in the agriculture, construction, mining and catering sectors through seasonal guest-worker employment programmes. Perhaps one of the most cited examples of bilateral agreements was the German *Gastarbeiter* programme, which brought around 3.6 million workers to Germany from Italy, Greece, Turkey and Yugoslavia in the period 1960–1966 (OECD, 2004).

The mid-1970s became a turning point for bilateral labour agreements. The number of bilateral recruitment schemes concluded by European countries considerably declined after the oil crisis in 1973. Restrictive measures in the regulation of labour immigration were introduced in response to a reduced demand for labour in many European countries following the economic downturn (Abella, 2004).

The re-emergence of bilateral labour agreements in Europe occurred in the 1990s and early 2000s, although with less intensity than during the recruitment drives of the 1950s and 1960s. The growth of labour migration in Europe in the early 1990s was facilitated by the opening of borders with Central and Eastern European countries. Among the most active co-signers of these "second generation" bilateral agreements were Germany, Spain, France and countries of Central and Eastern Europe – Poland, the Czech Republic, Slovakia and Hungary (OECD, 2004). Apart from the European integration and enlargement agenda, this recovery period in signing bilateral labour agreements was reinforced with the ethical recruitment discourse. The latter, in particular, has become one of the key issues in policy debates on the health worker mobility.

At that time, the United Kingdom, one of the pioneer countries among EU Member States considering ethical dimensions in the international recruitment of health workers, introduced an ethical recruitment policy where bilateral labour agreements, alongside the Code of Practice (2001, revised in 2004), became one of its tools. In the early 2000s, the British Government led negotiations on health worker migration with several source countries within the EU (Spain, Germany, Italy, France) as well as with non-EU states: India, the Philippines, South Africa, China and Indonesia.

Information about other bilateral labour agreements negotiated in the health sector in the early 2000s elsewhere in the world is rather limited. Some references appear in the policy documents and working papers of the OECD, International Organization for Migration and the International Labour Organization (International Organization for Migration, 2004; Wickramasekara, 2006; Dumont & Zurn, 2007).

In this chapter the list of agreements, based on data collected from international policy reports, is not exhaustive but attempts to map government agreements negotiated since the early 2000s worldwide in the international recruitment of health workers. Although these identified bilateral schemes demonstrate a vast geographical scope, diverse purposes for negotiation as well as various administrative arrangements, the majority of agreements on health professions predominantly referred to nurses. Some of these agreements initially negotiated to recruit nurses from overseas were extended to recruitment of foreign doctors, for example the agreement between the United Kingdom and Spain (Table 14.1). These agreements in the early 2000s reflected the growing demand for nurses but also the increasing cross-border mobility of nurses (Kingma, 2006; Hendel, 2008) compared with the 1970s when mainly physicians moved across borders in response to international recruitment drives (Meija, 1978).

As Table 14.1 indicates, there are various bilateral and regional agreements set up within the EU to facilitate the movement of health workers. For example, in 2005, an agreement on cooperation of health services in the border region was negotiated between the French and German Ministries of Health. As reported by the Federal Ministry of Health and Social Security (2005, cited by Wiskow, 2006, p. 27): "The agreement aims at facilitating the use of ambulances and emergency staff on foreign territory, in order to improve emergency care in accidents. Further, it facilitates the cooperation of hospitals in the border regions through partnerships and exchange of personnel and knowledge. The

**Table 14.1** Examples of bilateral agreements negotiated to facilitate health worker mobility

| Countries | Date | Focus on the health workforce | Key points |
|---|---|---|---|
| *Within Europe* | | | |
| United Kingdom–Spain | 2000 | Nurses (extended to doctors in 2001) | Recruitment |
| United Kingdom (Scotland)–Malawi | 2005 | Nurses, midwives | Cooperation |
| Spain–France | 2002 | Nurses | Recruitment |
| Poland–Netherlands | 2002 | Nurses | Recruitment, capacity building |
| France–Germany | 2005 | Ambulances, emergency staff | Cooperation in the border regions |
| Romania–Italy | 2002 | Nurses | Recruitment |
| *Outside Europe* | | | |
| United Kingdom–South Africa | 2003 | Nurses and doctors | Cooperation/personnel exchange |
| United Kingdom–China | 2005 | Nurses | Restricted recruitment (only through approved agencies) |
| United Kingdom–Philippines | 2002/ 2003 | Nurses | Recruitment stimulation; strengthening ethical recruitment |
| United Kingdom–India | 2002 | Nurses | Restricted recruitment (excluding regions: Andhra Pradesh, Madhya Pradesh, Orissa, West Bengal) |
| United Kingdom–Indonesia | 2002 | Nurses | Pilot project on recruitment |
| United Kingdom–Egypt | 2001 | Doctors | Education/training exchange |
| China–Singapore | 1995 | Nurses | Recruitment |
| Kenya–Namibia | n/a | Nurses | Recruitment |

*Sources*: OECD, 2004; Buchan & Perfilieva, 2006; Dumont & Zurn, 2007; Aspen Institute, 2011.

overall goal is to improve access to continuous care for the population in the region."

Another example is the cross-border cooperation in the field of health care between Spain and France, which was formally established in 2005 to manage health services in the cross-border region of Cerdanya. The objective of the project was to ensure the provision of medical care for the local population and tourists coming into the region. For this purpose, a cross-border hospital is being set up under a joint administration and management system in Puigcerdá (Scheres, 2006; Mission Opérationnelle Transfrontalière, 2007; Wismar et al., 2011). Prior to this inter-regional cooperation, a bilateral recruitment agreement was reached with France to recruit nurses from Spain in 2002. The agreement led to the recruitment of 1 364 nurses and was closed in 2004 (Dumont & Zurn, 2007).

Apart from the regional cooperation and small-scale recruitment projects, the other type of bilateral agreement negotiated within Europe in the early 2000s aimed to enhance labour mobility between the "old" EU members and the EU candidates and/or new EU members. During the active enlargement process in the early 2000s, these agreements were negotiated to speed up integration across Europe. For example, an agreement between Poland and the Netherlands called the Covenant on Migrant Health Workers (CAZ) was signed in 2002. This project became a part of the integration programme for Poland and ended in 2004 when it became an EU Member State. The project addressed the nurse shortage in the Dutch health services and aimed to improve the competencies of Polish nurses and promote recognition of their diplomas at the European level. In total, 91 Polish nurses were employed by the project. The International Organization for Migration monitored and evaluated the programme (International Organization for Migration, 2005).

Another bilateral labour agreement in health was negotiated between two EU Member States in 2002. The Autonomous Region of Friuli-Venezia-Giulia in Italy initiated a programme to recruit nurses from Romania to address nurse shortages in Italy (Barbin, 2004). To improve and secure the recruitment process, an association (Association de Préparation et de Perfectionnement Professionnel) was established under Romanian law to improve the quality of recruitment. In particular, the established association was involved in evaluation of candidates, preparation of successful candidates for expatriation and retraining of individuals (OECD, 2004).

Patchy information is available on labour agreements in the health sector negotiated in the early 2000s outside Europe. Identified examples include agreements between Kenya and Namibia and between China and Singapore. In response to the HIV/AIDS crisis, Namibia's public health sector has been carrying out a comprehensive strategy to hire and deploy professional and non-professional health workers with the aim of providing comprehensive care. In addition to the policies adopted at the national level, the Namibian Government initiated a project on the recruitment of foreign health workers under which 100 nurses were recruited from Kenya in the early 2000s (Frelick & Mameja, 2006).

Bilateral relations between China and Singapore in the health sector began approximately two decades ago when the Chinese Government sent a group of English-speaking nurses to work in Singapore and Saudi Arabia. The Chinese Government charged around 10–15% of each nurse's annual salary as the "handling fee" for employment through the government arrangement. The contracts under this agreement usually lasted two to three years, and most nurses returned to work in their original hospitals afterwards (Fang, 2007).

These examples of bilateral agreements negotiated within and outside Europe indicate diverse styles, contents and reasons for developing agreements, which are not limited to labour recruitment as they were mainly perceived to cover in the 1960s. Today, these agreements cover a broad array of functions including regional cooperation and integration, training of foreign health personnel, personnel exchange, restriction or stimulation of recruitment (depending on a country's circumstances) and finally, promotion of ethical principles in recruitment of health workers, at least on paper.

These observed changes indicate the diversification of bilateral labour agreements, in terms of both their format and functions. This transformation has led contemporary policy analysts to address the problem of evaluation of such various forms of agreements.

## 14.3 Policy discourse on the role of bilateral agreements

The role of bilateral agreements has become one of the topical themes in contemporary policy discourse on regulation of health worker migration. There are a number of policy reports produced by international organizations as well as individual studies that examine the impact of these agreements. These projects explore practices of single countries (Blitz, 2005; International Organization for Migration, 2005; Ollier, 2007), cross-country experience in negotiation of such agreements (Hars, 2003; Wiskow, 2006; Chanda, 2008, 2009; Aspen Institute, 2011) and also propose a framework for evaluation of their impact (OECD, 2004; Go, 2007).

The OECD, for example, identifies a number of dimensions that could be applied in the evaluation of bilateral labour agreements. This includes the narrow perspective, which looks largely at the economic impacts of agreements on the labour market, and a broader view on the political effects of such agreements in the arena of international relations, migration policies, development aid provision and regional integration. An alternative dimension is analysis of bilateral agreements from the perspective of source and destination countries (OECD, 2004).

For source countries, it is recognized that, in economic terms, agreements are valuable in a number of ways. Yet it is also important to note that policy reports that consider the role of bilateral agreements often do not separate economic impacts of labour migration in general from bilateral agreements as one of its channels (Bobeva & Garson, 2004). Therefore, the following points, presented in these policy reports about economic effects, refer to both foreign labour migration and bilateral labour agreements. First, bilateral agreements contribute to reducing the unemployment rate by sending the labour surplus abroad. Second, agreements become one of the means of increasing migrant remittances, which are crucial to the national economies of many developing countries. A typical example would be agreements negotiated by the Philippines, a traditional source country (Go, 2007). However, if agreements become a part of the national strategy, such as is the case in the Philippines, concern arises about the dependency of developing countries on sending their health professionals abroad and the possibility that this reduces incentives to create jobs and improve working conditions locally.

The impact of bilateral labour agreements on the labour market in receiving countries is evident at two levels. At one level, these agreements can resolve the problem of the labour shortage in destination countries in the short term. At another level, there is a concern, similar to that for source countries, that these agreements may build up a dependency in destination countries on foreign labour and lead to an inability to train and retain a sufficient number of native workers (Bach, 2004).

On a broader scale of economic consequences of agreements on both receiving and source countries, policy analysts recognize the positive effects of these policy tools in facilitating trade and business relations between countries (Bobeva & Garson, 2004). However, it should be mentioned that the labour market impact of bilateral agreements is decreasing. Currently, the largest labour movement between countries takes place outside the channel of bilateral agreements (through recruitment agencies, family links and social networks), and, in this sense, bilateral agreements are considered to be old-fashioned instruments. For example, as indicated in the Royal College of Nursing labour market review (Buchan & Seccombe, 2004), the proportion of registered nurses who were recruited in the early 2000s to Britain from the Philippines through bilateral agreements was significantly smaller than the number of Filipino nurses who came through other channels, such as private recruiting agencies. Moreover, a comprehensive approach based on generic immigration rules is considered to be more effective than bilateral agreements in the longer term (OECD, 2004).

Contrary to the labour market effects of bilateral labour agreements, which generally correspond with the impacts of labour migration, there are a number of distinctive political and sociocultural outcomes produced by these policy tools. It is recognized that bilateral agreements could potentially improve international relations, assist in the management of migration, provide means for the implementation of development policies in poor world regions, provide social protection of foreign labour abroad and facilitate regional integration between regions/countries (OECD, 2004). For example, bilateral agreements could be used as regulatory tools to control and channel foreign labour migration by reducing the need to utilize commercial recruitment agencies, thus ensuring a more predictable and transparent process for both parties and shifting the cost of migration from individual migrants to employers and governments of a recipient country (Bach, 2003). However, a number of weak points are also recognized in reports on the implementation of bilateral agreements. Predominantly these refer to the financial costs and organizational burden of recruiting health workers from overseas for public institutions when the recruitment is centralized at the government level and the public authorities take part in facilitation of administrative procedures, such as recognition of diplomas of foreign health workers, evaluation of the professional abilities of candidates and the integration of foreign health workers into the broader sociocultural environment (Garson, 2006). An illustrative example would be the agreement signed between the United Kingdom and Spain (2000) on recruitment of nurses, where the English Department of Health played an active role in the coordination, administration and financial provision for the recruitment process in Spain. The contrary example would be the agreement between the United Kingdom and the Philippines (2003), where the Department of Health did not have to fulfil recruitment functions as the infrastructure of public and private agencies specializing on recruitment of Filipino nurses was well established and did not require substantial financial and/or administrative assistance from the British Government (Plotnikova, 2011).

Recognition of the drawbacks or weaknesses of bilateral labour agreements is also expressed by international trade and financial institutions, such as the World Trade Organization. From the neoliberal perspective, bilateral labour agreements are considered to be inefficient, bureaucratic and time-consuming mechanisms. They promote exclusive labour market access to service providers based on nationality and profession, which is inconsistent with the non-discriminatory principle of the "most favoured nations" (Nielson, 2006). The latter is a basic principle of the World Trade Organization system, which requires that all trade partners are treated equally. If one of the partners is granted more benefits (e.g. reduced tariffs on certain goods or favourable access for certain service providers) then all other trade partners shall receive the same treatment (World Trade Organization, 2012).

In summary, the few attempts to evaluate bilateral labour agreements have primarily focused on developing a common framework for their analysis. This framework includes economic, political and sociocultural criteria and the perspectives of both receiving and source countries. This may well be a good starting point; however, understanding the role of bilateral agreements is perhaps a more complex exercise where application of a standard set of criteria is not always appropriate. It rather requires contextualized policy analysis that pays attention to the policy setting, the policy actors involved in negotiation and implementation of agreements, their intentions, and the expected and latent consequences.

The next section of this chapter develops further this approach by analysing the United Kingdom practice in negotiation of bilateral agreements.

## 14.4 Analysis of the United Kingdom and its contribution to understanding bilateral agreements

In the early 2000s, the United Kingdom was one of the pioneer countries to introduce bilateral agreements in the framework of ethical recruitment of foreign health workers. Previously, negotiation of bilateral labour agreements was not a typical practice in British labour migration policy (Rollason, 2004). In the 1950s and 1960s, the British Government sponsored a number of programmes to attract foreign medical professionals from the West Indies. However, such programmes were implemented through the introduction of a number of favourable conditions for overseas health workers to obtain visas and professional registration rather than through direct negotiation with the governments of source countries (Smith, 1981). It is for this reason that the negotiation of bilateral labour agreements in the early 2000s attracted research attention and encouraged analysis of their role in the British recruitment policy, with consideration of the policy context in which these agreements originated, the perceptions of these agreements by policy actors involved in the negotiations, and the broader debate of recruitment of foreign health workers to the United Kingdom. The findings described here are based on analysis of policy documents and interviews with experts in international organizations, officials in the Department of Health (England), recruitment officers in the source countries and professional organizations and trade unions in the United Kingdom.

Agreements with four countries – Spain, the Philippines, India and South Africa – were selected as the units of analysis. These agreements were negotiated in different formats, including recruitment contracts and health personnel exchange schemes, memorandum of understanding and verbal agreements (Table 14.2).

The recruitment contracts were signed with Spain (2000) and the Philippines (2002) to organize a centralized government-led campaign where the government bodies were directly involved in recruiting nurses.

Another type of agreement was negotiated with the Philippines (2003) and India (2001). Contrary to the agreement with Spain, these agreements were negotiated to set up a framework and inform the relevant stakeholders in both

**Table 14.2** Types of bilateral labour agreements with illustrations

| Type of agreement and example | Format | Number of recruits/ placements | Typical characteristics of the agreement type |
|---|---|---|---|
| *Recruitment agreement* | | | |
| United Kingdom– Philippines, 2002 | Contract-like document | Total number is not available; fragmental evidence points at 186 Filipino nurses who were employed in the NHS via this recruitment agreement[a] | Precise wording<br><br>Quantitative target (optional)<br><br>Defined conditions on recruitment, recognition of professional qualification and employment<br><br>Assigned financial and organizational responsibilities to both parties: stakeholders in source and destination countries<br><br>Acknowledged by lawyers from each country (optional) |
| United Kingdom–Spain, 2000 | Contract-like document | Approx 1 300 | |
| *Framework agreement on recruitment issues* | | | |
| United Kingdom–India, 2001 | Exchange of letters/verbal agreement | 9 972[b] | A framework for encouraging/slowing down recruitment (depending on both countries' needs)<br><br>Setting ethical recruitment standards |
| United Kingdom– Philippines, 2003 | Memorandum of Understanding | 24 135[b] | A framework for encouraging/slowing down recruitment (depending on both countries' needs)<br><br>Setting ethical recruitment standards |
| *Framework agreement on co-operation and personnel exchange* | | | |
| United Kingdom–South Africa, 2003 | Memorandum of understanding | 18 South African nurses in United Kingdom (2003)<br><br>70 United Kingdom health workers in RSA (2003–2004)<br><br>259 United Kingdom health workers in RSA (2004–2005) | Establishment of opportunities and channels for cooperation and exchange of knowledge and health personnel between two countries |

*Notes*: NHS, National Health Service; [a]Buchan and Seccombe, 2004; [b]Estimated using data from Nursing and Midwifery Council registration from 2000 to 2005; there is no distinction between recruitment through the government agreements and individual applications through private agencies for these data.

countries about the opportunities and conditions on which recruitment was eligible.

Finally, the agreement with South Africa (2003) was not principally about recruitment but rather the establishment of channels for cooperation and exchange of knowledge and health personnel between two countries.

The various formats of these agreements reflect the diverse positions of source countries on the recruitment of their nurses. These positions were framed in the language of human rights, and reinforced by the Millennium Development Goals and the New Labour Government's ethical agenda in foreign policy. On the one hand, international recruitment was recognized as a factor undermining the right to health of citizens in developing countries, but, on the other hand, the potential restriction on international recruitment was portrayed as a violation of the right to freedom of movement for health workers. There were a number of interplaying layers behind this formulation, including conflicting interests between and within political actors. For example, some source countries (such as South Africa) criticized active recruitment campaigns organized by employers and agencies from the United Kingdom (Khan & Nixson, 2002) while other countries actively sending health personnel abroad, such as India and the Philippines, were interested in continuing the practice of international recruitment (except from some regions with a critical nurse shortage). The reason for this position of promoting the outflow of nurses was that the remittances sent home by health workers working abroad represented a significant contribution to the national economies of these countries (Buchan, 2003; Stilwell et al., 2004).

Ambivalent positions on international recruitment were expressed by professional organizations and trade unions in both source countries and the United Kingdom. In source countries, these bodies supported the right of migrants to freedom of movement and protection from exploitation; in this way, they secured overseas career opportunities for health workers and protected their working conditions abroad (Jordan, 2001). Nonetheless, these organizations also became concerned about the constant outflow of skilled workers to developed countries and therefore joined others in criticizing the active recruitment strategies of developed countries including the United Kingdom (Healey, 2006).

Trade unions and professional organizations in the United Kingdom also expressed a duality of interests in international recruitment. While they showed solidarity with their counterparts in source countries and in principle supported the right of overseas health workers to work in the United Kingdom, they also criticized the heavy reliance of national health care institutions on foreign workers. They pointed out the reasons for this dependency, namely poor remuneration and working conditions that discouraged local talent (Bach, 2004).

International organizations tried to counterbalance this debate, appealing to both groups of rights. Initially prioritizing the right to health in source countries, they also acknowledged the rights of health workers to freedom of movement and decent employment conditions abroad (WHO, 2004; International Organization for Migration, 2008).

As for the United Kingdom Government, it found itself in a policy trap. The New Labour Government needed to continue international recruitment in order to fill the gap in the national workforce and fulfil a commitment to the expansion of public health services by bringing more doctors and nurses into practice. However, it also had to slow down active recruitment from developing countries to stop accusations of "stealing" health workers (Deeming, 2004).

To balance the conflicting claims of many stakeholders at both ends of the migratory process, the United Kingdom Government introduced an ethical recruitment policy, in which government-to-government agreements with Spain, India, the Philippines and South Africa became an important component. The role of these agreements on cross-border mobility of health professionals was to contain conflicting interests between and within political actors in order to legitimize the recruitment of foreign nurses and other health professionals in the context of adverse publicity about the United Kingdom's contribution to the "brain drain" problem in developing countries.

## 14.5 Discussion and conclusion

A number of lessons for further successful implementation of bilateral labour agreements can be learnt from an analysis of the United Kingdom recruiting practices from four source countries: India, the Philippines, Spain and South Africa.

From the perspective of the destination country, negotiation with a source country requires prior research into a number of dimensions that might facilitate, or challenge, the implementation of agreements, such as institutional factors, characteristics of recruited personnel and employers' needs. From the institutional perspective, considerations include:

- postcolonial and other historical and cultural links between source and destination countries, which could ensure similarity in educational programmes and the language proficiency of recruited personnel;

- the position on the outflow of health professionals of the government in the source country, as well as the perspectives of other relevant political actors such as professional organizations and trade unions; and

- whether there is a recruitment infrastructure, organized either centrally by the government of the source country (such as in the Philippines) or by private agencies.

Further, particular attention should be paid to the characteristics of personnel available in the source country for overseas employment. Such characteristics include their qualifications, language proficiency, motivations for taking up jobs overseas, expectations and future career plans. Finally, employers' expectations and needs in the destination country should be considered to ensure a good match with the recruited personnel from abroad.

The key conclusion is that the role of bilateral labour agreements has gradually been transforming since the 1960s, from primarily tools for labour recruitment to tools with a broader array of functions. Agreements have become tools that can potentially reinforce regional integration, establish economic links, strengthen cultural ties, protect the welfare of migrant workers and ensure that workers return home after contracts expire. In addition, the study of the British experience in negotiation of bilateral agreements reveals a further role as a component of an ethical recruitment policy, which could legitimize the practice of international recruitment and balance a contradictory policy discourse by appeasing various stakeholders.

The case study of British practice, as well as evidence from other countries, contributes to an understanding of the meaning of contemporary bilateral labour agreements in the contentious context of cross-border labour mobility today and facilitates projections about the future prospects for such agreements. A series of observations can be made.

First, the efficiency of bilateral labour agreements, as recruitment schemes, is much in doubt because such types of agreement are costly, time consuming and place an administrative burden on the civil services of the countries involved. Furthermore, as a tool of labour recruitment, bilateral labour agreements face challenges and competition from the expanding global labour market, where the dominating role is taken by private agencies and individuals themselves since information technology facilitates international job searches. Private agencies have been shown to have more flexible, adaptive and cost-effective strategies, although their high level of competitiveness is often maintained by using "grey" and even illegal practices in recruitment. Rather than issues of how to "compete" with private agencies for foreign labour in the global market using government-to-government agreements, policy-makers at the national level have the more substantial regulatory problem of how to monitor and control the activities of such private agencies to ensure their compliance with national and international laws.

Second, these agreements, despite their decreasing economic role as recruitment tools, have already demonstrated their role in international relations as diplomatic instruments promoting good relations between governments.

Third, for the destination country, in this case the United Kingdom, the negotiation of bilateral agreements was a temporary measure taken to respond to and counter accusations of stimulating the "brain drain".

Finally, while bilateral labour agreements remain an important component of the diplomatic etiquette in international relations, they are losing their position in the recruitment business as private agencies have successfully occupied this niche; this does not exclude the possibility of small-scale, temporary recruitment programmes between countries to target specific problems in the short term. If such recruitment programmes are to be introduced, then government positions should be agreed prior to their conclusion, and also the needs and expectations of employers in destination countries and qualifications and career aspirations of recruited personnel in source countries should be explored to ensure that international recruitment brings a "win–win" solution for stakeholders at both ends of the migration process.

## Acknowledgement

This study forms part of a PhD thesis at the University of Edinburgh, 2011: Plotnikova E, *Recruiting Foreign Nurses for the UK: the Role of Bilateral Labour Agreements*.

## References

Abella M (2004). *Cooperation in managing labour migration in a globalizing world*. Geneva, International Labour Organization (http://eforum.jil.go.jp/foreign/event_r/event/documents/2004sopemi/2004sopemi_e_all.pdf#page=102, accessed 3 January 2014).

Aspen Institute (2011). *Databank of bilateral agreements*. (http://www.aspeninstitute.org/policy-work/global-health-development/news/hwmi-databank-bilateral-agreements, accessed 3 January 2014).

Bach S (2003). *International migration of health workers: labour and social issues*. Geneva, International Labour Organization.

Bach S (2004). *Overseas recruitment of health workers sparks controversy*. Dublin, European Industrial Relations Observatory (http://www.eurofound.europa.eu/eiro/2004/07/feature/uk0407107f.htm, accessed 3 January 2014).

Barbin JG (2004). Recruitment of nurses in Romania by the Friuli-Venezia-Giulia Region in Italy. In OECD, ed. *Migration for employment: bilateral agreements at a crossroads,* Ch. 13. Paris, Organisation for Economic Co-operation and Development.

Blitz BK (2005). "Brain circulation": the Spanish medical profession and international medical recruitment in the United Kingdom. *Journal of European Social Policy,* 15(4):363–379.

Bobeva D, Garson J-P (2004). Overview of bilateral agreements and other forms of labour recruitment. In OECD, ed. *Migration for employment: bilateral agreements at a crossroads.* Paris, Organisation for Economic Co-operation and Development.

Bomba M (2009). Exploring legal frameworks to mitigate the negative effects of international health-worker migration. *Boston University Law Review,* 89(1130):1130–1135.

Buchan J (2003). Here to stay? International nurses in the UK. London, Royal College of Nursing (http://www.rcn.org.uk/__data/assets/pdf_file/0011/78563/001982.pdf, accessed 3 January 2014).

Buchan J, Perfilieva G (2006). *Health worker migration in the European Region: country case studies and policy implications.* Copenhagen, WHO Regional Office for Europe.

Buchan J, Seccombe I (2004). *Fragile future? A review of the UK nursing labour market in 2003.* London, Royal College of Nursing.

Chanda R (2008). *Low-skilled workers and bilateral, regional and unilateral initiatives lessons for the GATS mode 4 negotiations and other agreements.* Geneva, United Nations Development Programme (UNDP Report).

Chanda R (2009). Mobility of less-skilled workers under bilateral agreements: lessons for the GATS. *Journal of World Trade,* 43(3):479–506.

Connell J, Buchan J (2011). The impossible dream? Codes of practice and the international migration of skilled health workers. *World Medical and Health Policy,* 3(3):1–17.

Deeming C (2004). Policy targets and ethical tensions: UK nurse recruitment. *Social Policy and Administration,* 38(7):775–792.

Dumont JC, Zurn P (2007). Immigrant health workers in OECD countries in the broader context of highly skilled migration. In OECD, ed. *International migration outlook,* 2nd edn. Paris, Organisation for Economic Co-operation and Development:161–228.

Fang ZZ (2007). Potential of China in global nurse migration. *Health Services Research*, 42(3):1419–1428.

Federal Ministry of Health and Social Security (2005). *Deutsch–französisches Rahmenabkommen über grenzüberschreitende Zusammenarbeit im Gesundheitsbereich [German–French framework agreement on cross-border cooperation in the health sector].* Berlin, Bundesministerium für Gesundheit und Soziale Sicherung (Press Release 159, 22 July) (http://www.france-allemagne. fr/Deutsch-franzosisches,618.html, accessed 3 January 2014).

Frelick G, Mameja G (2006). *Health workforce innovative approaches and promising practices study. Strategy for the rapid start-up of the HIV/AIDS program in Namibia: outsourcing the recruitment and management of human resources for health.* Chapel Hill, NC, IntraHealth for the Capacity Project (http:// www.intrahealth.org/files/media/strategy-for-the-rapid-start-up-of-the-hivaids- program-in-namibia-outsourcing-the-recruitment-and-management-of-human- resources-for-health/promising_practices_namibia.pdf, accessed 3 January 2014).

Garson JP (2006). Bilateral agreements and other forms of labour recruitment: some lessons from OECD countries' experiences. *Workshop on international migration and labour market in Asia, Tokyo, 17 February.*

Go SP (2007). Asian labor migration: the role of bilateral labor and similar agreements. *Regional informal workshop on labor migration in Southeast Asia: what role for parliaments Manila, 21–23 September.*

Hars A (2003). *Channelled east–west labour migration in the frame of bilateral agreements.* Hamburg, Hamburg Institute of International Economics (http:// www.migration-research.org/EastWest/dokumente/Flowenla13.pdf, accessed 3 January 2014).

Healey M (2006). *Outsourcing care: ethics and consequences of the global trade in Indian nurses.* (http://www.sueztosuva.org.au/south_asia/2006/Healey.pdf, accessed 20 October 2010).

Hendel T (2008). Nurse migration: the donor perspective. In Tschudin V, Davis AJ, eds. *The globalisation of nursing.* Abingdon, UK, Radcliffe:91–103.

International Council of Nurses (2001). *Position statement: ethical nurse recruitment.* Geneva, International Council of Nurses (http://www.icn.ch/ psrecruit01.htm, accessed 3 January 2014).

International Organization for Migration (2003). Illustration of multilateral, regional and bilateral cooperative arrangements in the management of migration. In Aleinikoff TA, Chetail V, eds. *Migration and international legal norms*. The Hague, TMC Asser Press:305–333.

International Organization for Migration (2004). *Labour migration management: current trends, practices and policy issues. The case of health workers*. Geneva, International Organization for Migration (http://www.mofa.go.jp/policy/economy/fta/sympo0407-3.pdf, accessed 3 January 2014).

International Organization for Migration (2005). *Bilateral labour agreements for managing migration*. Geneva, International Organization for Migration (http://www.colomboprocess.org/follow_sub2/session%201/Bilateral%20Labour%20Agreements%20for%20Managing%20Migration.pdf, accessed 3 January 2014).

International Organization for Migration (2008). *World migration report 2008: managing labour mobility in the evolving global economy*. Geneva, International Organization for Migration.

Jordan B (2001). *Nurses face emigration tax*. Durban, Health Systems Trust (http://www.hst.org.za/news/nurses-face-emigration-tax, accessed 3 January 2014).

Khan F, Nixson M (2002). *South Africa takes strain as doctors lured to Britain*. Durban, Health Systems Trust (http://www.hst.org.za/news/south-africa-takes-strain-doctors-lured-britain, accessed 3 January 2014).

Kingma M (2006). *Nurses on the move: migration and the global health care economy*. Ithaca, NY, Cornell University Press.

Meija A (1978). Migration of physicians and nurses: a world-wide picture. *International Journal of Epidemiology*, 7:207–215.

Mission Opérationnelle Transfrontalière (2007). Espaces transfrontaliers. *Proceedings of the European conference on cross-border territories: day-to-day Europe*. Paris, Mission Opérationnelle Transfrontalière (http://www.espaces-transfrontaliers.org/Colloque/ACTES_EN.pdf, accessed 8 October 2013).

Mullan B (1998). The regulation of international migration: the US and Western Europe in comparative historical perspective. In Bocker A et al., eds. *Regulation of migration: international experiences*. Amsterdam, Het Spinhuis: 27–45.

Nielson J (2006). Promoting labor mobility: international migration and trade agreements. *The UNITAR/UNFPA/IOM/ILO Key Migration Workshop Series, 15 March 2006*, New York, United Nations Institute for Training and Research.

OECD (2004). *Migration for employment: bilateral agreements at a crossroads.* Paris, Organisation for Economic Co-operation and Development.

OECD (2010). *International migration of health workers. Improving international co-operation to address the global health workforce crisis.* Paris, Organisation for Economic Co-operation and Development (Policy Brief, February).

Ollier L (2007). *Evaluating the impact and effectiveness of the Department of Health's bilateral cooperation agreements and memoranda of understanding.* London, DH Publications.

Plotnikova E (2011). *Recruiting foreign nurses for the UK: the role of bilateral labour agreements.* Edinburgh, University of Edinburgh Press.

Rollason N (2004). Labour recruitment for skill shortages in the United Kingdom. In OECD, ed. *Migration for employment: bilateral agreements at a crossroads*, Ch. 8. Paris, Organisation for Economic Co-operation and Development.

Scheres J (2006). Coordinating structures in cross-border care. *Seminar on cross-border activities: good practice for better health, Bielefeld, 20–21 January.*

Smith R (1981). Overseas doctors coming to Britain. *British Medical Journal,* 282(6296):1045–1047.

Stilwell B et al. (2004). Migration of health-care workers from developing countries: strategic approaches to its management. *Bulletin of the World Health Organization,* 82(8):595–600.

WHO (1995). *General agreement on trade in services (GATS).* Geneva, World Health Organization (http://www.who.int/trade/glossary/story033/en/index.html, accessed 3 January 2014).

WHO (2004). *Recruitment of health workers from the developing world.* Geneva, World Health Organization (Report by the Secretariat, 114th Session, Provisional agenda item 4.3) (http://apps.who.int/gb/archive/pdf_files/EB114/B114_5-en.pdf, accessed 12 January 2014).

WHO (2010). *WHO global code of practice on the international recruitment of health personnel.* Geneva, World Health Organization (Sixty-third World Health Assembly, WHA63.16) (http://www.who.int/hrh/migration/code/WHO_global_code_of_practice_EN.pdf, accessed 1 October 2013).

Wickramasekara P (2006). Labour migration in Asia. Role of bilateral agreements and MOUs. *Workshop on international migration and labour market in Asia, Tokyo, 17 February.*

Wiskow C, ed. (2006). *Health worker migration flows in Europe: overview and case studies in selected CEE countries: Romania, Czech Republic, Serbia and Croatia.* Geneva, International Labour Organization (Working Paper 245) (http://www.ilo.org/wcmsp5/groups/public/---ed_dialogue/---sector/documents/publication/wcms_161162.pdf, accessed 14 December 2013).

Wismar M et al. (2011). *Cross-border health care in the European Union.* Copenhagen, WHO Regional Office for Europe on behalf of the European Observatory on Health Systems and Policies (Observatory Studies Series 22).

World Trade Organization (2012). *Understanding the WTO: basics. Principles of the trading system.* Geneva, World Trade Organization (http://www.wto.org/english/thewto_e/whatis_e/tif_e/fact2_e.htm#seebox, accessed 3 January 2014).

# Chapter 15

# Creating good workplaces: retention strategies in health-care organizations

*Elisabeth Jelfs, Moritz Knapp, Paul Giepmans and Peter Wijga*

## 15.1 Introduction

Sustainable and accessible health care services substantially depend on their workforce, in terms of both availability and quality (Dubois, Nolte & McKee, 2006). With shortages of health professionals projected by the European Commission to reach nearly 1 million in the EU by 2020 (cited in Sermeus & Bruyneel, 2010), gaps in the health workforce are expected to have a significant impact on the future organization and quality of health care delivery. Although these shortages affect some regions, hospitals or health professions more than others, this is an issue of importance for the health systems of every Member State across the EU.

Health workforce issues have gained increasing attention from EU policy-makers in recent years, with major research projects, council conclusions and the start of Joint Action on Workforce Planning early in 2013. The accent of the debate on professional mobility at European level has often been on the flows of health professionals from one Member State to another at the macro-level. However, as the debate has developed, the discussion has expanded to include the role of employers at local organizational level. This has also been mirrored in the growing body of EU-funded research on the health workforce. As the PROMeTHEUS project has progressed, the results (particularly from the policy dialogues) have pointed towards the importance of action at local organizational level for professional mobility, and specifically the need to develop organizations that convince workers to stay. In line with this, the 12-country Registered Nurse Forecasting (RN4CAST) study has shown that there is promising evidence that improving work environments can improve both nurse retention and quality of care (Aiken, 2011; Sermeus et al., 2011). A review in 2010 on improving access to health workers in remote and rural areas carried out by the WHO has highlighted the importance of human resource management and organizational capacity, and the need for "individuals with strong management and leadership skills, particularly at the facility level" (WHO, 2010, p. 15).

Taken together with the increasing attention for the organizational level, these studies pose a number of questions. What do we know about retention at organizational level and measures to improve it? What are health care organizations in Europe doing to respond to the challenges of staff retention? And where can action at different levels of the health system add most value? Building on the existing literature, this chapter looks at a broad sweep of measures to retain staff through case studies from three different hospitals in the public sector, with a particular emphasis on nursing retention. To give context to these case studies, the chapter starts with a look at the literature (focusing on Europe, but also drawing on relevant North American studies), pulling together some findings from existing research. The chapter also seeks to provide suggestions for some potential pathways for action at EU, national and local levels in these areas.

## 15.2 What do we know about retention strategies in health care?

### 15.2.1 Insights from the literature

Staff turnover is a natural and necessary process in all health care organizations. However, when turnover reaches high levels it can have a detrimental effect on quality of care (Gray & Phillips, 1996; Tai, Bame & Robinson, 1998; Shields & Ward, 2001; Gunnarsdóttir et al., 2009; Buchan, 2010; Simon, Müller & Hasselhorn, 2010), as well as being costly (Jones, 2004; Waldman et al., 2004; O'Brien-Pallas et al., 2006). Further problems arise when employees leave not only the organization but the health workforce itself. In a sector that is already suffering from shortages, employees are often difficult to replace. For the sake of clarity, we use the term "turnover" for employees leaving the organization and "attrition" for employees leaving the health workforce. As the chapter focuses at organizational level, the emphasis is on initiatives to maintain appropriate levels of turnover. However, where strategies to prevent attrition overlap with strategies to manage turnover, these are reflected in the discussion. The chapter focuses on the health professional (and particularly nursing) workforce rather than the health workforce in general because of the weight of current research evidence on which the case study framework has been built.

## 15.2.2 Influencing staff retention: causes and responses

The literature identifies a range of factors that are reported to have an impact on retention within the health workforce (WHO, 2010). Within this wider scope of recommendations, which includes interventions in education (e.g. Frenk et al., 2010) and regulation, this section focuses on interventions on an organizational level, and hospitals in particular as evidence shows the positive effect of good working environments on retention (Hinno, Partanen & Vehvilainen-Julkunen, 2011). From this perspective, differentiation is usually made between external factors (e.g. the general economic situation and the labour market), individual factors (e.g. educational level, length of service, non-professional commitments) and organizational factors (those relating to the way in which a health care organization is managed) (Hayes et al., 2006); the last is the main focus of this chapter.

To provide a framework for the case studies, the organizational factors are divided into three dimensions, based on the work of Wiskow, Albrecht and De Pietro (2010) (Table 15.1):

* employment quality

* work quality

* organizational quality.

Wiskow, Albrecht and De Pietro (2010) recognized employment and work quality, while organizational quality and a number of elements resulting from the literature review have been added here. The dimensions are chosen to focus on interventions on an organizational level. Employment quality refers to the contractual relationships between employer and employee, work quality the material characteristics of the tasks that employees carry out and the work environment in which they act, and organizational quality the measure wherein the organization is able to adapt to changes in the outside world.

### *Employment quality*

Studies show that although wages are often seen as one of the most obvious factors influencing staff retention, it is difficult to draw firm conclusions on the effects of improving remuneration. For nurses, an OECD Working Paper concluded that: "the impact of pay increases on the nurses' labour market is not easy to define … The least what [sic] can be said is that the pay increases

**Table 15.1** Organizational factors for case studies

| Dimension | Elements |
| --- | --- |
| Employment quality | Wages |
| | Type of contract, e.g. permanent, temporary |
| | Working hours, including work schedules and family–work balance |
| | Social benefits |
| Work quality | Professional development (training and skills development) |
| | Work organization, including teamwork, division of work, staffing adequacy, administrative burden |
| | Safety |
| | Pace of work and stress |
| | Social work environment |
| | Access to technology/appropriate facilities to get one's job done |
| Organizational quality | Leadership (management, participation in decision-making processes)[a] |
| | Culture |
| | Quality (improvement programmes, complaints committees, innovation) |
| | Appropriate professional autonomy |

*Source*: adapted from Wiskow, Albrecht & De Pietro, 2010.

[a] This chapter considers management as being the organization and coordination of the activities of an organization in order to achieve defined objectives; leadership is the activity of leading a group of people or an organization.

had a favourable effect on the number of new potential entrants in nursing education" (Buchan & Black, 2011, p. 4). Tai, Bame and Robinson (1998) concluded that higher salaries are rarely a successful measure for retention although there is some indication from some studies on nurse supply of a weak positive correlation between wage and labour supply (Antonazzo et al., 2003; Chiha & Link, 2003; Shields, 2004).

Health care professionals often undertake shift, night and weekend work, with evidence suggesting that professionals carrying out this type of work often suffer from increased levels of stress and fatigue (Costa, 2003; Schernhammer & Thompson, 2010). This has been associated by Aiken et al. (2002) with threats to patient safety. Irregular working hours also impact the work–life balance of health care professionals, particularly for female employees, with women still carrying the major part of family responsibilities (van der Heijden, Demerouti & Bakker, 2008).

Social benefits are an important part of the employment quality dimension. Contractual relationships that allow for pension schemes, flexible retirement policies, childcare provisions, and so on have shown to be factors influencing job quality (Wiskow, Albrecht & De Pietro, 2010; Muñoz de Bustillo et al., 2009). Carraher and Buckley (2008), however, found only a weak relationship between attitudes towards benefits (although these are not clearly defined) and turnover. Although contract type is sometimes included in retention typologies, there was little evidence in the literature surveyed on the impact of different types of contract (e.g. permanent or temporary) on retention.

### *Work quality*

The definition of work quality most often used at European level is that of Muñoz de Bustillo et al. (2009, p. 14): "how the activity of work itself and the conditions under which it takes place can affect the well-being of workers: the work intensity, social environment, physical environment, etc."

Work quality, therefore, includes a number of variables around inappropriate or unsafe work. For example, high levels of administrative burden (such as non-patient care duties for clinical staff) have been shown to have a negative effect on retention (Aiken et al., 2001). In addition to this, there are many studies on the negative effects of work-related stress in health care, particularly from high workload.[1] Empirical studies have found burn-out rates of around 35% and job dissatisfaction of 35% (the average of a sample of nurses from nine countries; Aiken et al., 2009). Studies show that the consequences of continued high levels of stress for health care professionals include not only absenteeism, reduced productivity, accidents and errors but also high staff turnover (European Agency for Occupational Safety and Health, 2009; van Wyk & van Wyk, 2010).

The impact of health and safety incidents on affected staff is similar to that of stress: resulting in high staff turnover (Di Martino, 2002). Needlestick injuries, heavy physical work (such as lifting patients), physical violence or intimidation and exposure to patients with communicable diseases are but a few of these risks. In a study by Estryn-Behar et al. (2008), 22% of nurses reported exposure to frequent violent events from patients or relatives, and those exposed to violence also had higher levels of stress and burn-out and reported more intentions to leave the profession or organization. Initiatives addressing the safety and health of health care professionals, in addition to being a moral and legal responsibility, can therefore be significant in improving retention of staff.

The literature also suggests that the social working environment (such as support from colleagues or nurse–doctor relations; Gunnarsdóttir et al., 2009) may also be of some importance to retention, although evidence is not as complete as for some other factors (van der Heijden & Kuemmerling, 2003). Rosenstein (2002) found that nurse–doctor relationships play an important role in nurse satisfaction and retention. Tai, Bame and Robinson (1998) have proposed that an increased perceived climate of personal and work group support reduces the

---

1 The European Agency for Occupational Safety and Health defines work-related stress as the inability of the worker to cope with or control the demands of the work environment.

likelihood of turnover. In particular, their research found that high levels of support from supervisors were shown to be strongly inversely correlated with turnover.

The importance of CPD (the opportunities organizations provide to their employees to continuously evolve professionally and personally, such as training, mentoring and lifelong learning) was also represented in the literature. In particular, Shields and Ward (2001) found that dissatisfaction with promotion and training opportunities has a stronger impact on nurse turnover than workload or pay.

Lastly, a number of typologies suggest that access to technology and appropriate facilities (availability of resources for effective working; Wiskow, Albrecht & De Pietro, 2010) is an important factor in retention. Although the literature surveyed for this study did not identify strong evidence for or against this, the focus groups carried out in the framework of the PROMeTHEUS study (see Chapter 7) support this suggestion.

### *Organizational quality*

In the domain of organizational quality, the literature on retention has a particular emphasis on the relationship between leadership and staff satisfaction. Indeed dissatisfaction with management styles has been shown to be a major driver in nurse job dissatisfaction and turnover (Bratt et al., 2000; Hayes et al., 2006). On the one hand, health professionals have reported dissatisfaction with their level of influence over their work, the perception of not being heard, disconnection between management and the work floor, lack of shared decision-making and lack of recognition (OECD, 2008). On the other hand, participation in decision-making processes, where representation in management is ensured (e.g. through a nurse advisory committee), has been found to enhance job satisfaction (Jones et al., 1993; Nakata & Saylor, 1994; Moss & Rowles, 1997; Yeatts & Seward, 2000). In a similar vein, a facilitative rather than directive management style has positive effects on retention, as does a leadership style that values staff contribution (Hayes et al., 2006). Aiken, Smith and Lake (1994) and Buchan (1994) have found positive effects of a decentralized organizational structure on retention. For doctors, evidence from Janus et al. (2008) suggests that decision-making and recognition are particularly important.

Along these lines, a number of studies have also argued that professional autonomy, the "freedom to act on what one knows" (Gunnarsdóttir & Rafferty, 2006), is a central factor for job satisfaction. Employer–worker arrangements such as self-governance, self-control, appropriate freedom and control over resources can give health professionals enough room to act and improve their perception of empowerment (Hayes et al., 2006). Kramer and Schmalenberg (2003) have found a strong relationship between the degree of nurse autonomy and ratings of job satisfaction (exact definition varying in the literature) and quality of care. Levels of job satisfaction are again correlated with intention to leave (which is associated with levels of turnover; Irvine & Evans, 1995; Coomber & Barriball, 2007), although a direct link was not established in the study by Hayes et al. (2006). Table 15.2 summarizes possible interventions with a positive effect on staff retention.

**Table 15.2** Possible interventions with a positive effect on staff retention

| Issue | Recommended interventions |
|---|---|
| *Employment quality* | |
| Wages | Fair wages using wage grids recognizing different education/experience levels; renegotiate work terms following skills upgrading |
| Type of contract (e.g. permanent, temporary) | Monitor individuals' wishes; allow for decisions on individual level |
| Working hours, including work schedules and family–work balance | Flexible working hours with family-oriented core times; maternity and parental leave; child-care provisions; reduction of work recalls; national policies on working times and flexibility; restrictions on work during night shifts; self-scheduling strategies |
| Social benefits | Leave and compensation benefits; health insurance schemes; pension schemes; flexible retirement policies |
| *Work quality* | |
| Professional development (training and skills development) | Career development programmes; mentorship programmes; make professional development part of budget planning |
| Appropriate autonomy | Allow for organizational units (e.g. wards) to shape their work based on direct feedback from staff, possibly varying from organizational line |
| Work organization (including teamwork, division of work, staffing, administrative burden) | Task shifting; work reorganization; job redesign; interdisciplinary staffing; adapted workload levels for pregnant workers and the older workforce |
| Health and safety | *Violence*: training, better teamwork; zero-tolerance policies; support programmes |
| | *Injuries*: awareness-raising, protective equipment; designing ergonomically sound work environments |
| Pace of work and stress | Caseload management database; make use of support personnel |
| Social work environment | Open and timely communication within team and between employer and worker; improving nurse–physician relationships |
| Access to technology/appropriate facilities/resources | To allow the job to get done |

**Table 15.2** contd

| Issue | Recommended interventions |
|---|---|
| *Organizational quality* | |
| Leadership (management, participation) | Decentralized organizational structure; shared governance; facilitating rather than directing management style; accessible management ("open door") |
| Culture | Motivating, service and safety climates; cross-disciplinary collaboration; organizational trust |
| Quality | Improvement programmes; complaints committees |

*Source*: adapted from Tran et al. (2008) and supplemented by results from the case studies and literature review.

## 15.3 Case studies

### 15.3.1 Introduction and methodology

In order to explore retention approaches and strategies at organizational level, interviews were carried out with staff from three hospitals: Canisius Wilhelmina Ziekenhuis (CWZ), Nijmegen, the Netherlands; Landeskrankenhaus Feldkirch (LKH), Austria, and the Children's Hospital, Vilnius, Lithuania (Table 15.3).

**Table 15.3** Case study hospitals

| | Canisius Wilhelmina Ziekenhuis | Landeskrankenhaus Feldkirch | Children's Hospital Vilnius |
|---|---|---|---|
| Country | Netherlands | Austria | Lithuania |
| City | Nijmegen | Feldkirch | Vilnius |
| Type of hospital | Top clinical hospital | Federal Academic Teaching Hospital | Children's hospital |
| Number of beds | 649 | 606 | n/a |

*Note*: n/a: Not available.

The aim was to find hospitals active in working to retain staff but doing so within their existing resources. None were in receipt of specific funding from external sources to develop retention strategies except for some limited funding for CPD in Lithuania through the European structural funds. The hospitals were chosen to illustrate approaches to retention in diverse health system contexts, and in particular to reflect different professional mobility contexts. As the case studies carried out through the PROMeTHEUS project have shown (Wismar et al., 2011), the Netherlands is typically a destination country for health professionals, Lithuania is typically a source country, and Austria is both a source and destination country. The hospitals in Austria and the Netherlands are located in semi-urban rather than urban areas and are located close to a border (Switzerland and Liechtenstein and Germany, respectively).

These case studies are not intended to provide comparative material but rather to test findings of the literature review against practice within health care organizations. The case studies explore both the underlying motivations behind why hospitals have a focus on retention, and also the types of approach and strategy used.

Within these three hospitals, human resources managers and general directors were interviewed (four interviews in total) by the authors using a structured interview approach. The template used consisted of a number of sections covering the three dimensions identified in the literature review: motivations for retention strategies, characteristics of the strategy, outcomes and the capacity to implement.

### 15.3.2 Case 1: CWZ, Nijmegen, the Netherlands

The CWZ is a top clinical hospital with 649 beds, 200 medical specialists and 3 698 other staff (detailed numbers for other groups such as nurses are not publically available). The annual budget is €227.4 million. In 2010, CWZ had 73 271 clinical admissions and 366 500 outpatient visits. The interviewees for CWZ were a human resources manager and an adviser.

#### *The health workforce situation*

Staff turnover in 2010 was 4.5% (corrected for short-term personnel, e.g. holiday staff). In the Netherlands, there was an annual gross mobility of nurses of 10–12% in the period 2002–2009, with 6% moving to another organization in the sector and 6% moving out (Arbeidsmarkt Zorg en Welzijn (Labour, Health and Welfare research programme)). Competition in the local labour market is relatively low: the only other hospital in Nijmegen is a large academic hospital with a very different profile to CWZ.

#### *Approaches to retention*

In the previous three to four years, CWZ had paid increasing attention to turnover and staff retention. In 2010, a new strategy was developed by the hospital to focus on personalizing patient care, which in terms of human resources strategy was translated to give a focus on "bind and captivate". In the view of CWZ, high-quality care is a means of attracting and retaining personnel. The strategy, developed with employees' input, was particularly targeted at nurses and medical support staff – core functions where there were typically shortages in the labour market – and groups that have high turnover within the organization. Parallel to the development of this strategy, CWZ developed the "excellent care programme" with six other hospitals in the Netherlands. This programme focuses on the quality of patient care as well as the quality of the working environment, and it promotes individual career development pathways; direct, near real-time, feedback of relevant patient outcomes to clinical staff; and evidence-based working. The initiative allows data and learning experiences to be shared and compared between the participating hospitals.

### Characteristics of the strategies employed

#### Employment quality

The hospital's approach to retention is not particularly focused on many of the "classic" dimensions of employment quality. For example, wages are oriented at what is normal in the market and there is no particular innovation in contracts. CWZ provides some minor social and fiscal benefits but these are not considered the focus of the strategy.

#### Work quality

By contrast, CWZ has invested significantly in elements with a positive impact on work quality. Continuous training is offered and career development plans are in place. Nurses are considered to have "room to influence" their work rather than full autonomy, while feedback of patient outcomes in near real-time gives significant information on performance that allows nurses to have more control over their practice. The hospital also has a "flex office" with employees that provide additional support to departments experiencing peaks in workload. If a team or department shows higher levels of absence because of sickness, actions are taken in the organization and workload of the team. Regarding technology, the hospital does not focus per se on primary technological innovations but rather on the smart application of technology that has proven itself elsewhere. Having introduced several technological innovations as the first hospital in the Netherlands, CWZ also sees itself as a frontrunner in this matter.

#### Organizational quality

In addition to actions that impact on work quality, CWZ has a particular focus on organizational and care quality. The core values and strategy of the hospital were developed together with hospital personnel. This engagement of staff is also carried into governance of the hospital; for example, nurse representatives act as an advisory body and also chair the Excellent Care Programme. Although it remains difficult to draw clear causal links between quality of care and attractiveness for personnel, in an evaluation of personnel satisfaction CWZ scored higher on loyalty and recognition of company values than any other hospital in the review. The hospital has consistently scored the top ranking in quality rankings of Dutch hospitals.

### 15.3.3 Case 2: Landeskrankenhaus, Feldkirch, Austria

LKH Feldkirch (Federal Academic Teaching Hospital Feldkirch) is part of a holding of public hospitals in the State of Vorarlberg. The hospital has a budget of €185 million and 606 beds. Its staff consists of 276 physicians, 110 medical assistants, 753 nurses and 387 technicians and administration: a total of 1 526. On average annually, 38 000 inpatients spend 166 500 nights in the hospital. It covers the treatment of 60 000 outpatients with 150 000 visits per year. The annual staff turnover rate is 7.5%. The Administrative Director of LKH was interviewed for the case study.

#### The health workforce situation

Although Vorarlberg is wealthier than other Austrian regions, it borders prosperous Switzerland and Liechtenstein. It is therefore in competition for staff with these countries. LKH started to experience workforce shortages from 2007, finding it harder to fill vacancies and to replace retiring doctors and nurses. In 2010, LKH commissioned a specific study that confirmed projected shortages, particularly of doctors, and recommended that specific steps be taken to retain and attract staff.

#### Approaches to retention

Following the identification of workforce shortages, LKH management carried out a survey of all staff to identify retention factors. Five areas were particularly highlighted: adequate and fair compensation, working hours/work–life balance, childcare, CPD and other benefits such as housing or staff cafeteria facilities.

#### Characteristics of the strategies employed

##### Employment quality

It is difficult for LKH to intervene on some of the key elements of employment quality, particularly wages. As a public employer, LKH is obliged to follow official wage tables that are negotiated and agreed through a political and administrative process at the state level. LKH senior management have therefore been working with the state government to influence necessary adjustments. However, in other areas LKH has more freedom of action. As the largest hospital within the holding, LKH has considerable influence over policies at holding level (e.g. working hours and CPD), as well as policies decided at hospital level (e.g. childcare facilities and local housing). LKH owns residential properties and facilities that it can offer to existing or incoming staff at subsidized prices or for free (for a short time). LKH provides in-house childcare facilities.

*Work quality*

The interviewee highlighted that for LKH staff work quality is strongly related to provision of childcare facilities and management of the family–work balance. The trend of increasing female preponderance of the clinical workforce (*Medizin wird weiblich*) was underlined as a strong impetus for tailored support. LKH has therefore undertaken targeted surveys with young female professionals to identify issues affecting employment quality.

*Organizational quality*

In order to devise and implement its retention strategy, LKH management engaged in a series of consultations with clinical staff. Clinical staff have been supportive of the initiatives and participated in a number of informal work groups that operated in addition to the formal structures for employee participation, such as the clinical advisory council (*Ärztlicher Beirat*) or the medical chamber (*Ärztekammer*). Work groups met to deal with particular issues and when these had been resolved the groups were disbanded.

### 15.3.4 Case 3: Children's Hospital, Vilnius, Lithuania

The Children's Hospital Vilnius (Affiliate of Vilnius University Hospital Santariskiu Klinikos) has a budget of approximately €26 million and is staffed by 280 doctors and 530 nurses. The hospital has more than 25 000 inpatient admissions and around 140 000 outpatient consultations every year. The hospital is a specialist paediatric hospital located in Lithuania's capital city. The head of the human resources department and the hospital's deputy management director were interviewed for the case study.

### *The health workforce situation*

Although Lithuania is considered a source country for health professional migration, the interview highlighted internal migration over migration to other EU Member States. Most nurses had moved to work for other hospitals within Lithuania in order to benefit from higher wages. Despite these pressures, the Children's Hospital has succeeded in retaining most of its staff.

### *Approaches to retention*

Because of time and resource pressures, the Children's Hospital has taken a step-by-step approach to dealing with retention issues, using an ad hoc approach rather than developing an overall strategy. It was recognized within the interview that a cohesive strategy would add value as it would "allow setting a long-term policy rather than a 'one problem at a time' approach". However, resources available for retention interventions were generally low. The hospital retention interventions have also focused more on nurse retention than doctors because the hospital experiences more nurses leaving the workplace than doctors.

### Characteristics of the strategies employed

#### Employment quality

The Children's Hospital is free, within a given framework, to set wages. According to the interviewee, this has been instrumental in retaining staff, both keeping them at the Children's Hospital rather than moving to other hospitals and, perhaps, stopping them from leaving the sector altogether. The hospital's focus on wages can be further explained by the choice of many nurses to work more than one full-time equivalent as a single wage is considered insufficient.

#### Work quality

As a consequence of its links to the university, the Children's Hospital emphasizes CPD. Each employee has 10 paid days per year for CPD; the courses are organized by the university and hospitals and are sometimes financed through the European structural funds. The CPD courses include how to cope with stress and manage conflict, a course established to address workload issues specifically for staff in accident and emergency and intensive care units.

#### Organization quality

There is evidence of senior management working to create a culture of shared problem solving and agenda setting with staff. Hospital management tries to address upcoming issues in cooperation with internal representatives including in areas such as improving staff safety, for example in the context of an increasing risk of hepatitis. The interview also underlined the hospital's reputation as an academic centre, which has had the consequence of both attracting and retaining staff.

## 15.3.5 Analysis of the case studies

The diversity of practice illustrated in the case studies highlights the importance of local context for understanding how to retain staff. However, when taken together, the case studies confirm and complement a number of findings within the literature review.

On employment quality, the case studies reflect the diversity within the literature on the importance of wages. These ranged from an environment where it was one of the most significant retention factors (Lithuania) through to Austria, where wages were in part an issue (but difficult to change on an organizational level), to the Netherlands, where changes to wages were not a strategic focus. There are indications that the difficult economic conditions facing the Children's Hospital in Lithuania may have made wages particularly important, given that almost half the hospital staff worked more than one full-time equivalent (the reported average was 1.25 full-time equivalents worked). The importance of wages was also strongly driven by the specific local context of the hospitals: in the case of LKH this was a cross-border wage competition; for the Children's Hospital in Lithuania most wage competition reported for nurses was with other Lithuanian hospitals. Concerning the question of family–work balance, the hospitals took different approaches. In line with findings from van der Heijden, Demerouti and Bakker (2008), LKH had identified pressure on family–work balance, particularly for women, as a central issue and had deployed specific initiatives in response. However, the other hospitals had not specifically targeted women or family–work conditions, with CWZ, in particular, focusing more on work quality in general.

On work quality, all three hospitals saw CPD as an important factor in retention. At LKH, it was one of the top five priorities, and CWZ had instituted individual career development pathways. At the Children's Hospital, the 10 paid days for CPD for staff members ensured that it was a strong priority, with courses specifically tailored to support the working environment. There was, however, a mixed approach to the question of autonomy despite its strength in the literature. Of the three hospitals, CWZ offered the most immediate near real-time feedback to nursing staff, allowing nurses to shape their practice and perhaps giving a greater element of control. The other hospitals did not highlight autonomy, which is interesting given that it is considered an important factor in the literature. How hospitals can best translate concepts of professional autonomy into practice remains an area for exploration.

On organizational quality, in line with findings from the literature, all three hospitals had invested significant time in developing participatory styles of management and leadership. Although their exact strategies differed, early and meaningful participation from staff, monitoring and addressing emerging issues, and creating a culture of deliberation with staff were regarded as highly important for staff retention in all three hospitals. The CWZ and the Children's Hospital both noted that their organization had a particular "brand" vis-à-vis other hospitals. For the Children's Hospital, this was attributed to well-respected professors who have their names connected to the institution, which according to their staff attracts health workers. The CWZ shares the "market" with a university hospital but argues that they do not need to compete for staff as some people prefer not to work for this university hospital given its specific patient population and more hierarchical organizational structure.

Either intentional or not, "branding" of hospitals may be an important factor in creating a culture with which staff workers can identify themselves.

Moving beyond individual factors, the hospital case studies raise questions on how strategies are developed at organizational level, how national and regional policies frame these strategies, and the role of robust research evidence in shaping them. At LKH, an external analysis had been undertaken and priorities assessed with staff; at CWZ, the strategy had been likewise developed with staff members. At the Children's Hospital, an ad hoc approach was taken, although the value of a strategic approach was recognized. However, none of the interviewees mentioned access to policy recommendations (e.g. WHO, 2010) or external evidence on the effectiveness of different interventions or cost–benefit analysis. From the case studies, it is clear that the input from health workers is of key importance, which implies the importance of input mechanisms to include their input.

Organizational strategies and actions might also illustrate the view of hospital managers on workforce challenges, which remains limited to their local situation, and each of the interviewees considered different challenges important to them. CWZ linked actions to the improvement of patient quality in a coherent strategy that linked to the emerging evidence on the relation between patient care quality and staffing adequacy and quality; LKH felt the pressure of regional mobility while the Children's Hospital Vilnius was trying to control emerging issues that were in their scope of action. In all three cases, hospitals appear to succeed by applying a range of managerial responses; however, this range of action is subject to national and regional policy frameworks.

## 15.4 Discussion and conclusions

Recognition of the role of retention within workforce mobility debates has increased significantly in recent years. The findings from recent EU research further emphasize the importance of moving beyond knowledge of how many health care professionals move and where they move to. Increasing understanding of why people leave, or stay in, organizations or the profession gives a broader and necessary frame for local management and national policy-makers to develop appropriate responses for recruitment and retention. Possibilities and options for successfully changing conditions and working environments are possible responses at organizational and policy level to mitigate the impact of an ageing workforce and reducing workforce shortages.

### 15.4.1 Research gaps

Attempting to push beyond an analysis of individual retention factors towards analysing their impact and developing strategic approaches reveals significant gaps in current knowledge. Although the literature is strong in identifying a wide variety of factors, there is relatively little literature evaluating the impact of particular retention initiatives, particularly their cost–effectiveness (also seen in findings of the WHO-commissioned realist review and synthesis of retention studies for health workers in rural and remote areas; Dieleman et al., 2011). Indeed the literature rarely discusses strategic approaches to retention (i.e. combining different initiatives tailored to a health care organization's particular need). While it is one thing to identify factors that have a large impact on retention, it is another to develop coherent retention strategies. Coherent organizational strategies, however, have the potential to align with policy "packages" that are required to address workforce challenges (WHO, 2010), which would allow for better interaction between policy initiatives and organizational practice. Even focusing on the literature on nurse retention, which is significantly more developed than for other health professions, there is only limited material on coherent strategies that specifically aim at retaining personnel.

There is, therefore, a need for research studies that move beyond looking at individual factors and possible responses to strategic approaches that link and prioritize interventions, evaluating their impact.[2] Research that explores the interaction between factors is needed, not only for decision-makers at organizational level (as their scope of action is limited as well) but also for policy-makers setting the frameworks in which organizations operate. With most policy-makers and managers facing difficult decisions on priorities and an increased squeeze on resources, it is particularly important that cost–effectiveness is considered.

If these knowledge gaps are substantial at hospital level, there are even more substantial gaps in looking at the non-medical workforce and beyond hospitals into primary care. The emerging policy drive to shift care away from hospitals and into community or primary care settings also suggests that retention outside hospital environments will become increasingly important in order to manage potential workforce shortages.

### 15.4.2 Organizational level interventions

As this chapter has demonstrated, action at the organization level is central. Although some actions are often carried out at other levels (e.g. wage

---

2 Please note that since this chapter was completed a study on this subject has started in January 2014, mapping recruitment and retention practices across the Euopean Union.

agreements), a number of critical elements that affect staff retention, including organizational and work quality, are primarily located at organization level and many interventions can only work if they are enacted locally.

Developing the existing typologies for assessing retention factors, both the literature and the case studies underline the importance of "organizational quality": the framing governance and management of organizations that shape the environment in which employees work. In particular, the case studies emphasize the need to know what employees want and to develop participatory leadership and management models that engage with staff and preserve an ongoing culture of deliberation and discussion. It is interesting to note that these changes do not necessarily imply significant extra resource investment, although culture change is not in itself without difficulty.

### 15.4.3 Regional and national level interventions

Although there is much that can be done at organization level, the literature and case studies suggest that there are particular domains where regional and national levels are of primary importance. In many EU Member States, wages are set not within the organization but beyond it, and there is a need for regional and national governments to engage (possibly through workers' representatives) with local employers, perhaps by allowing border regions experiencing considerable pressure from mobility to adapt their wages. In addition to bargaining higher wages, regional or local governments can also play an important role by supporting health providers and their staff with other social benefits, including reduced housing costs or childcare, and setting a retention-supporting context and framework in which organizations can operate. Regional and national levels also have a potential role in developing programmes that support organizational quality. In the Netherlands, for example, the *In voor Zorg!* (*In for Care!*) programme, an initiative from the Dutch Ministry for Health, Science and Sport and Vilans (Centre of Expertise for Long-term Care), aims to support care providers to make their work processes supportive to health workers: making knowledge available on existing solutions and providing support for organizations to run change projects.

### 15.4.4 EU interventions

The EU has a number of potential avenues available for increasing knowledge on retention and for facilitating the exchange of good practice at national, regional and organizational level. First, the EU's research programme Horizon2020, which includes funding for health services research projects, may support workforce research that gives organizations knowledge on effective strategic approaches to retain their staff. This will be an important component of strengthening the health workforce for the future, safeguarding quality of care even within times of resource constraint and higher demand for services. Second, the European Commission's Public Health Programme also offers potential ways to support and strengthen workforce retention, for example through the exchange of good practice in implementing retention measures, particularly through coherent strategies. Lastly, the revision of the structural funds programme provides a potential opportunity to support retention in order to ensure staffing adequacy as a priority within the funding for health. In particular, the structural funds may allow regions to direct resources to local levels to encourage the development of effective training and CPD, factors shown through this chapter to be of high importance for hospitals addressing retention issues across very different health system contexts.

## References

Aiken LH (2011). RN4CAST: Evidence from Europe and the US for improving nurse retention and patient outcomes. *International Society for Quality in Health Care 28th International Conference, Hong Kong, 14–17 September.*

Aiken LH, Smith HL, Lake ET (1994). Lower Medicare mortality among a set of hospitals known for good nursing care. *Medical Care*, 32(8):771–787.

Aiken LH et al. (2001). Nurses' reports on hospital care in five countries. *Health Affairs*, 20(3): 43–53.

Aiken LH et al. (2002). Hospital nurse staffing and patient mortality, nurse burnout, and job dissatisfaction. *Journal of the American Medical Association*, 288(16):1987–1993.

Aiken LH, Cheung RB, Olds DM (2009). Education policy initiatives to address the nurse shortage in the United States *Health Affairs*, 28(4):646–656.

Antonazzo EA et al. (2003). The labour market for nursing: a review of the labour supply literature. *Health Economics*, 12:465–478.

Bratt MM et al. (2000). Influence of stress and nursing leadership on job satisfaction of paediatric intensive care unit nurses. *American Journal of Critical Care*, 9:307–317.

Buchan J (1994). Nursing shortages and human resource planning. *International Journal of Nursing Studies*, 31(5):460–470.

Buchan J (2010). The benefits of health workforce stability. *Human Resources for Health*, 8:29.

Buchan J, Black S (2011). *The impact of pay increases on nurses' labour market: a review of evidence from four OECD countries.* Paris, Organisation for Economic Co-operation and Development (OECD Health Working Paper No. 57) (http://www.eurofedop.org/IMG/pdf/OECD_publication_-_The_impact_of_pay_increases_on_nurses_labour_market_2011_09_23_EN_FR_PUB. pdf, accessed 8 October 2013).

Carraher SM, Buckley MR (2008). Attitudes towards benefits and behavioral intentions and their relationship to absenteeism, performance, and turnover among nurses. *Academy of Health Care Management Journal,* 4(2):89–105.

Chiha YA, Link CR (2003). The shortage of registered nurses and some new estimates of the effects of wages on registered nurses labour supply: a look at the past and a preview of the 21st century. *Health Policy,* 64(3):349–375.

Coomber B, Barriball KL (2007). Impact of job satisfaction components on intent to leave and turnover for hospital-based nurses: a review of the research literature. *International Journal of Nursing Studies,* 44(2):297–314.

Costa G (2003). Shift work and occupational medicine: an overview. *Occupational Medicine,* 53:83–88.

Di Martino V (2002). Workplace violence in the health sector: country case studies Brazil, Bulgaria, Lebanon, Portugal, South Africa, Thailand and an additional Australian study – Synthesis report. *ILO/ICN/WHO/PSI joint programme on workplace violence in the health sector.* Geneva, International Labour Office (http://www.who.int/violence_injury_prevention/injury/work9/en/index3.html, accessed 2 January 2014).

Dieleman M et al. (2011). *Realist review and synthesis of retention studies for health workers in rural and remote areas.* Geneva, World Health Organization.

Dubois C-A, Nolte E, McKee M (2006). Analysing trends, opportunities and challenges. In Dubois C-A, Nolte E, McKee M, eds. *Human resources for health in Europe.* Maidenhead, UK, Open University Press:15–40.

Estryn-Behar MB et al. (2008). Violence risks in nursing: results from the European 'NEXT' Study. *Occupational Medicine,* 58:107–114.

European Agency for Occupational Safety and Health (2009). *OSH in figures: stress at work: facts and figures.* Luxembourg, Office for Official Publications of the European Communities (https://osha.europa.eu/en/publications/reports/TE-81-08-478-EN-C_OSH_in_figures_stress_at_work, accessed 8 October 2013).

Frenk J et al. (2010). Health professionals for a new century: transforming education to strengthen health systems in an interdependent world. *Lancet,* 376(9756):1923–195

Gray AM, Phillips VL (1996). Labour turnover in the British National Health Service: a local labour market analysis. *Health Policy*, 36:273–289.

Gunnarsdóttir S, Rafferty AM (2006). Enhancing working conditions. In Dubois C-A, Nolte E, McKee M, eds. *Human resources for health in Europe*. Maidenhead, UK, Open University Press:155–172.

Gunnarsdóttir S et al. (2009). Front-line management, staffing and nurse–doctor relationships as predictors of nurse and patient outcomes. *International Journal of Nursing Studies*, 4(7):920–927.

Hayes LJ et al. (2006). Nurse turnover: a literature review. *International Journal of Nursing Studies*, 43:237–263.

Hinno S, Partanen P, Vehvilainen-Julkunen K (2011). Hospital nurses' work environment, quality of care provided and career plans. *International Nursing Review*, 58:255–262.

Irvine DM, Evans MG (1995). Job satisfaction and turnover among nurses: integrating research findings across studies. *Nursing Research*, 44(4):246–253.

Janus K et al. (2008). Job satisfaction and motivation among physicians in academic medical centres: insights from a cross-national study. *Journal of Health Politics, Policy and Law*, 33(6):1133–1167.

Jones CB (2004). The costs of nurse turnover. *Journal of Nursing Administration*, 34(12):562–566.

Jones CB et al. (1993). Shared governance and the nursing practice environment. *Nursing Economics*, 11(4):208–214.

Kramer M, Schmalenberg C (2003). Securing "good" nurse–physician relationship. *Nursing Management*, 34(7):34–38.

Moss R, Rowles CJ (1997). Staff nurse job satisfaction and management style. *Nursing Management*, 28(1):32–34.

Muñoz de Bustillo R et al. (2009). *Indicators of job quality in the European Union*. Brussels, European Parliament.

Nakata JA, Saylor C (1994). Management style and staff nurse satisfaction in a changing environment. *Nursing Administration Quarterly*, 18(3):51–57.

O'Brien-Pallas L et al. (2006). The impact of nurse turnover on patient, nurse, and system outcomes: a pilot study and focus for a multicenter international study. *Policy, Politics, and Nursing Practice*, 7:169–179.

OECD (2008). *The looming crisis in the health workforce. How can OECD countries respond?* Paris, Organisation for Economic Co-operation and Development

(OECD Health Policy Studies) (http://www.who.int/hrh/migration/looming_crisis_health_workforce.pdf, accessed 15 December 2013).

Rosenstein AH (2002). Nurse–physician relationships: impact on nurse satisfaction and retention. *American Journal of Nursing*, 102(6):26–34.

Schernhammer EA, Thompson CA (2010). Light at night and health: the perils of rotating shift work. *Occupational Environmental Medicine*, 68(5):310–311.

Sermeus W, Bruyneel L (2010). *Investing in Europe's health workforce of tomorrow: scope for innovation and collaboration, summary report of the three policy dialogues.* London, European Observatory on Health Systems and Policies (http://www.healthworkforce4europe.eu/downloads/Report_PD_Leuven_FINAL.pdf, accessed 8 October 2013).

Sermeus W et al. (2011). Nurse forecasting in Europe (RN4CAST): rationale, design and methodology. *BMC Nursing*, 10(6):1–9.

Shields M (2004). Addressing nurse shortages: what can policy makers learn from the econometric evidence on nurse labour supply? *Economic Journal*, 114:464–498.

Shields MA, Ward M (2001). Improving nurse retention in the National Health Service in England: the impact of job satisfaction on intentions to quit. *Journal of Health Economics*, 20(5):677–701.

Simon M, Müller BH, Hasselhorn HM (2010). Leaving the organization or the profession: a multilevel analysis of nurses' intentions. *Journal of Advanced Nursing*, 66(3):616–626.

Tai T, Bame S, Robinson C (1998). Review of nursing turnover research, 1977–1996. *Social Science and Medicine*, 47(12):1905–1924.

Tran D et al. (2008). Identification of recruitment and retention strategies for rehabilitation professionals in Ontario, Canada: results from expert panels. *BMC Health Services Research*, 8:249.

van der Heijden B, Kuemmerling A. (2003). Social work environment and nurses' commitment. In Hasselhorn HM, Tackenberg P, Müller BH, eds. *Working conditions and intent to leave the profession among nursing staff in Europe.* Stockholm, National Institute for Working Life:46–52 (http://nile.lub.lu.se/arbarch/saltsa/2003/wlr2003_07.pdf, accessed 8 October 2013).

van der Heijden B, Demerouti E, Bakker AB (2008). Work–home interference among nurses: reciprocal relationships with job demands and health. *Journal of Advanced Nursing*, 62(5):572–584.

van Wyk BE, van Wyk VP (2010). Preventive staff-support interventions for health workers. *Cochrane Database of Systematic Reviews* 2010, 3.

Waldman, J, Kelly F, Arora S, Smith HL (2004). The shocking cost of turnover in health care. *HealthCare Management Review*, 29(1):2–7.

WHO (2010). *Increasing access to health workers in remote and rural areas through improved retention: global policy recommendations.* Geneva, World Health Organization.

Wiskow C, Albrecht T, De Pietro C (2010). *How to create an attractive and supportive working environment for health professionals.* Copenhagen, WHO Regional Office for Europe.

Wismar M et al. (2011). *Health professional mobility and health systems. Evidence from 17 European countries.* Copenhagen, WHO Regional Office for Europe on behalf of the European Observatory on Health Systems and Policies.

Yeatts DE, Seward RR (2000). Reducing turnover and improving health care in nursing homes: the potential effects of self-managed work teams. *Gerentologist,* 40(3):358–363.

# Chapter 16
# Lessons from retention strategies outside Europe

*Carmen Mihaela Dolea*

## 16.1 Introduction

Globally, rural population represents half of the world population on average, but it is served by less than a quarter of the world's doctors, and by about a third of the world's nurses (Fig. 16.1). Geographical maldistribution of health workers is a constant feature of the health labour market in virtually every country in the world. At the country level, the imbalances are even more prominent. For example, in Bangladesh, 30% of nurses are located in four metropolitan districts where only 15% of the population lives (Zurn et al., 2004). In South Africa, rural areas are inhabited by 46% of the total population, but only 12% of doctors and 19% of nurses are working there (Hamilton & Yau, 2004).

**Fig. 16.1** *Rural/urban worldwide distribution of physicians, nurses and population*

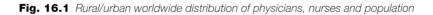

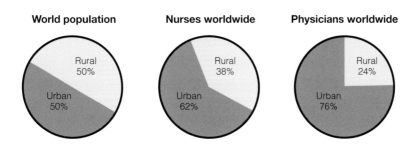

*Sources*: WHO, 2006, 2010a (nurses, physicians); United Nations, 2008 (population).

These inequalities are not only a feature of low-income or middle-income countries. Richer countries have long battled with the inability to cover, recruit and retain qualified health personnel in rural and remote areas. In the United States, for example, 9% of registered physicians practise in rural areas, whereas 20% of the population live in rural areas (Rickets, Hart & Pirani, 2000). In France, there are also large inequalities in the density of GPs, with well-off areas of the south of France and metropolitan Paris being much more endowed than the centre or north (Cash & Ulmann, 2008). While rural Canada covered 99.8% of the nation's territory, and accounted for 24% of the Canadian population in 2006, this only represents 9.3% of the physician workforce (Dumont et al., 2008).

To address the long-standing issue of internal and external migration of health personnel, WHO has adopted a two-pronged approach. On the one hand, since 2006 it has facilitated intergovernmental negotiations on a *Global Code of Practice for International Recruitment of Health Personnel*. This was eventually adopted by the World Health Assembly in 2010 and represents now the only global legal framework (albeit voluntary) that sets the general principles for managing migration of international health workers (WHO, 2010c).

WHO has also established a programme of work to address the rural–urban internal migration of health workers (WHO, 2009). The programme was launched in February 2009 and had three aims: (1) to build the evidence base of what works in attracting and retaining health workers in remote and rural areas; (2) to produce evidence-based global recommendations for increasing retention in these areas (these were eventually launched in September 2010; WHO, 2010a); and (3) to provide technical assistance to member countries in addressing the challenges of rural health workforce retention, as part of the overall support for health workforce strengthening.

This chapter will present an overview of the WHO global policy recommendations and will highlight some of the evidence coming out of the WHO-commissioned case studies, as well as other reviews of the evidence.

## 16.2 The WHO recommendations

Through this programme, the WHO has put together a group of 30–40 international experts who met several times between 2009 and 2010 to review current evidence in this area and develop recommendations. The process was in line with the requirements of the WHO Guidelines Review Committee for transparency, systematic review of the evidence and disclosure of conflict of interest of experts involved (WHO, 2012). The guidelines development group graded the quality of evidence as high, medium, low or very low, based on a set of standard criteria. In addition, the group considered other elements related to the design and implementation of proposed policy interventions, such as values and preferences, benefits and harms, feasibility and resource use. Based on these, the group agreed on a set of recommendations, which were graded as "strong" when evidence was of high quality and/or there was little variability across the other elements, and "weak" when evidence was very low and/or a large variability existed across the other four elements (WHO, 2010a, 2012).

After several expert group consultations and country consultation, the WHO *Global Policy Recommendations on Increasing Access to Health Workers in Remote and Rural Areas* document was launched in September 2010 in South Africa (WHO, 2010a). The document contained 16 evidence-based recommendations, grouped in four categories: education, regulation, financial incentives and personal and professional support (Table 16.1). These interventions have been proven to be effective in improving attraction, recruitment and retention of health workers in remote and rural areas and were agreed by the expert group as a necessary bundle of approaches to improve the distribution of health workers in such areas. The document also proposes a set of guiding principles and a

**Table 16.1** Effective interventions to improve rural recruitment and retention

| Category of intervention and examples | Quality of the evidence | Strength of the recommendation |
|---|---|---|
| *A. Education* | | |
| A1 Students from rural backgrounds | Moderate | Strong |
| A2 Health professional schools outside major cities | Low | Conditional |
| A3 Clinical rotations in rural areas during studies | Very low | Conditional |
| A4 Curricula that reflect rural health issues | Low | Strong |
| A5 Continuous professional development for rural health workers | Low | Conditional |
| *B. Regulation* | | |
| B1 Enhanced scope of practice | Very low | Conditional |
| B2 Different types of health worker | Low | Conditional |
| B3 Compulsory service | Low | Conditional |
| B4 Subsidized education for return of service | Low | Conditional |
| *C. Financial incentives* | | |
| C1 Appropriate financial incentives | Low | Conditional (strong in short term) |
| *D. Personal and professional support* | | |
| D1 Better living conditions | Low | Strong |
| D2 Safe and supportive working environment | Low | Strong |
| D3 Outreach support | Low | Strong |
| D4 Career development programmes | Low | Strong |
| D5 Professional networks | Low | Strong |
| D6 Public recognition measures | Low | Strong |

*Source*: WHO, 2010a.

framework to support the design, implementation, monitoring and evaluation of these strategies, taking due account of the specific context of each country (see Discussion below).

### 16.2.1 Recommendations

#### Education

Evidence suggests that targeting the admission of students from a rural background into medical schools is the single factor most strongly associated with rural practice (Grobler et al., 2009). Some studies have shown they continue to practise in those areas for at least 10 years (De Vries & Reid, 2003; Laven & Wilkinson, 2003; Woloshuk & Tarrant, 2004; Rabinowitz et al., 2005). It is true that students from rural areas may need more financial assistance during their studies, as rural families often have significantly lower incomes than urban families. They may also need more academic and social support, because of the transition from a rural to an urban area. But when students from rural backgrounds are trained in schools that are also located in rural areas, using curricula that are adapted for rural health needs, they are even more likely to return to work in those areas. Hence, it is important for policy-makers to bundle together at least these three interventions for a better result (A1 bundled together with A2 and A3; see Table 16.1).

Large observational studies from high- and low-income countries show that medical schools located in rural areas are likely to produce more physicians working in rural areas than urban located schools (Wang, 2002; Mathews, Rourke & Park, 2008; Longombe, 2009; Wilson et al., 2009). Some evidence is emerging about the benefits of locating schools for other health professions in rural areas in developing countries as well (Codjia, Jabot & Dubois, 2010; Zurn, Codjia & Lamine Sall, 2010), but the effects need to be better studied. There is emerging evidence about the importance of promoting a social accountability framework for medical education in underserved areas to better respond to the needs of these communities. As a response, for example, several need- and outcome-driven medicals schools in remote or rural areas in Australia, Canada, the Philippines and South Africa formed a network of institutions that "are committed to achieving health equity through medical education, research and service that is responsive to the priority needs of communities. Together as a community of practice, and partnering with others, THEnet seeks to transform medical education, build institutional capacity and shape policy so as to make health systems around the world more equitable" (Training for Health Equity Network, 2013).

A key factor in influencing the choice of practice location is the exposure of students to various contexts and practice environments during their training years. Typically, undergraduate education, particularly for physicians, is conducted in tertiary care institutions using the latest available technology and diagnostic tools. Consequently, young graduates have no or limited skills to deal with health service situations in areas where advanced technology and tools are not available. Clinical placements in rural areas during undergraduate studies are therefore an effective way to expose students to the health issues and conditions of service within rural communities and may further influence their subsequent choices of rural practice location (Courtney et al., 2002; Smucny et al., 2005; Capstick, Beresford & Gray, 2008; Halaas et al., 2008).

This is also linked to the relevance of the content of their education to the health needs of rural populations, and the adaption of curricula to those contexts. There is, some evidence that education with a primary care focus or a generalist perspective is conducive to producing practitioners willing and able to work in rural areas (Kaye, Mwanika & Sewankambo, 2010).

Finally, in order to maintain their competence and improve their performance, health workers in remote and rural areas often have to travel to urban locations. There is however, ample supportive evidence that if CPD programmes are delivered in rural areas, and if they are focused on the expressed needs of rural health workers, they are likely to improve the competence of rural health workers, make them feel part of a professional group and increase their desire to remain and practise in those areas (Humphreys et al., 2007; White et al., 2007).

### Regulation

Task shifting has been widely used as a measure to address the shortage of health workers, particularly in the context of HIV/AIDS (WHO, 2008). Health workers serving rural and remote communities may often have to provide services beyond the remit of their formal training because of the absence of other more qualified health workers. Some studies have shown that enhanced scope of practice for rural practitioners may lead to improved job satisfaction, but whether or not this has actually contributed to retention of health workers is unclear from the current evidence (Hoodless & Bourke, 2009).

Another way to address shortages has been to train different types of health worker specifically for rural practice. A recent survey of sub-Saharan African countries found non-physician clinicians were active in 25 out of the 37 countries investigated and concluded: "Low training costs, reduced training duration, and success in rural placements suggest that non-physician clinicians could have substantial roles in the scale-up of health workforces" (Mullan &

Frehywot, 2007, p. 2158). For example, Mozambique began to educate and train assistant medical officers with surgical skills in 1987. A study found that these *técnicos* performed 92% of all major obstetrical surgical interventions in rural hospitals; in addition, 20 years after the initiation of the programme, 88% of all these graduates were still working in district hospitals, compared with only 7% of medical officers (Pereira et al., 2007). Very recently, India has initiated a special medical education programme for rural doctors, but it is too early to comment on its impact on retention (Kinra & Ben-Shlomo, 2010).

One of the most commonly employed and equally controversial interventions to address the rural–urban imbalance is compulsory service, or bonding. This is usually an obligation for young graduates to serve a number of years in remote and rural areas in exchange for obtaining their licence, when financed by public funds, or in exchange for loans for their studies. A comprehensive review of compulsory service schemes undertaken as part of the development of the WHO recommendations found that approximately 70 countries have previously used or are currently using compulsory service (Frehywot et al., 2010). The duration varies from country to country, from a minimum of one year to a maximum of nine years, and the policies have targeted almost all types of health worker. Despite the popularity of compulsory service, very few evaluations of such schemes have been conducted; the results show mostly improved job satisfaction, with little influence on retention of health workers in the long run, and often difficulties in administering the schemes (Cavender & Alban, 1998; Reid, 2001).

However, some countries rely heavily upon graduates who do comply with their compulsory service obligations to deliver services in rural areas. For example, in Thailand, 28 years after the implementation of a national compulsory service strategy, almost half of doctors in rural district hospitals were new graduates completing their compulsory service requirements (Wongwatcharapaiboon, Sirikanokwilai & Pengpaiboon, 1999; Wibulpolprasert & Pengpaibon, 2003). In Japan, 30 years after the implementation of a "home prefecture recruitment scheme" within Jichi Medical University, almost 70% of the graduates remained in their home prefectures for at least six years after their obligatory service (Matsumoto, Inoue & Kajii, 2008). This programme contained a severe pay-back clause whereby students who breached the contract of serving nine years after graduation in their home prefecture, of which six years would be in remote areas, would have to pay back all their expenses for medical education in one lump sum.

When compulsory service is tied to receiving financial incentives for education (return of service schemes), retention rates seem to be higher. A systematic review analysing the effectiveness of such programmes found that the proportion of participants who remained in the underserved area after completing their obligated period of service ranged from 12% to 90% (Bärnighausen & Bloom, 2009). However, many studies included in this systematic review had serious methodological flaws and therefore these findings should be interpreted with some caution.

### Financial incentives

Financial incentives are very common and most of the time tend to be used as a "first-aid" measure to address the problem of rural retention of health workers. However, effects of such interventions are usually mixed. In Australia, for example, one programme providing financial incentives for long-serving physicians in remote and rural areas succeeded in achieving a 65% retention rate of physicians after five years (Gibbon & Hales, 2006; Mason, 2013). Other studies have also shown positive effects of financial incentives on increased attractiveness of rural areas (Reid, 2004; Koot & Martineau, 2005). In Niger, however, two years after the implementation of a financial incentives scheme for rural areas, the proportion of health workers choosing to go to these areas had not changed significantly (from 42% at the start to 46% after two years) (Ministry of Public Health, Niger, 2008). Because these schemes tend to be costly, and in many low-income countries they tend to be donor dependent and therefore less predictable and sustainable, significant analysis needs to be done prior to implementing such schemes in order to fully understand the opportunity costs of working in remote and rural areas. Feasibility studies, such as discrete choice experiments and labour market analysis, are essential to inform the design of an appropriate package of interventions, including financial incentives, so that they are matched to the demands and expectations of health workers.

### Personal and professional support

When health workers are asked what are the main factors deterring them from taking up a rural position, invariably the top reasons include a sense of isolation, lack of social and physical infrastructure, and lack of opportunities for professional development. Therefore, the interventions that would most likely result in improved retention rates for rural and remote areas have to do with ensuring professional and personal support.

Usually these interventions tend to take more time to implement, cut across other sectors, such as infrastructure and rural development and are more expensive. But the expected benefits can also last longer. For example, improving rural infrastructure is part of the overall economic development of rural and remote areas. It is an investment that will help to improve health worker retention, but it can have similarly beneficial effects on workers from other public sectors, such as teachers and policemen, and in the long term can also create a more attractive environment for private sector activities in all economic sectors.

The evidence of effectiveness of such intervention is usually scarce, as often these interventions are part of an overall package of health systems reforms or a bundle of interventions and it is difficult to attribute the observed results to the specific professional and personal support interventions. For example, there is no direct evidence that outreach support programmes improve rural or remote retention. However, there is supportive evidence that such programmes can improve competencies and job satisfaction of rural health workers, can contribute to improving quality of care and can reduce feelings of professional isolation (Watanabe, Jennett & Watson, 1999; Gruen et al., 2003; Como de Corral et al., 2005; Gagnon et al., 2006). They are likely to be more beneficial in settings where there is a critical shortage of health workers, limited infrastructure or very sparse populations, as it provides a service that otherwise would not be available (e.g. mobile clinics or fly-in services) (Gagnon et al., 2007; De Roodenbecke et al., 2010).

"Soft" interventions, such as the existence of professional associations or public recognition measures, can prove beneficial in the long term as they respond to concerns related to professional isolation and intrinsic motivation. For example, in Mali, young doctors who were supported by the professional association *Association des Médecins de Campagne* remained in rural areas for an average of four years; the retention rate was lower for those who did not have this support (Codjia, Jabot & Dubois, 2010). The Rural Doctors Society and Foundation in Thailand was one of the key drivers of rural development and improvement in health services in rural areas (Wibulpolprasert & Pengpaibon, 2003).

### 16.2.2 Implementation issues

The WHO policy recommendations also proposed a set of guiding principles when deciding to implement the most appropriate package of incentives to address the issue of shortages in remote and rural areas (Box 16.1).

Before embarking on any policy to address a maldistribution of health workers, disease patterns and health needs of the rural populations need to be understood. The health system structure, as well as the structure and needs of the health workforce, should also be understood. A comprehensive health labour market analysis should be carried out in order to identify mismatches between supply and demand factors. This can help to quantify the levels of urban versus rural unemployment, underemployment or dual employment of health workers; the

---

**Box 16.1** *Principles to guide the design, implementation, monitoring and evaluation of appropriate rural retention strategies*

- Focus on health equity
- Ensure rural retention policies are part of the national health plan
- Understand the health workforce
- Understand the wider context
- Strengthen human resource management systems
- Engage with all relevant stakeholders from the beginning of the process
- Get into the habit of evaluation and learning.

---

wage differentials between rural and urban areas; and the sources of inflows and outflows of health workers within the public and private health sectors.

Another important element in deciding on the set or bundle of interventions is a clear understanding of the factors that influence the decisions/choices of health workers to go to stay in or to leave rural areas. These factors are very complex, spanning a range covering personal factors, health system characteristics and the overall social, economic and political environment. The interplay of these factors is also complex and strongly influenced by the underlying motivation, be this economic, social, cultural, religious and so on. To some extent, answers for these questions can be obtained through assessments of job preferences of health workers. These kinds of assessment will explore the relative importance of desirable features of a rural job for health workers, as well as the willingness to pay for different characteristics; "discrete choice experiments" have the potential to be a precise and reliable technique to identify and weigh these features (Mangham, Hanson & McPake, 2008; Lagarde & Blaauw, 2009).

### 16.2.3 Uses of the WHO global policy recommendations by countries

Since their publication in 2010, the WHO global policy recommendations have been disseminated through several subregional workshops in Africa, Asia and Eastern Europe (Buchan et al., 2013). Some countries, such as South Africa, have adapted the recommendations to their context and have included them in the national health workforce development plan (National Department of Health, 2011; Rural Health Advocacy Project, 2011). In Asia, a regional professional association, the Asia-Pacific Action Alliance on Human Resources for Health (AAAH), has initiated multi-country policy assessments of rural retention policies based on the WHO recommendations. Five countries (China, Lao PDL, Sri Lanka, Thailand and Vietnam) used a policy analysis tool to map the existing retention strategies and to assess or predict outcomes. The most common set of strategies across the five countries incuded recruitment of students from a rural background, mandatory rural service and the use of financial and non-financial incentives (Buchan et al., 2013). In Africa, under the coordination of the African Development Bank Group, a multi-country study was planned to assess the effectiveness of rural retention interventions in these countries, again based on the WHO guidelines (Atef El-Maghraby, personal communication). Last but not least, the World Bank has developed a guidance note for its Bank Task Team Leaders, providing more detailed technical information on the necessary steps for the assessment, design and implementation of rural retention strategies based on the WHO global policy recommendations (Akiko Maeda, personal communication).

## 16.3 Lessons learnt from country case studies

As part of the process of evidence gathering, WHO commissioned a series of country case studies and systematic reviews of rural retention interventions. The country case studies used a similar template and were intended to identify current experiences and challenges with rural retention in a variety of settings. Additional evidence was published in a special theme issue of the *Bulletin of the World Health Organization* in May 2010 (WHO, 2010b). In addition, a review of compulsory service strategies and outreach services identified some further country experiences (Frehywot et al., 2010), while a realist review identified the mechanism and contextual factors that influence the effects of such interventions (Dieleman et al., 2011).

### 16.3.1 "Small" does not mean any easier: Samoa and Vanuatu

The case studies from Samoa and Vanuatu are illustrative of the challenges faced by small island states in recruiting and retaining health workers for remote and rural areas (Buchan, Connell & Rumsey, 2011). Geography is one of the main challenges, with large distances between cities and villages, mostly over water but sometimes with mountainous areas with difficult access. Lack of physical as well as socioeconomic infrastructure is a major deterrent for professional health workers to take up positions in these remote areas. In addition, because of the large outmigration of doctors, or increased reluctance of doctors to take up rural posts, these countries rely heavily on nurses to cover remote and rural areas. For example, Samoa has developed a nurse-led model of community services and outreach, whereas Vanuatu has used mobile nurse teams to reach remote areas. Training capacity for additional nursing staff is limited in both countries, and neither can train its own doctors; some efforts to use technology for distance-based continuous education have been ongoing for some years now in Samoa through the Pacific Open Learning Health Net (POLHN, 2013).

Several policies have been implemented or proposed to address these challenges in the two small states. In the education category, both Vanuatu and Samoa have included a remote posting as part of the clinical placement for nurses during training. In the regulation category, task shifting has been implemented, as a reaction to the reluctance of doctors to take up rural posts. The clinical nurse consultant has been established as an advanced role for nurses, and current regulatory reforms may further support an initiative to provide prescribing rights to clinical nurse consultants. In terms of financial incentives, no specific interventions were found in either country. At the time of the study though, the Government of Samoa was about to announce a review of salary structures, with a view to changing pay rates for rural workers. With regards to professional and personal support, it is worth mentioning the initiative in Samoa, where the national health service has purchased cars for all district hospitals to give nurses improved access to rural communities. Some innovative outreach strategies were also explored in Vanuatu, building on previous models, where a boat equipped for minor surgery was used to increase access to remote areas. In addition, funding from the Australia Agency for International Development has recently enabled a clinical team rotation model that would allow a team of clinical specialist and support workers from the main hospital in the capital to visit the rural hospitals on a weekly basis.

These two case studies illustrate the extent to which the overall human resources for health context is problematic in the Pacific Islands States. Because of weak economies and high dependence on overseas aid, lack of or insufficient capacity to train their own doctors, coupled with high outmigration, the policy focus in these countries seems to be on reducing the acute shortages, before a more equitable distribution of health workers can be conceived.

### 16.3.2 Contracting experience in Senegal: Plan Cobra

Like most sub-Saharan African countries, Senegal is experiencing a critical health workforce shortage, in particular in remote and rural areas. Over the past few years, the Ministry of Health of Senegal adopted measures to improve the posting process and the recruitment and retention of health workers in rural and remote areas (Zurn, Codjia & Lamine Sall, 2010). Among them was the introduction of an innovative special contracting system for recruiting health workers: Plan Cobra.

Under this system, the health worker enters into a contractual arrangement with the Ministry of Health for a specific post in a particular location and for a specific length of time, usually a year. Like health workers recruited in the civil service by the Ministry of Public Services, health workers who are contracted by the Ministry of Health in Plan Cobra are also entitled to special benefits when working in remote and rural areas. For example, nurses heading a health post receive a house, while other contracted workers receive various motivation or hardship allowances. In the context of Plan Cobra, 122 health outposts were reopened in Senegal. This contributed substantially to reinforcing health district teams. Overall, 365 contracts were issued between 2006 and 2008, including 59 for physicians, 155 for nurses and 151 for midwives.

Plan Cobra showed the positive role that a flexible contracting system can play in improving health workforce recruitment and deployment to rural and remote areas, as well as in redressing the imbalance in health worker distribution between geographical regions. Unfortunately, the funds allocated to this project had been used up by the end of 2009, so no other contracting has been possible since. Although its overall impact has been positive, the contracting system was obviously not enough to redress geographical health worker imbalances in Senegal. Other strategies should be and have also been considered to improve health workforce recruitment and retention. For example, new training centres were created in a number of remote regions of Senegal that allowed for more locally recruited students to be trained. Specific financial support measures were also provided, for example grants for seventh-year medical students wishing to do internships in remote or rural areas.

### 16.3.3 Setting up a rural practice by young medical graduates: Mali

The initiative to set up medical practices in rural areas in Mali appeared during the early 1990s, when the country began decentralization of health services, with an aim to improving access to care and use of services for rural populations (Codjia, Jabot & Dubois, 2010). At the same time, many young medical graduates became unemployed or underemployed because the country was producing too many doctors, and structural adjustment policies were capping recruitment in the public sector. After the decentralization and administrative reform (1999–2002), a programme of social and health development resulted in the revitalization of community health centres, which were primary structures responsible for providing a minimum package of services for rural populations; they covered 5 000 inhabitants within a radius of 15 km and were managed by community associations and local councils.

Because of lack of career prospects in the civil service, young doctors came gradually to settle in rural areas, offering their services privately to these community health centres. With support from an NGO, Santé-Sud, young physicians who were willing to establish a private practice in these centres were provided with an installation package (medical kit, solar panel – these areas had no electricity and no running water), and a six-month training programme in community medicine. Some of these doctors eventually organized themselves into a professional organization, the Association of Community Medicine (Association de Medicine Communautaire). These young doctors signed a contract with the community health associations and local councils for the provision of their services that was similar to a "pay for performance" contract.

The evaluation of this initiative, commissioned by WHO, found that more than 100 doctors had settled in rural areas over the past decade, encouraged by the combination of strategies supported by the Health Facilities Project South and the Mali Government. Physicians based in rural areas tended to be younger and they stayed an average of four years in those practices. Those affiliated with the Association of Community Medicine benefited from additional support measures, such as additional training and regular professional exchanges, and tended to stay for longer periods in their rural practices. The success of this initiative was possible because of a combination of strategies: opportunities for medical students to study in rural areas (or young graduates to study community medicine), support for installation (the installation package), the formalization of a contract of employment, including social security and retirement scheme, and last but not least, the affiliation to a professional association. However, despite these supportive measures, the living and working conditions in the areas assessed remained precarious, which was incompatible with a long-term career.

A good sign was the fact that many actors have partially or totally appropriated the strategies for recruiting young doctors in remote and rural areas. The Association of Community Medicine has incorporated these strategies in its annual plan to conduct them routinely. The Medical School also plans to integrate training modules in its rural health curricula. However, the institutionalization of these strategies is still limited, and their integration into the activities of the organizations primarily concerned (local councils and community health centres) depends on the financial and management capacities of the latter. The financial benefits for doctors, which were one of the key conditions for long-term stay, depended also on the utilization of the centres and the financial capacities of the populations. If mechanisms to increase the affordability of services by the population are not adopted, rural doctors are unlikely to remain in rural areas.

## 16.4 Discussion

One of the key messages coming out of this study is that the 16 interventions are more effective when they are implemented in complementary bundles. For example, in Thailand during the last 30 years a combination of interventions, ranging from rural recruitment, training and hometown placement, compulsory public service and various financial incentives, has led to a steady increase of the density of rural doctors (Wibulpolprasert & Pengpaibon, 2003).

Except for Mali, most case studies did not find evaluation or impact assessments. The thinking is mainly at the level of identifying factors and measuring the extent of the problem. Financial incentives seem to be attractive for policy-makers, but there are no assessments of costs and future implications, or of opportunity costs for choosing one intervention over another.

Last but not least, one of the key factors to sustain success of these interventions is the engagement of all stakeholders, across sectors and ministries. This will ensure, for example, buy-in for investing in long-term infrastructure programmes, support from professional associations on education and training initiatives, or engaging unions and NGOs for fair labour contracts.

---

**Box 16.2** *Research gaps and priorities*

*Effectiveness and impact evaluation*

- How do different types of retention intervention work? What makes them successful or not and what key contextual factors influence their success?
- Which individual or bundle of interventions has had the most effective impact?
- Is there any evidence of improved health outcomes as a result of the implementation of the recommendations?

*Implementation issues*

- Feasibility analysis on the recommendations from political viability, economic feasibility, technical feasibility and social feasibility
- Spending, fiscal funding, and costing analysis for the interventions
- What are the best methods for accurately identifying the actual incentives and motivations of health workers for going to and remaining in rural and remote underserved areas? (Discrete choice experiment and alternative methods.)

*Specific interventions for future exploration*

- What are the effects of dual practice regulations on rural retention?
- What are the effects of facilitating the establishment of rural practices in rural areas?
- What are the effects of health financing reforms, including universal health coverage, on the right types of incentives to stay in rural areas?

---

Moving forward, many questions remain unanswered (Box 16.2). More needs to be known about the impact of these interventions in the long term, the extent to which they contribute to improved health outcomes and the enabling factors contributing to their success. Also, some specific interventions will need to be better understood, for example the effects of regulation allowing dual practice in remote and rural areas, as well as the effects of financial reforms, including universal health coverage, on the right types of incentives to serve in rural areas.

## 16.5 Conclusions

In conclusion, regardless of the level of socioeconomic development, all countries experience serious imbalances in health worker distribution between rural and urban areas, and all have difficulties in attracting and retaining health workers in rural and remote areas. The factors that influence the decisions of health workers to stay or leave underserved regions are similar across countries and regions, and they have to do with feelings of isolation, both professionally and socially; a lack of infrastructure, with poor working conditions; and few prospects for professional development. Many countries have introduced various policies and interventions to address these problems, but little evaluation of the impact of such interventions has been conducted (Dolea, Stormont & Braichet, 2010).

The case studies presented here are illustrative of the challenges present in many countries. Despite anecdotal evidence, or in many countries even more concrete evidence of the impact that such shortages in rural areas can have on the health of rural populations, policy responses still lag behind. Even when policies or interventions are being implemented, assessment of their impact is often lacking. The WHO global policy recommendations identified a set of 16 evidence-based effective strategies that have been used by countries to address the issue of health workforce shortages in remote and rural areas. These recommendations will have to be adapted to country-specific contexts and implemented based on local needs. Assessing the impact of these interventions in the long term will contribute to common learning and knowledge sharing and will result in further adaptation of these interventions so that they can better respond to the needs of populations and health workers themselves.

Implementing such interventions to improve recruitment and retention of health workers in remote and rural areas can eventually address the imbalances observed today within countries between urban and rural areas. These interventions also offer insights for addressing the issue of international migration of health workers. For example, solutions related to education, regulation, financial and personal and professional support might also be considered to improve retention of health workers in their home countries, and thus reduce the international outflow of health workers. In addition, health professional education based on national curricula and relevant to country-specific needs is more likely to keep health workers in their home country than an internationally based curriculum. Potential avenues to increase health workers' professional satisfaction and thus reduce the desire to leave their source country include training the types of health worker that respond best to the national burden of disease of home countries, paying adequate and timely salaries, creating financial incentives, implementing effective management and providing professional support measures. This does not preclude maintaining a right to leave one's country but it will provide health workers in these source countries with more reasons to stay than to leave.

## References

Bärnighausen T, Bloom D (2009). Financial incentives for return of service in underserved areas: a systematic review. *BMC Health Services Research*, 9:86.

Buchan J, Connell J, Rumsey M (2011). *Recruiting and retaining health workers in remote areas: Pacific Island case-studies*. Geneva, World Health Organization.

Buchan J et al. (2013). Early implementation of the WHO recommendations for the retention of health workers in remote and rural areas. *Bulletin of the World Health Organization*, 91:834–840.

Capstick S, Beresford R, Gray A (2008). Rural pharmacy in New Zealand: effects of a compulsory externship on student perspectives and implications for workforce shortages. *Australian Journal of Rural Health*, 16:150–155.

Cash R, Ulmann P (2008). *Projet OCDE sur la Migration des Professionnels de Santé: Le Cas de la France*. Paris, Organisation for Economic Co-operation and Development (OECD Health Working Paper No. 36).

Cavender A, Alban M (1998). Compulsory medical service in Ecuador: the physician's perspective. *Social Science and Medicine*, 47(12):1937–1946.

Codjia L, Jabot F, Dubois H (2010). *Evaluation du programme d'appui à la médicalisation des aires de santé rurales au Mali [An evaluation of the support programme for the medicalization of rural health areas in Mali]*. Geneva, World Health Organization (Accroître l'accès aux personnels de santé dans les zones rurales ou reculées, étude de cas No. 2).

Como del Corral MJ et al. (2005). Utility of a thematic network in primary health care: a controlled interventional study in a rural area. *Human Resources for Health*, 3(4):1–7.

Courtney M et al. (2002). The impact of rural clinical placement on student nurses' employment intentions. *Collegian*, 9(1):12–18.

De Roodenbecke E et al. (2010). *Outreach services as a strategy to increase access to health workers in remote and rural areas*. Geneva, World Health Organization.

De Vries E, Reid S (2003). Do South African medical students of rural origin return to rural practice? *South African Medical Journal*, 93(10):783–793.

Dieleman et al. (2011). *Realist review and synthesis of retention studies for health workers in rural and remote areas*. Geneva, World Health Organization.

Dolea C, Stormont L, Braichet JM (2010). Evaluated strategies to increase attraction and retention of health workers in remote and rural areas. *Bulletin of the World Health Organization*, 88:379–385.

Dumont J-C et al. (2008). *International mobility of health professionals and health workforce management in Canada: myths and realities*. Paris, Organisation for Economic Co-operation and Development (OECD Health Working Paper No. 40).

Frehywot S et al. (2010). Compulsory service programmes for recruiting health workers in remote and rural areas: do they work? *Bulletin of the World Health Organization*, 88:364–370.

Gagnon M-P et al. (2006). Exploring the effects of telehealth on medical human resources supply: a qualitative case study in remote regions. *BMC Health Services Research*, 7(6):1–9.

Gagnon M-P et al. (2007). Implementing telehealth to support medical practice in rural/remote regions: what are the conditions for success? *Implementation Science*, 1(18):1–8.

Gibbon P, Hales J (2006). *Review of the rural retention program: final report*. Canberra, Australian Government Department of Health and Ageing.

Grobler L et al. (2009). Interventions for increasing the proportion of health professionals practising in rural and other underserved areas. *Cochrane Database of Systematic Reviews*, 21(1):CD005314.

Gruen RL et al. (2003). Specialist outreach clinics in primary care and rural hospital settings. *Cochrane Database of Systematic Reviews*, (4):CD003798.

Halaas GW et al. (2008). Recruitment and retention of rural physicians: outcomes from the rural physician associate program of Minnesota. *Journal of Rural Health*, 24(4):345–352.

Hamilton K, Yau J (2004). *The global tug-of-war for health care workers*. Washington, DC, Migration Policy Institute (http://www.migrationinformation. org/Feature/print.cfm?ID=271, accessed 16 December 2013).

Hoodless M, Bourke L (2009). Expanding the scope of practice for enrolled nurses working in an Australian rural health service: implications for job satisfaction. *Nurse Education Today*, 29(4):432–438.

Humphreys J et al. (2007). *Improving primary health care workforce retention in small rural and remote communities: how important is ongoing education and training?* Canberra, Australian Primary Health Care Research Institute.

Kaye DK, Mwanika A, Sewankambo N (2010). Influence of the training experience of Makerere University medical and nursing graduates on willingness and competence to work in rural health facilities. *Rural and Remote Health*, 10:1372.

Kinra S, Ben-Shlomo Y (2010). Rural MBBS degree in India. *Lancet*, 376(9749):1284–1285.

Koot J, Martineau T (2005). *Zambian health workers retention scheme (ZHWRS) 2003–2004: mid-term review*. Lusaka, Government of Zambia (http://www. hrhresourcecenter.org/hosted_docs/Zambian_Health_Workers_Retention_ Scheme.pdf, accessed 16 December 2013).

Lagarde M, Blaauw D (2009). A review of the application and contribution of discrete choice experiments to inform human resources policy interventions. *Human Resources for Health*, 7:62.

Laven G, Wilkinson D (2003). Rural doctors and rural backgrounds: how strong is the evidence? A systematic review. *Australian Journal of Rural Health*, 11:277–284.

Longombe AO (2009). Medical schools in rural areas: necessity or aberration? *Rural and Remote Health*, 9:1311.

Mangham LJ, Hanson K, McPake B (2008). How to do (or not to do) … Designing a discrete choice experiment for application in a low-income country. *Health Policy and Planning*, 24(2):151–155.

Mathews M, Rourke JTB, Park A (2008). The contribution of Memorial University's medical school to rural physician supply. *Canadian Journal of Rural Medicine*, 13(1):15–21.

Matsumoto M, Inoue K, Kajii E (2008). Long-term effect of the home preference recruiting scheme of Jichi Medical University Japan. *Rural and Remote Health*, 8:1–15.

Ministry of Public Health, Niger (2008). *Impact des mesures d'incitation financière accordées aux médecins, pharmaciens et chirurgiens dentistes [Impact of financial incentive measures for doctors, pharmacists and dentists].* Niamey, Ministère de la Santé Publique.

Mullan F, Frehywot S (2007). Non-physician clinicians in 47 sub-Saharan African countries. *Lancet*, 370:2158–2163.

National Department of Health (2011). *Human resources for health South Africa 2030.* Pretoria, National Department of Health.

Pereira C et al. (2007). Meeting the need for emergency obstetric care in Mozambique: work performance and histories of medical doctors and assistant medical officers trained for surgery. *BJOG: An International Journal of Obstetrics and Gynaecology*, 114:1530–1533.

POLHN (2013). *Pacific Open Learning Health Net.* [website]. Suva, Fiji Islands, WHO Regional Office for the Western Pacific (http://polhn.com/, accessed 16 December 2013).

Rabinowitz HK et al. (2005). Long-term retention of graduates from a program to increase the supply of rural family physicians. *Academic Medicine*, 80:728–732.

Reid SJ (2001). Compulsory community service for doctors in South Africa: an evaluation of the first year. *South African Medical Journal*, 91(4):329–335.

Reid SJ (2004). *Monitoring the effect of the new rural allowance for health professionals: research project report.* Durban, Health Systems Trust (http://healthlink.org.za/uploads/files/rural_allowance.pdf, accessed 16 December 2013).

Ricketts TC, Hart LG, Pirani M (2000). How many rural doctors do we have? *Journal of Rural Health*, 16(3):198–207.

Rural Health Advocacy Project (2011). *The WHO global policy recommendations on increasing access to health care workers in remote and rural areas through improved recruitment and retention: the South African context.* Braamfontein, Rural Health Advocacy Project.

Smucny J et al. (2005). An evaluation of the Rural Medical Education Program of the State University of New York Upstate Medical University, 1990–2003. *Academic Medicine*, 80:733–738.

Training for Health Equity Network (2013). [web site]. Brussels, (http://thenetcommunity.org/about-thenet/, accessed 16 December 2013).

United Nations (2008). *World urbanization prospects: the 2007 revision*. New York, United Nations Department of Economic and Social Affairs.

Wang L (2002). A comparison of metropolitan and rural medical schools in China: which schools provide rural physicians? *Australian Journal of Rural Health*, 10:94–98.

Watanabe M, Jennett P, Watson M (1999). The effect of information technology on the physician workforce and health care in isolated communities: the Canadian picture. *Journal of Telemedicine and Telecare*, 5(Suppl. 2):11–19.

White CD et al. (2007). Making a difference: education and training retains and supports rural and remote doctors in Queensland. *Rural and Remote Health*, 7:700.

WHO (2006). *Working together for health: world health report 2006*. Geneva, World Health Organization.

WHO (2008). *Task shifting: global recommendations and guidelines*. Geneva, World health organization (http://www.who.int/workforcealliance/knowledge/resources/taskshifting_globalrecommendations/en/index.html, accessed 16 December 2013).

WHO (2009). *WHO rural health worker retention programme*. Geneva, World Health Organization (flyer) (http://www.who.int/hrh/migration/retention_flyer/en/index.html, accessed 16 December 2013).

WHO (2010a). *Global policy recommendations on increasing access to health workers in remote and rural areas through improved retention*. Geneva, World Health Organization.

WHO (2010b). Special theme issue of retaining health workers in remote and rural areas. *Bulletin of the World Health Organization*, 88(5):321–400 (http://www.who.int/bulletin/volumes/88/5/en/index.html, accessed 16 December 2013).

WHO (2010c). *WHO global code of practice on the international recruitment of health personnel*. Geneva, World Health Organization (Sixty-third World Health Assembly, WHA63.16) (http://www.who.int/hrh/migration/code/WHO_global_code_of_practice_EN.pdf, accessed 1 October 2013).

WHO (2012). *Handbook for guideline development*. Geneva, World Health Organization (http://www.who.int/kms/guidelines_review_committee/en/index.html, accessed 16 December 2013).

Wibulpolprasert S, Pengpaibon P (2003). Integrated strategies to tackle the inequitable distribution of doctors in Thailand: four decades of experience. *Human Resources for Health*, 1:12.

Wilson NW et al. (2009). A critical review of interventions to redress the inequitable distribution of healthcare professionals to rural and remote areas. *Rural and Remote Health*, 9:1060.

Woloschuk W, Tarrant M (2004). Do students from rural backgrounds engage in rural family practice more than their urban-raised peers? *Medical Education*, 38:259–261.

Wongwatcharapaiboon P, Sirikanokwilai N, Pengpaiboon P (1999). The 1997 massive resignation of contracted new medical graduates from the Thai Ministry of Health: what reasons behind? *Human Resources for Health Development Journal*, 3(2):147–156.

Zurn P, Codjia L, Lamine Sall F (2010). *La fidélisation des personnels de santé dans les zones rurales ou reculées [The retention of health workers in rural and remote areas]*. Geneva, World Health Organization, 2010 (Accroître l'accès aux personnels de santé dans les zones rurales ou reculées, étude de cas No. 1).

Zurn P et al. (2004). Imbalance in the health workforce. *Human Resources for Health*, 2:13.